Recent Titles in This Series

30 **Eric Todd Quinto, Margaret Cheney, and Peter Kuchment, Editors,** Tomography, impedance imaging, and integral geometry, 1994

29 **Eugene L. Allgower, Kurt Georg, and Rick Miranda, Editors,** Exploiting symmetry in applied and numerical analysis, 1993

28 **Christopher R. Anderson and Claude Greengard, Editors,** Vortex dynamics and vortex methods, 1990

27 **Werner E. Kohler and Benjamin S. White, Editors,** Mathematics of random media, 1989

26 **Eugene L. Allgower and Kurt Georg, Editors,** Computational solution of nonlinear systems of equations, 1988

25 **Randolph E. Bank, Editor,** Computational aspects of VLSI design with an emphasis on semiconductor device simulation, 1987

24 **G. S. S. Ludford, Editor,** Reacting flows: combustion and chemical reactors, Parts 1 and 2, 1982

23 **Basil Nicolaenko, Darryl D. Holm, and James M. Hyman, Editors,** Nonlinear systems of partial differential equations in applied mathematics, Parts 1 and 2, 1982

22 **B. Engquist, S. Osher, and R. C. J. Somerville, Editors,** Large-scale computations in fluid mechanics, Parts 1 and 2, 1982

21 **Moshe Flato, Paul Sally, and Gregg Zuckerman, Editors,** Applications of group theory in physics and mathematical sciences, 1982

20 **Norman R. Lebovitz, Editor,** Fluid dynamics in astrophysics and geophysics, 1981

19 **Frank C. Hoppensteadt, Editor,** Mathematical aspects of physiology, 1980

18 **Christopher I. Brynes and Clyde F. Martin, Editors,** Algebraic and geometric methods in linear systems theory, 1979

17 **Frank C. Hoppensteadt, Editor,** Nonlinear oscillations in biology, 1978

16 **Richard C. DiPrima, Editor,** Modern modeling of continuum phenomena, 1975

15 **Alan C. Newell, Editor,** Nonlinear wave motion, 1972

14 **William H. Reid, Editor,** Mathematical problems in the geophysical sciences. 2. Inverse problems, dynamo theory, and tides, 1970

13 **William H. Reid, Editor,** Mathematical problems in the geophysical sciences. 1. Geophysical fluid dynamics, 1970

12 **George B. Dantzig and Arthur F. Veinott, Jr., Editors,** Mathematics of the decision sciences, Part 2, 1967

11 **George B. Dantzig and Arthur F. Veinott, Jr., Editors,** Mathematics of the decision sciences, Part 1, 1967

10 **Jürgen Ehlers, Editor,** Relativity theory and astrophysics. 3. Stellar structure, 1965

9 **Jürgen Ehlers, Editor,** Relativity theory and astrophysics. 2. Galactic structure, 1965

8 **Jürgen Ehlers, Editor,** Relativity theory and astrophysics. 1. Relativity and cosmology, 1965

7 **J. Barkley Rosser, Editor,** Space mathematics. Part 3, 1963

6 **J. Barkley Rosser, Editor,** Space mathematics. Part 2, 1963

5 **J. Barkley Rosser, Editor,** Space mathematics. Part 1, 1963

4 **R. Jost,** Quantum mechanics, 1960

3 **K. O. Friedrichs,** Perturbation of spectra in Hilbert space, 1960

2 **I. E. Segal with G. W. Mackey,** Mathematical problems of relativistic physics, 1960

1 **G. E. Uhlenbeck and G .W. Ford with E. W. Montroll,** Lectures in statistical mechanics, 1960

3A **L. Bers, F. John, and M. Schechter,** Partial differential equations, 1964

2A **S. Goldstein and J. M. Burgers,** Lectures on fluid mechanics, 1960

Lectures in APPLIED MATHEMATICS

Volume 30

Tomography, Impedance Imaging, and Integral Geometry

1993 AMS-SIAM Summer Seminar on
the Mathematics of Tomography,
Impedance Imaging, and Integral Geometry
June 7–18, 1993
Mount Holyoke College, Massachusetts

Eric Todd Quinto
Margaret Cheney
Peter Kuchment
Editors

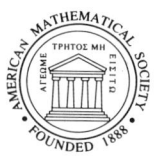

American Mathematical Society
Providence, Rhode Island

The Proceedings of the 1993 AMS-SIAM Summer Seminar on the Mathematics of Tomography, Impedance Imaging, and Integral Geometry were prepared by the American Mathematical Society with support from the National Science Foundation, Grant DMS-9220809.

1991 *Mathematics Subject Classification.* Primary 92C55, 35R30, 44A12.

Library of Congress Cataloging-in-Publication Data
AMS-SIAM Summer Seminar on the Mathematics of Tomography, Impedance Imaging, and Integral Geometry (1993 : Mount Holyoke College)
  Tomography, impedance imaging, and integral geometry : 1993 AMS-SIAM Summer Seminar on the Mathematics of Tomography, Impedance Imaging, and Integral Geometry, June 7–18, 1993, Mount Holyoke College, Massachusetts / Eric Todd Quinto, Margaret Cheney, Peter Kuchment, editors.
    p. cm. — (Lectures in applied mathematics, ISSN 0075-8485 ; v. 30)
  Includes bibliographical references.
  ISBN 0-8218-0337-9
  1. Integral geometry—Congresses. 2. Inverse problems (Differential equations)—Congresses. 3. Tomography—Mathematics—Congresses. I. Quinto, Eric Todd, 1951– . II. Cheney, Margaret, 1955– . III. Kuchment, Peter, 1949– . IV. American Mathematical Society. V. Title. V. Series: Lectures in applied mathematics (American Mathematical Society) ; v. 30.
  QA672.A47 1993
  616.07′57′01515353—dc20   94-28800
                                                                          CIP

Copying and reprinting. Individual readers of this publication, and nonprofit libraries acting for them, are permitted to make fair use of the material, such as to copy an article for use in teaching or research. Permission is granted to quote brief passages from this publication in reviews, provided the customary acknowledgment of the source is given.

Republication, systematic copying, or multiple reproduction of any material in this publication (including abstracts) is permitted only under license from the American Mathematical Society. Requests for such permission should be addressed to the Manager of Editorial Services, American Mathematical Society, P.O. Box 6248, Providence, Rhode Island 02940-6248. Requests can also be made by e-mail to reprint-permission@math.ams.org.

The appearance of the code on the first page of an article in this publication indicates the copyright owner's consent for copying beyond that permitted by Sections 107 or 108 of the U.S. Copyright Law, provided that the fee of $1.00 plus $.25 per page for each copy be paid directly to the Copyright Clearance Center, Inc., 222 Rosewood Drive, Danvers, Massachusetts 01923. This consent does not extend to other kinds of copying, such as copying for general distribution, for advertising or promotional purposes, for creating new collective works, or for resale.

© Copyright 1994 by the American Mathematical Society. All rights reserved.
The American Mathematical Society retains all rights
except those granted to the United States Government.
Printed in the United States of America.
⊗ The paper used in this book is acid-free and falls within the guidelines
established to ensure permanence and durability.
♻ Printed on recycled paper.
All articles in this volume were printed from copy prepared by the authors.
Some articles were typeset using $\mathcal{A}_{\mathcal{M}}\mathcal{S}$-TEX or $\mathcal{A}_{\mathcal{M}}\mathcal{S}$-LATEX,
the American Mathematical Society's TEX macro systems.

10 9 8 7 6 5 4 3 2 1   99 98 97 96 95 94

Contents

Preface ... ix

An inversion formula for the horocyclic Radon transform on the real hyperbolic space
    CARLOS A. BERENSTEIN AND ENRICO CASADIO TARABUSI ... 1

Image reconstruction and dense subspaces in the range of the radon transform
    W. K. CHEUNG AND ANDREW MARKOE ... 7

On a spatial limited angle model for X-ray computerized tomography
    ARLENE CORREA, RODNEY CRUZ, AND PABLO M. SALZBERG ... 25

The backpropagation method in inverse acoustics
    GIOVANNI F. CROSTA ... 35

Some nonlinear aspects of the radon transform
    LEON EHRENPREIS ... 69

Spherical tomography and spherical integral geometry
    SIMON GINDIKIN, JIM REEDS, AND LARRY SHEPP ... 83

That kappa operator: Gelfand-Graev-Shapiro inversion and radon transforms on isotropic planes
    E. L. GRINBERG ... 93

On uniqueness in the inverse conductivity problem with one boundary measurement
    VICTOR ISAKOV ... 105

A method for finding discontinuities of functions from the tomographic data
    A. I. KATSEVICH AND A. G. RAMM ... 115

Probability measure estimation using "weak" loss functions in positron emission tomography
    ALVIN KURUC ... 125

On stability estimates in the exterior problem for the radon transform
    SERGUEI LISSIANOI ... 143

Data correction and restoration in emission tomography
    SERGE J. LVIN ... 149

On problems of integral geometry in the non-convex domains
    R. MUKHOMETOV   157

Recent developments in X-ray tomography
    F. NATTERER   177

Some mathematical aspects of 3D X-ray tomography
    V. P. PALAMODOV   199

A note on consistency conditions in three dimensional diffuse tomography
    S. K. PATCH   211

Radon transforms on curves in the plane
    ERIC TODD QUINTO   231

Inverse boundary value problems for first order perturbations of the Laplacian
    GUNTHER UHLMANN   245

Multidimensional analogue of the Erdélyi lemma and the radon transform
    ALEXANDER I. ZASLAVSKY   259

On the Willmore deficit of convex surfaces
    JIAZU ZHOU   279

Preface

One of the most exciting features of tomography is the strong relationship between high-level pure mathematics (such as harmonic analysis, partial differential equations, microlocal analysis, and group theory) and applications to medical imaging, impedance imaging, radiotherapy, and industrial non-destructive evaluation.

The 1993 AMS Summer Seminar on Tomography, Impedance Imaging, and Integral Geometry at Mount Holyoke College in South Hadley, Massachusetts, had the following general goals: to communicate research at the forefront of the fields, to strengthen the connection between the pure and applied aspects of these areas, and to provide a productive opportunity for new and more established researchers to meet and share ideas. To this end, the first three days of the conference were devoted to introductory talks by researchers in the field. Over thirty graduate students and other newcomers to the field attended.

Common themes became apparent at the conference and are represented in these proceedings. Group theory is fundamental both to tomographic sampling theorems and to pure Radon transforms. Microlocal and Fourier analysis are important for research in all three fields. "Applied" theorems need to be tested on real data in real situations. Radon transforms can be used to model impedance imaging problems. Several significant cross-fertilizations occurred, including Gindikin's use of the Kappa operator to simplify the Shepp and Reeds' spherical tomographic inversion method.

These proceedings include exciting results from the conference in all three fields. These articles have been refereed and are in final form; no article will be submitted for publication elsewhere.

The applied articles in these proceedings are in fields as diverse as acoustics and diffuse and emission tomography. They include a new inversion method for spherical tomography [Gindikin, Reeds, and Shepp], using sampling to improve X-ray tomographic reconstructions [Natterer], a probabilistic method for emission tomography [Kuruc], a method for finding discontinuities of functions [Katsevich and Ramm]. Consistency conditions are used to improve inversion in diffuse [Patch], emission [Lvin], and X-ray [Cheung and Markoe] tomography. Stability estimates are given for exterior tomography [Lissianoi]. New theoretical results in impedance imaging, acoustics, and conductivity problems are presented in these proceedings [Crosta], [Isakov], [Uhlmann], and intriguing reconstructions from real impedance data were presented at the conference.

Integral geometry provides theoretical underpinnings of tomograhy and is beautiful pure mathematics. Mathematical aspects of 3-D tomography [Palamodov], integral geometry along geodesics [Mukhometov], non-linear aspects of Radon transforms [Ehrenpreis], and support theorems for curved Radon transforms [Quinto] are presented in these proceedings. Geometric aspects of integral geometry [Zaslavsky] [Zhou], inversion formulas for the horocycle Radon transform [Berenstein and Tarabusi], and finite limited angle Radon tomography [Correa, Cruz, and Salzberg] are also represented. The Kappa operator [Gindikin, Reeds, and Shepp] [Grinberg] played an important role during the conference.

The conference coorganizers, Margaret Cheney, Simon Gindikin, Peter Kuchment, Todd Quinto, and Larry Shepp, thank the National Science Foundation for their generous support without which the conference would have been impossible. We thank James Maxwell, Associate Director of the American Mathematical Society for his assistance and support throughout this process and, in particular, for getting International Science Foundation support. This allowed us to support beginners more generously. We are indebted to Donna Salter, AMS Conference Coordinator, for being cheerful and helpful to the participants and for making our job much easier. The proceedings editors thank Donna Harmon, Alison Buckser, and the technical staff of the AMS for doing such an efficient and careful job putting these proceedings together. We thank the article referees for their conscientious, thoughtful evaluations. Finally, we thank the conference participants who made the conference stimulating and fun, and without whom the proceedings would have been quite slim.

Margaret Cheney
Peter Kuchment,
Todd Quinto
May 20, 1994

An inversion formula for the horocyclic Radon transform on the real hyperbolic space

CARLOS A. BERENSTEIN AND ENRICO CASADIO TARABUSI

ABSTRACT. Let R be the Radon transform which integrates over horocycles of the real hyperbolic space. Reducing it to an Abel-type transform, we prove an inversion formula for R in terms of the 'distance p' dual Radon transform considered by Helgason. Such formula is in some sense the 'continuous' analog of a similar one recently proved for trees.

1. Introduction

There are striking analogies between real hyperbolic spaces and (homogeneous) trees in the study of Radon transforms. Some have already been pointed out in, e.g., [**C**], [**BCP**], both for the totally geodesic and for the horocyclic Radon transform, which integrate functions along geodesics (or totally geodesic submanifolds), respectively along horocycles. Several inversion formulas are known for the latter transform on the n-dimensional hyperbolic space $\mathbf{H}^n$, such as Gel′fand's so-called Fourier-slice (a special case of [**H1**]), as well as that due to Gel′fand and Graev [**GGV**, Chapter V, §2.3]. In this paper we shall prove one which corresponds to a certain extent to the inversion formula established for trees in [**CCP**, p. 379], and makes use of Helgason's 'distance p' dual Radon transform [**H3**].

1991 *Mathematics Subject Classification*. Primary 44A12; Secondary 44A15, 53C65.

Key words and phrases. Radon transform, real hyperbolic space, horocycles, Abel-type transform.

The first author was partially supported by NSF grants DMS9225043 and CDR8803012.

This paper is in final form and no version of it will be submitted for publication elsewhere.

2. Preliminaries

We shall be using the notation of [**BC**]. In particular, as a model for $\mathbf{H}^n$ we take the unit ball $\mathbf{B}^n$ of $\mathbf{R}^n$ with the metric

$$ds^2 = \frac{4dx^2}{(1-\|x\|^2)^2};$$

the relation between the distance $d(\,\cdot\,,o)$ from the origin o and the Euclidean norm $\|\cdot\|$ is given by

$$\|x\| = \tanh\frac{d(x,o)}{2}.$$

The horocycles are the Euclidean spheres tangent to $\partial\mathbf{B}^n$ internally: let Ξ be their space. With a slight abuse of notation we shall write $d(\xi,x)$ for the *signed* distance between ξ, x: since the geodesic joining x with its closest point $x_0 \in \xi$ shares one boundary point b with the horocycle ξ, the sign of $d(\xi,x)$ will be positive exactly when x_0 lies between x and b.

The horocyclic Radon transform Rf on $\mathbf{H}^n$ of a function f, say, in $\mathcal{S}(\mathbf{H}^n)$ is given by

$$Rf(\xi) = \int_\xi f(x)\,dm_\xi(x) \qquad \text{for every } \xi \in \Xi,$$

where dm_ξ is the $(n-1)$-volume measure on ξ induced by the metric. For $p \in \mathbf{R}$, the 'distance p' dual Radon transform $R_p^*\phi$ of a function ϕ on Ξ is given by

$$R_p^*\phi(x) = \int_{d(\xi,x)=p} \phi(\xi)\,d\mu_{x,p}(\xi) \qquad \text{for every } x \in \mathbf{H}^n,$$

where $d\mu_{x,p}$ is the normalized measure on $\{\xi \in \Xi : d(x,\xi) = p\}$ which is invariant by the isotropy group of x. In particular, with $p=0$ we obtain the usual Radon transform R^*.

The geodesics of $\mathbf{H}^n$ are the arcs of circles orthogonal to $\partial\mathbf{B}^n$, and, in general, the k-dimensional totally geodesic submanifolds of $\mathbf{H}^n$ (for $k < n$) are the intersections with $(k+1)$-planes through o of spherical caps orthogonal to $\partial\mathbf{B}^n$. Correspondingly are defined the k-dimensional totally geodesic Radon transform and its 'distance p' dual. For later comparison we record here an inversion formula for the former.

THEOREM 2.1. [**H3**, Theorem 3.1] *Setting $U = \operatorname{sech} u$, the k-dimensional totally geodesic Radon transform $X = X^k$ on $\mathbf{H}^n$ is inverted by*

$$f(x) = \frac{2^k \Gamma((k+1)/2)}{\pi^{(k+1)/2}(k-1)!} \frac{d^k}{d(T^2)^k} \left[\int_0^T (T^2-U^2)^{k/2-1} X_u^* Xf(x)\,dU\right]\bigg|_{T=1}$$

(Γ *is the Euler Gamma function*). □

We conclude this section by recalling the tree analog for Theorem 3.1 below (we refer the reader to [**CCP**] for definitions and literature).

THEOREM 2.2. [**CCP**, p. 379] *The horocyclic Radon transform R on a $(q+1)$-homogeneous tree T is inverted by*

$$f(x) = R_0^* Rf(x) + (1-q)\sum_{j=1}^{\infty} R_{2j}^* Rf(x). \quad \square$$

3. Derivation of the inversion formula

For $k < n$, the k-volume of a k-dimensional geodesic sphere (i.e., the intersection of a geodesic sphere with a $(k+1)$-dimensional totally geodesic submanifold through its center) of radius u is

$$c_k \sinh^k u, \qquad \text{where } c_k = \frac{2\pi^{(k+1)/2}}{\Gamma((k+1)/2)}.$$

Let $M = M_o$ be the radializing operator with respect to o, i.e.,

$$Mf(u) = \frac{1}{c_{n-1}\sinh^{n-1} u} \int_{d(x,o)=u} f(x)\, d\nu_u(x) \qquad \text{for every } u \geq 0,$$

where $d\nu_u$ is the $(n-1)$-volume measure on the geodesic sphere of radius u centered at o: in other words, $Mf(u)$ is the average of the values of f taken at distance u from o. Obviously $Mf(0) = f(o)$; regarding Mf as a function on $\mathbf{H}^n$ by the abuse of notation $Mf(x) = Mf(d(x,o))$ for all $x \in \mathbf{H}^n$, we get $R_p^* R M f(o) = R_p^* Rf(o)$. Therefore there is no loss of generality in assuming f to be radial, i.e., $f = Mf$. In this case $R_p^* Rf(o) = Rf(\xi)$ where ξ is any horocycle at (signed) distance p from o—such value can be computed by integrating on each intersection of ξ with the geodesic sphere of center o and radius $u \geq |t|$, then summing on u. So (recalling that the metric is conformal to the Euclidean one)

$$R_t^* Rf(o) = Rf(\xi) = \int_{|t|}^{\infty} \frac{1}{\cos\psi} c_{n-2} (\sinh u \sin\gamma)^{n-2} f(u)\, du,$$

where ψ, γ are the angles between the geodesic $\overline{ox}$ (if $x \in \xi$ is such that $d(o,x) = u$) with the horocycle ξ, respectively with the geodesic $\overline{ob}$, if b denotes the boundary point of ξ. The quantities $U = \tanh u/2$, $T = \tanh t/2$ (so t, T can be negative) are the Euclidean distances from o of x, respectively of ξ. By elementary trigonometry applied to the Euclidean triangle oxc, where c is the Euclidean center of ξ, we get

$$\cos\psi = \frac{\sqrt{(1-U^2)(U^2-T^2)}}{U(1-T)},$$

$$\sin\gamma = \frac{\sqrt{(1-U^2)(U^2-T^2)}}{U(1+T)};$$

since $\sinh u = 2U/(1-U^2)$, we have

(3.1) $\qquad R_t^* Rf(o) = 2^{n-1} c_{n-2} \frac{1-T}{(1+T)^{n-2}} \int_{|T|}^{\infty} (U^2 - T^2)^{(n-3)/2} F(U)\, dU,$

having set
$$F(U) = \begin{cases} \dfrac{U}{(1-U^2)^{(n+1)/2}} f(u) & \text{for } 0 \le U < 1, \\ 0 & \text{for } U \ge 1. \end{cases}$$

Identity (3.1) is an Abel-type integral equation, which can be solved explicitly. For $n = 3$ it becomes
$$\int_{|T|}^{\infty} \frac{U}{(1-U^2)^2} f(u) \, dU = \frac{1}{8\pi} \frac{1+T}{1-T} R_t^* R f(o)$$

(observe that the left-hand side is an even function of T): since the integrand is independent of T, the solution is simply
$$f(u) = -\frac{(1-U^2)^2}{8\pi U} \frac{d}{dU}\left(\frac{1+U}{1-U} R_u^* R f(o)\right)$$
$$= -\frac{(1+U)^2}{4\pi U} \left[R_u^* R f(o) + \frac{d}{du} R_u^* R f(o)\right].$$

The quantity in square brackets vanishes at $u = 0$, it being (obtained from) the derivative at 0 of an even function (see above): evaluation at $u = 0$ hence yields
$$f(o) = -\frac{1}{2\pi} \left(\frac{d}{du} + \frac{d^2}{du^2}\right) R_u^* R f(o) \bigg|_{u=0}.$$

For general odd $n = 2m+1$, differentiating $m-1$ times the integral in (3.1) with respect to T^2, then once with respect to T, we obtain
$$F(U) = \frac{U}{(-4\pi)^m} \frac{d^m}{d(U^2)^m} \left[\frac{(1+U)^{2m-1}}{1-U} R_u^* R f(o)\right],$$

so that
$$f(o) = \frac{1}{(-4\pi)^m} \frac{d^m}{d(U^2)^m} \left[\frac{(1+U)^{2m-1}}{1-U} R_u^* R f(o)\right]\bigg|_{u=0}.$$

For even $n = 2m$, an $(m-1)$-fold differentiation of the integral in (3.1) with respect to T^2 yields the equation
$$\int_{|T|}^{\infty} \frac{F(U)}{\sqrt{U^2 - T^2}} dU = \frac{1}{4(-4\pi)^{m-1}} \frac{d^{m-1}}{d(T^2)^{m-1}} \left[\frac{(1+T)^{2m-2}}{1-T} R_t^* R f(o)\right],$$

that is equivalent to the standard Abel integral equation, and is solved by
$$F(U) = \frac{2}{(-4\pi)^m U} \int_U^1 \frac{1}{\sqrt{T^2 - U^2}} \left(T + T^2 \frac{d}{dT}\right) \frac{d^{m-1}}{d(T^2)^{m-1}}$$
$$\left[\frac{(1+T)^{2m-2}}{1-T} R_t^* R f(o)\right] dT$$

(the integrand vanishes for $T \geq 1$). Solving for $f(u)$ and evaluating at $u = 0$, which involves a double differentiation of the integral with respect to U, we get

$$f(o) = \frac{1}{(-4\pi)^m} \int_0^1 \left(\frac{\partial}{\partial T} + \frac{\partial}{\partial U}\right)^2 \left(\frac{1}{\sqrt{T^2 - U^2}}\left(T + T^2 \frac{d}{dT}\right)\frac{d^{m-1}}{d(T^2)^{m-1}}\left[\frac{(1+T)^{2m-2}}{1-T} R_t^* Rf(o)\right]\right)\bigg|_{u=0} dT.$$

For all values of n we can now drop the assumption that f be radial, and replace o by an arbitrary $x \in \mathbf{H}^n$ in each formula. We have thereby proved the following:

THEOREM 3.1. *Setting $U = \tanh u/2$, $T = \tanh t/2$, the horocyclic Radon transform R on $\mathbf{H}^{2m+1}$ (with $m \geq 1$) is inverted by*

$$f(x) = \frac{1}{(-4\pi)^m} \frac{d^m}{d(U^2)^m}\left[\frac{(1+U)^{2m-1}}{1-U} R_u^* Rf(x)\right]\bigg|_{u=0};$$

in particular, if $m = 1$ we have

$$f(x) = -\frac{1}{2\pi}\left(\frac{d}{du} + \frac{d^2}{du^2}\right) R_u^* Rf(x)\bigg|_{u=0}.$$

While that on $\mathbf{H}^{2m}$ is inverted by

$$f(x) = \frac{1}{(-4\pi)^m} \int_0^1 \left(\frac{\partial}{\partial T} + \frac{\partial}{\partial U}\right)^2 \left(\frac{1}{\sqrt{T^2 - U^2}}\left(T + T^2 \frac{d}{dT}\right)\frac{d^{m-1}}{d(T^2)^{m-1}}\left[\frac{(1+T)^{2m-2}}{1-T} R_t^* Rf(x)\right]\right)\bigg|_{u=0} dT. \quad \square$$

REFERENCES

[BC]   C. A. Berenstein, E. Casadio Tarabusi, *Inversion formulas for the k-dimensional Radon transform in real hyperbolic spaces*, Duke Math. J. **62** (1991), 613–631.

[BCCP]   C. A. Berenstein, E. Casadio Tarabusi, J. M. Cohen, M. A. Picardello, *Integral geometry on trees*, Amer. J. Math. **113** (1991), 441–470.

[BCP]   C. A. Berenstein, E. Casadio Tarabusi, M. A. Picardello, *Radon transforms in hyperbolic spaces and their discrete counterparts*, Telesio Courses in Math. (to appear).

[C]   E. Casadio Tarabusi, *Inversion of the X-ray transform: continuous vs. discrete*, Contemp. Math. **113** (1990), 31–39.

[CCP]   E. Casadio Tarabusi, J. M. Cohen, M. A. Picardello, *The horocyclic Radon transform on non-homogeneous trees*, Israel J. Math. **78** (1992), 363–380.

[GGV]   I. M. Gel'fand, M. I. Graev, N. Ya. Vilenkin, *Generalized functions, V: Integral geometry and representation theory*, Academic Press, New York, 1966.

[H1]   S. Helgason, *Radon-Fourier transforms on symmetric spaces and related group representations*, Bull. Amer. Math. Soc. **71** (1965), 757–763.

[H2]   _____, *Groups and geometric analysis: integral geometry, invariant differential operators, and spherical functions*, Pure and Appl. Math., vol. 113, Academic Press, Orlando, 1984.

[H3]   _____, *The totally-geodesic Radon transform on constant curvature spaces*, Contemp. Math. **113** (1990), 141–149.

[H4] _____, *Radon transforms for double fibrations: examples and viewpoints*, 75 years of Radon transform (S. G. Gindikin, P. Michor, eds.), International Press, Hong Kong, 1993, pp. 163–168.

DEPARTMENT OF MATHEMATICS AND INSTITUTE FOR SYSTEMS RESEARCH, UNIVERSITY OF MARYLAND, COLLEGE PARK, MARYLAND 20742, U.S.A.

E-mail address: cab@math.umd.edu, carlos@src.umd.edu

DIPARTIMENTO DI MATEMATICA "G. CASTELNUOVO", UNIVERSITÀ DI ROMA "LA SAPIENZA", PIAZZALE A. MORO 2, 00185 ROMA, ITALY

E-mail address: casadio@itnvax.science.unitn.it, casadio@itncisca.bitnet

Image Reconstruction and Dense Subspaces in the Range of the Radon Transform

W. K. CHEUNG AND ANDREW MARKOE

April 19, 1994

ABSTRACT. We investigate some aspects of doing image reconstruction in the range of the Radon transform by giving a characterization of dense subspaces of the range. We also extend results of B.F. Logan and P. Maass for the finite x-ray transform and A.K. Louis for the finite Radon Transform. We give Sobolev norm estimates for the reconstruction error in the case that the projections are approximately equal. These estimates depend on the closeness of the projections from finitely many directions, a term involving noise in the projection data (singular values) and the Logan-Louis-Maass estimates. But, there are no asymptotic constants in the estimates.

1. Introduction

We investigate some aspects of doing image reconstruction in the range of the Radon transform. We do not give an algorithm for doing image reconstruction in the range of the Radon transform. References [18], [10], [1] and [3] provide several methods of doing this, the idea being to gather projection data from finitely many directions and then to seek an element of the range of the Radon transform which is as close as possible to the given data in the given directions. Then one inverts the element of the range (or just keeps track of where it came from). We do give a general criterion for approximating functions in the range of the Radon transform, i.e., a characterization of dense subspaces of the range of the Radon transform. The dense subspaces considered here consist of linear combinations of products of spherical harmonics (in the angular direction) with functions of the radial variable.

1991 *Mathematics Subject Classification.* Primary 92A05, 44A12.
Key words and phrases. Radon transform, x-ray transform, image reconstruction, Logan's uncertainty principle
This paper is in final form and no version of it will be submitted for publication elsewhere.

We also give estimates for how close the reconstruction is to the object generating the projection data. In the case that the projections are exactly equal from finitely many directions, B.F. Logan [11], in the case of the finite x-ray transform with dimension $n = 2$, P. Maass [17], in the case of the finite x-ray transform with arbitrary dimension and A.K. Louis [13], in the case of the finite Radon transform with arbitrary dimension have shown by an analysis of the frequency behavior in the null space, that the transform determines a low frequency object in the following sense: two low frequency moderately massive objects with *exactly* the same transforms from finitely many directions must be extremely close to each other (in L^2 - norm). We extend these results in two ways: first the objects can have *approximately* the same transforms from finitely many directions: two low frequency moderately massive objects with approximately the same x-ray transforms from finitely many directions must be close modulo a direction dependent noise term and a direction independent term containing Logan's estimates and the normed difference of the objects. Secondly we generalize from the L^2 norm to the Sobolev norm. Similar results hold for the finite Radon transform, but in this case when the dimension is larger than 2, both terms are direction dependent. This result is angle independent for the x-ray transform or for the Radon transform in dimension $n = 2$. A corollary of this result gives a minor extension of the work of Logan, Louis and Maass, referred to above, in which the Sobolev norm replaces the L^2 norm.

As in references Louis-Natterer [15] and Natterer [19], we work in the context of Sobolev spaces.

There are many good general references on the Radon and x-ray transforms. Some of these are Helgason [7], Ludwig [16], Louis and Natterer [15], Natterer [19], Radon [20] and Smith, Solmon and Wagner [23]. Also Seeley [21] is a good reference on spherical harmonics.

Our notation conforms in the most part to that of Natterer [19] and Hörmander [8]. The major difference is that we use the following normalization of the Fourier transform: $\widehat{f}(\xi) = \int_{\mathbf{R}^n} f(x) \exp(-2\pi i x \cdot \xi) \, dx$. Also we sometimes use $\|\cdot\|_s$ in place of $\|\cdot\|_{H^s}$ for the Sobolev norm.

We begin with a study of what we term **Bochner-Riesz functions**. These will be used in the following two sections which present the results outlined above.

2. Bochner-Riesz Functions and Sobolev Spaces

The Radon transform of a function is generally smoother than the original function. Thus products of polynomials by the function $(1 - |x|^2)^\mu$ become important when taking the Radon transform of polynomials restricted to the unit ball. In this article we call these products **Bochner-Riesz** functions.

Bochner-Riesz functions arise in harmonic analysis as the means of the Bochner-Riesz summability method (c.f. Stein and Weiss [24] p. 171.)

DEFINITION 1. **Bochner-Riesz Functions** *The* **Bochner Riesz generator of order** μ *is the function* $br_\mu \colon \mathbf{R}^n \to \mathbf{R}$ *defined by* $br_\mu(x) = \begin{cases} (1 - |x|^2)^\mu & \text{, if } |x| \leq 1 \\ 0 & \text{, if } |x| > 1 \end{cases}$
The **space of Bochner Riesz functions** *of order μ is defined to be the set of*

products of br_μ by polynomials and is denoted by $BR^\mu(\Omega)$ where Ω is the unit ball of $\mathbf{R}^n$.

We begin with the following result.

LEMMA 2. *Let μ be a real number in $(0,1]$. Then $br_\mu \in C_0^\gamma$ for $0 \le \gamma \le \mu$. Here C_0^γ is the space of Hölder functions of order γ as defined in Hörmander [8] page 241.*

Proof. Let f denote br_μ. We handle the case $n = 1$ first. Since $\mu \le 1$, f is concave down and hence the following relation between secants holds for $x, y \in [-1, 1]$ with $x < y$:

$$\text{(1)} \qquad \left|\frac{f(x) - f(y)}{x - y}\right| \le \left|\frac{f(x) - f(1)}{x - 1}\right|$$

If now $0 \le \gamma \le 1$

$$\text{(2)} \qquad |x - y|^{1-\gamma} \le |x - 1|^{1-\gamma}$$

From (1) and (2) it follows that

$$\frac{|f(x) - f(y)|}{|x - y|^\gamma} = \left|\frac{f(x) - f(y)}{x - y}\right| |x - y|^{1-\gamma} \le \left|\frac{f(x) - f(1)}{x - 1}\right| |x - 1|^{1-\gamma}$$

$$= |1 - x|^{\mu - \gamma} |1 + x|^\mu.$$

for $0 \le \gamma \le \mu$ and $x, y \in [-1, 1]$. From this inequality it is obvious that $\frac{|f(x)-f(y)|}{|x-y|^\gamma}$ is bounded on $[-1,1]$. It easily follows that this is true also for any $x, y \in \mathbf{R}$, thus proving the lemma for the case $n = 1$.

Now let $n \ge 1$ and let $x, y \in \mathbf{R}^n$. Without loss of generality we may assume that at least one of $x, y \in \Omega$, so there exist $a, b \in \Omega$ such that x, y lie on the line through a, b. Then we may parametrize the line by $x(t) = \frac{1}{2}(1-t)a + (1+t)b)$. Define $u(t) = [\frac{1}{2}(1-t^2)(1 - a \cdot b)]^\mu$. An easy calculation shows that $f(x(t)) = u(t)$. If then $x = x(t)$ and $y = x(s)$ we have

$$\frac{|f(x) - f(y)|}{|x - y|^\gamma} = const \frac{|u(t) - u(s)|}{|s - t|^\gamma}.$$

The constant actually depends on $a \cdot b$. But $a, b \in \Omega$, so the constant is bounded for all $x, y \in \mathbf{R}^n$. Then, since u is a constant multiple of a 1-dimensional Bochner-Riesz generator, the case of general n follows from that of the case $n = 1$ already proved. $\square$

COROLLARY 3. *If $0 \le s < \mu$, then $BR^\mu(\Omega) \subset H_0^s(\Omega)$.*

Proof. It follows from the lemma that $BR^\mu(\Omega) \subset C_0^\mu$. But by result (7.9.6) of Hörmander [8], page 242, $C_0^\mu \subset H_0^s(\Omega)$, if $0 \le s < \mu$.

PROPOSITION 4. *Let $s \ge 0$ and $\mu > s$ and let $g \in C_0^\mu$. Then the map $G : C_0^\infty(\mathbf{R}^n) \to H_0^s(\mathbf{R}^n)$ defined by $u \mapsto g \cdot u$ is well defined and continuous.*

Proof. By definition of the topology of $C_0^\infty(\mathbf{R}^n)$ it suffices to prove that the map $G : C_0^\infty(K) \to H_0^s(\mathbf{R}^n)$ is continuous for any compact $K \subset \mathbf{R}^n$ ($C_0^\infty(K)$ has the topology of uniform convergence of derivatives on K). Let $s = k + t$ where $k = [s]$ and $t = s - k$. If $t > 0$ then the following is an equivalent norm for the Sobolev space $H_0^s(\Omega)$ (Hörmander [8], page 241):

$$\|u\|_{(s)} = \sum_{|\alpha|=0}^{k} \|\partial^\alpha u\|_0 + \left[\sum_{|\alpha|=k} \iint |\partial^\alpha u(x) - \partial^\alpha u(y)|^2 |x-y|^{-n-2s} \, dxdy \right]^{\frac{1}{2}}$$

Replacing u by $g \cdot u$ and using Leibniz's product formula we get

(3)
$$\|\partial^\alpha g \cdot u\|_0 \leq \sum_{|\beta| \leq |\alpha|} \binom{\alpha}{\beta} \|\partial^\beta g \cdot \partial^{\alpha-\beta} u\|_0$$
$$\leq \sum_{|\beta| \leq |\alpha|} \binom{\alpha}{\beta} \|\partial^\beta g\|_0 \|\partial^{\alpha-\beta} u\|_K \sqrt{meas(K)}$$
$$\leq C \sum_{|\beta| \leq |\alpha|} \|\partial^{\alpha-\beta} u\|_K$$

where C depends only on s, K and g. In a similar fashion:

$$\iint |\partial^\alpha g \cdot u(x) - \partial^\alpha g \cdot u(y)|^2 |x-y|^{-n-2s} \, dxdy$$
$$\leq C \sum_{|\beta| \leq |\alpha|} \binom{\alpha}{\beta} \iint |\partial^\beta g(x) \cdot \partial^{\alpha-\beta} u(x) - \partial^\beta g(y) \cdot \partial^{\alpha-\beta} u(y)|^2 |x-y|^{-n-2s} \, dxdy$$
$$\leq C \sum_{|\beta| \leq |\alpha|} \binom{\alpha}{\beta} \iint \left[\begin{array}{c} |\partial^{\alpha-\beta} u(x)|^2 |\partial^\beta g(x) \cdot - \partial^\beta g(y)|^2 \\ + |\partial^\beta g(y)|^2 |\partial^{\alpha-\beta} u(x) - \partial^{\alpha-\beta} u(y)|^2 \end{array} \right] |x-y|^{-n-2s} \, dxdy$$
$$\leq C \sum_{|\beta| \leq |\alpha|} \binom{\alpha}{\beta} \|g\|_{(s)}^2 \|\partial^{\alpha-\beta} u(x)\|_K^2 + \|\partial^\beta g(y)\|_\Omega^2 \|u\|_{(s)}^2$$
(4)

In (4) $\|\partial^\beta g(y)\|_\Omega$ is finite because $g \in C_0^\mu$. Also in (4) $\|u\|_{(s)}^2 \leq \|u\|_{(k+1)}^2 < \infty$ since $u \in C_0^\infty(K)$. But $\|u\|_{(k+0)}^2 \leq const \cdot \|u\|_{k+1}^2 \leq const \cdot \sum_{|\beta| \leq k+1} \|\partial^\beta u\|_K^2 \cdot meas(K)$. Combining this with (4) we arrive at

(5)
$$\iint |\partial^\alpha g \cdot u(x) - \partial^\alpha g \cdot u(y)|^2 |x-y|^{-n-2s} \, dxdy$$
$$\leq const \cdot \sum_{|\beta| \leq |\alpha|} \|\partial^{\alpha-\beta} u(x)\|_K^2 + \sum_{|\beta| \leq |\alpha|} \sum_{|\beta| \leq k+1} \|\partial^\beta u\|_K^2$$

Combining inequalities (3) and (5) we arrive at

$$\|g \cdot u\|_{(s)} \leq const \cdot \sum_{|\beta| \leq k+1} \|\partial^\beta u\|_K$$

which proves the proposition. $\square$

COROLLARY 5. *Let $s \geq 0$ and $\mu > s$. Then the map $G_\mu : C_0^\infty(\mathbf{R}^n) \to H_0^s(\mathbf{R}^n)$ defined by $g \longmapsto g \cdot br_\mu$ is well defined and continuous.*

THEOREM 6. *For $s < \mu$, the Bochner-Riesz space $BR^\mu(\Omega)$ is dense in the Sobolev space $H_0^s(\Omega)$.*

Proof. By the previous corollary we know that $BR^\mu(\Omega)$ is a subspace of $H_0^s(\Omega)$ for $s < \mu$. By the Hahn-Banach theorem it suffices to show that any continuous linear functional $\theta \in H_0^s(\Omega)'$ which vanishes on $BR^\mu(\Omega)$ also vanishes on $H_0^s(\Omega)$.

The functional $\tau : \mathcal{D} \to \mathbf{C}$ defined by $\tau(u) = \theta(u \cdot br_\mu)$ is well defined and continuous by corollary 5, i.e., τ is a distribution. Furthermore, τ is compactly supported since br_μ is compactly supported.

The Paley-Wiener-Schwartz theorem implies that the Fourier transform $\widehat{\tau}$ of τ is an entire analytic function. Then by the derivative theorem for Fourier transforms: $D^\alpha \widehat{\tau}(t) = (x^\alpha \tau)\widehat{\,}(t) = \tau(x^\alpha \exp(-2\pi i x \cdot t))$. If $t = 0$ this gives $D^\alpha \widehat{\tau}(0) = \tau(x^\alpha) = \theta(x^\alpha \cdot br_\mu(x)) = 0$, since this is θ evaluated on an element of $BR^\mu(\Omega)$. Hence every derivative of the analytic function $\widehat{\tau}$ vanishes. Thus $\widehat{\tau} = 0$ and with this also $\tau = 0$.

By the definition of τ, this means that $\theta(u \cdot br_\mu) = 0$ for any $u \in \mathcal{D}$. Hence given $\varphi \in \mathcal{D}(\Omega)$ we may define

$$u(x) = \begin{cases} \frac{\varphi(x)}{br_\mu(x)} & , \text{if } x \in \mathrm{supp}(\varphi) \\ 0 & , \text{elsewhere} \end{cases}$$

The function $u \in \mathcal{D}$ because br_μ is C^∞ on Ω and since br_μ does not vanish on $\mathrm{supp}(\varphi)$. Hence $\theta(\varphi) = \theta(br_\mu \cdot u) = 0$. This shows that the functional θ vanishes on $\mathcal{D}(\Omega)$. But $\mathcal{D}(\Omega)$ is dense in $H_0^s(\Omega)$ (by the result 4.3s, Th 1b in Triebel [25] .) Thus $\theta = 0$ on all of $H_0^s(\Omega)$ proving the theorem. □

3. Estimates for Reconstructions from Finitely Many Projections

In this section we consider a situation in which there are two objects f and g with approximately the same projections from finitely many directions. We derive an estimate for the difference in Sobolev norm of smoothed versions of f and g. This estimate depends on the L^2 weights of f and g and on the noise in the projections. This is done for both the finite x-ray transform and for the finite Radon transform. A consequence is that low bandwidth, moderately massive objects with approximately the same projections from finitely many directions must be themselves approximately the same.

A corollary of this result shows that two low bandwidth objects with identically the same x-ray projections from finitely many directions must be close in L^2 - norm if the number of directions is sufficiently large. Even as few as 100 directions will give extremely close estimates in this case. This may be considered in counterpoint to the famous, but pessimistic, result of Smith, Solmon and Wagner [23] that *A finite set of radiographs tells nothing at all.* They showed that two objects can have the same x-ray projections from a given finite number of directions yet be very different. Our result shows that for this to happen the difference between the objects must be an extremely highly oscillating function, i.e., a high bandwidth object. Khalfin and Klebanov [9] have achieved similar results but only in $\mathbf{R}^2$, only for positive functions and only for certain special directions, even in the case of identical and not approximate projections. In certain bandwidth-direction number ratios our estimates are better while in others theirs are. More details follow the proof of theorem 16.

DEFINITION 7 [Finite X-Ray Transform]. Let $W : \mathbf{R}^n \longrightarrow \mathbf{R}$ and $w_\theta : \theta^\perp \longrightarrow \mathbf{R}$ be weight functions. For $f \in L^2(\Omega, W)$ and $\theta \in \mathbf{S}^{n-1}$ define **the x-ray projection in direction θ**
$$P_\theta : L^2(\Omega, W) \longrightarrow L^2(\theta^\perp, w)$$
by
$$P_\theta f(\sigma \in \theta^\perp) = \int_{-\infty}^{\infty} f(\sigma + t\theta) dt$$
where the weights W and w are such that P_θ is a bounded operator.

Given a finite set of directions $\vartheta = \{\theta_1, \ldots, \theta_p\}$ let $L^2(\vartheta, w) \stackrel{def}{=} \bigoplus_{j=1}^{p} L^2(\theta_j^\perp, w)$. Then define **the finite x-ray transform**
$$P_\vartheta : L^2(\Omega, W) \longrightarrow L^2(\vartheta, w)$$
by
$$(P_\vartheta f)_j = P_{\theta_j} f$$
We also define Sobolev spaces $H^s(\mathbf{R}^n, W)$, $H_0^s(\Omega, W)$ and $H^s(\vartheta, w)$ in the obvious way for non-negative integral values of s (using weighted L^2-norms of derivatives). Then we use interpolation to define these Sobolev spaces for non-integral values. We consider $P_\vartheta : H_0^s(\Omega, W) \longrightarrow H^s(\vartheta, w)$ when the map is bounded in Sobolev norm.

DEFINITION 8 [Finite Radon Transform]. Let $W : \mathbf{R}^n \longrightarrow \mathbf{R}$ and $w : \mathbf{R} \longrightarrow \mathbf{R}$ be weight functions. For $f \in L^2(\Omega, W)$ and $\theta \in \mathbf{S}^{n-1}$ define **the Radon projection in direction θ**
$$R_\theta : L^2(\Omega, W) \longrightarrow L^2(\mathbf{R}, w)$$
by
$$R_\theta f(x \in \mathbf{R}) = \int_{\sigma \in \theta^\perp} f(x\theta + \sigma) d\sigma$$
where the weights W and w are such that R_θ is a bounded operator.

Also given a finite set of directions $\vartheta = \{\theta_1, \ldots, \theta_p\}$ define **the finite Radon transform**
$$R_\vartheta : L^2(\Omega, W) \longrightarrow \bigoplus_{j=1}^{p} L^2(\mathbf{R}, w)$$
by
$$(R_\vartheta f)_j = R_{\theta_j} f$$
As above we define Sobolev spaces and consider the map
$$R_\vartheta : H_0^s(\Omega, W) \longrightarrow \bigoplus_{j=1}^{p} H^s(\mathbf{R}, w)$$
when it is bounded in Sobolev norm.

The *Fourier transform* of a function f is denoted by $\mathcal{F}f$ or by $\hat{f}$ and is defined by

$$\mathcal{F}f(\xi) = \hat{f}(\xi) = \int_{\mathbf{R}^n} f(t) e^{-2\pi i t \cdot \xi} dt$$

Then the *inverse Fourier transform* is given by

$$\mathcal{F}^{-1} g(t) = \int_{\mathbf{R}^n} g(\xi) e^{2\pi i t \cdot \xi} d\xi$$

DEFINITION 9. ϕ_c denotes the characteristic function of the ball B_c of radius c centered at the origin of $\mathbf{R}^n$: $\phi_c(x) = 1$ if $x \in B_c$ otherwise $\phi_c(x) = 0$. Then the **ideal low bandpass filter** Φ_c is defined by

$$\Phi_c = \mathcal{F}^{-1} \phi_c$$

DEFINITION 10. For $f \in L^2(\mathbf{R}^n)$, define

$$\lambda(f; c) = \frac{\|\hat{f} \cdot \phi_c\|_{L^2}^2}{\|\hat{f}\|_{L^2}^2}$$

$\lambda(f; c)$ is the *percentage of energy of the function f in bandwidth c*.

DEFINITION 11.

$$\lambda_p(c) = \sup(\lambda(f; c) : f \text{ has } p \text{ vanishing x-ray projections})$$

The quantities $\lambda_p(c)$ and $\lambda(f; c)$ depend on the dimension n, but there will be no confusion by not referring to the dimension in the notation. We note that if $\vartheta = \{\theta_1, \ldots, \theta_p\}$ and $f_0 \in N(P_\vartheta)$, then an easy consequence of Parseval's theorem and this definition is that

$$\|f_0 * \Phi_c\| \leq \sqrt{\lambda_p(c)} \|f_0\|$$

THEOREM 12 [Logan's Uncertainty Principle]. (Logan [11] for n=2, Maass [17] for general n). For $\beta \in \mathbf{R}^+$,

$$\lim_{p \to \infty} \lambda_p(\beta(p + \frac{n}{2} - 1)) = \begin{cases} 0 \text{ if } \beta < 1 \\ 1 \text{ if } \beta > 1 \end{cases}$$

The meaning of this limit is that most of the energy of a ghost (from a sufficiently large number p of directions) must lie outside the bandwidth $p + \frac{n}{2} - 1$. This limit is a result of one of the many estimates for the quantities $\lambda_p(c)$ in Logan [11]. These estimates stem from the fact that $\lambda_p(c)$ is the maximum eigenvalue of a certain Hankel integral equation whose eigenfunction happens to be one of Slepian's generalized prolate spheroidal wave functions [22].

The analogous results for the Radon transform are due to Louis [13].

Condition V (Louis [13]) $\vartheta_p = \{\theta_1, \cdots, \theta_p\} \subset \mathbf{S}^{n-1}$ *satisifes condition V if there is an integer solution m to*
$$p = \binom{m+n-2}{n-1}$$
and there is no spherical harmonic q of degree $m-1$ such that $q(\theta_j) = 0$ for all $\theta_j \in \vartheta_p$.

DEFINITION 13 [Louis [13]].

$$\mu_p(c) = \sup(\lambda(f;c) : f \text{ has } p \text{ vanishing x-ray projections}$$
$$\text{from a set of directions } \vartheta_p \text{ such that } p \text{ and } \vartheta_p$$
$$\text{satisfy condition V})$$

The theorem for the finite Radon transform analogous to theorem 12 is

THEOREM 14 [Louis [13] theorem 4.1]. *Let condition V be fulfilled and let m be the integer corresponding to the number of directions p in condition V, $\alpha > 0$ and $\frac{1}{3} < \beta < 1$, then*
$$lim_{p\to\infty} \mu_p((m + \frac{n}{2} - 1) - \alpha(m + \frac{n}{2} - 1)^\beta) = 0$$

Note that for dimension $n = 2$ condition V imposes no restrictions on the set of directions. ϑ_p. However, it is clear that the uncertainty principle for the Radon transform is very dependent on the distribution of the directions in dimension $n > 2$. Here is a restatement of condition V and theorem 14 in the case $n = 3$.

Condition V (for $n = 3$) $\vartheta_p = \{\theta_1, \cdots, \theta_p\} \subset \mathbf{S}^{n-1}$ *satisifes condition V if p is the sum of an arithmetic progression $1 + \cdots + m$. In this case $8p + 1$ is a perfect square, $m = \frac{\sqrt{8p+1}-1}{2}$ and ϑ_p must not be in an algebraic subvariety of $\mathbf{S}^{n-1}$ of degree $\frac{\sqrt{8p+1}-1}{2} - 1$.*

THEOREM 15. *(Louis's theorem [14] for the case $n = 3$) Let condition V be fulfilled for $n = 3$ and let $\alpha > 0$ and $\frac{1}{3} < \beta < 1$, then*
$$lim_{p\to\infty} \mu_p((\frac{\sqrt{8p+1}}{2}) - \alpha(\frac{\sqrt{8p+1}}{2})^\beta) = 0$$

The next result gives the promised estimate for the difference between an object and its reconstruction.

THEOREM 16. *Let p be a positive integer, let ϑ be a set of p directions in $\mathbf{S}^{n-1}$ and let $c > 0$. Let w be a weight function for which the finite x-ray transform $P_\vartheta : L^2(\Omega) \longrightarrow L^2(\vartheta, w)$ has a singular value decomposition with singular values σ_i. Letting $\sigma = \inf_i \sigma_i$ we have for $f, g \in H^s(\Omega)$,*

$$\|f * \Phi_c - g * \Phi_c\|_{H^s(\mathbf{R}^n)} \leq \frac{1}{\sigma}\|P_\vartheta f - P_\vartheta g\|_{H^s(\vartheta,w)} + \sqrt{\lambda_p(c)}\|f - g\|_{H_0^s(\Omega)}$$

A similar result holds for the finite Radon transform. Here it is necessary that ϑ satisfy condition V and that $R_\vartheta : L^2(\Omega) \to \bigoplus_{j=1}^{p} L^2(\mathbf{R}, w)$ have a singular value decomposition with singular values μ_i. Let $\mu = \inf_i \mu_i$. Then for $f, g \in H^s(\Omega)$,

$$\|f * \Phi_c - g * \Phi_c\|_{H^s(\mathbf{R}^n)} \leq \frac{1}{\mu}\|R_\vartheta f - R_\vartheta g\|_{\bigoplus_{j=1}^{p} H^s(\mathbf{R},w)} + \sqrt{\mu_p(c)}\|f - g\|_{H_0^s(\Omega)}$$

REMARK

If $\sigma = 0$, then the right hand side is infinite and no information is given. However, we will see that there are choices of the weights which give singular value decompositions with $\sigma > 0$.

Proof. We are grateful to the referee for suggesting the following proof which is a vast improvement of our original one. We give the proof for the case of the finite x-ray transform. A similar proof works in the Radon case.

By linearity we prove the result for $f \in L^2(\Omega)$, assuming $g = 0$. All the norms in this proof are in $L^2(\Omega)$ or $L^2(\mathbf{R}^n)$ unless otherwise noted. The extension to the Sobolev norm is handled at the end.

Decompose $f = f_0 + f_1$ where $f_0 \in N(P_\vartheta)$ and $f_1 \in Range(P_\vartheta^*)$.

We observe that $P_\vartheta^{-1} : Range(P_\vartheta^*) \to L^2(\Omega, W)$ is well defined and bounded. In fact, by the properties of the singular value decomposition, $\|P_\vartheta^{-1}\| \leq \frac{1}{\sigma}$. From this and the fact that $f_1 \in Range(P_\vartheta^*)$, we easily obtain:

$$\|f_1 * \Phi_c\| \leq \|f_1\| = \|P_\vartheta^{-1} P_\vartheta(f_1)\| \leq \frac{1}{\sigma}\|P_\vartheta(f_1)\| \leq \frac{1}{\sigma}\|P_\vartheta(f)\|$$

From this and the remark in definition 11 we get

(6) $$\|f * \Phi_c\| \leq \|f_0 * \Phi_c\| + \|f_1 * \Phi_c\| \leq \frac{1}{\sigma}\|P_\vartheta(f)\| + \sqrt{\lambda_p(c)}\|f_0\|$$

which is the desired result for $f \in L^2(\Omega) = H_0^s(\Omega)$.

Now let s be an integer ≥ 0. Assume that $f \in H_0^s(\Omega)$. Then for every multi-index α with $|\alpha| \leq s$ we have from (6)

(7) $$\|(\partial^\alpha f) * \Phi_c\|_{L^2(\Omega)} \leq \frac{1}{\sigma}\|P_\vartheta(\partial^\alpha f)\|_{L^2(\vartheta,w)} + \sqrt{\lambda_p(c)}\|\partial^\alpha f\|_{L^2(\Omega)}$$

Since ∂^α factors out of P_ϑ we get

(8) $$\|\partial^\alpha (f * \Phi_c)\|_{L^2(\Omega)} \leq \frac{1}{\sigma}\|\partial^\alpha (P_\vartheta(f))\|_{L^2(\vartheta,w)} + \sqrt{\lambda_p(c)}\|\partial^\alpha f\|_{L^2(\Omega)}$$

Finally adding the norms in 8 as α varies with $|\alpha| \leq s$ gives the desired inequality in Sobolev norm. If $s > 0$ is not an integer, then the result follows by interpolation among the integer order spaces.

A similar proof works in the Radon case. The main difference is that when one gets to the analogue of inequality (8) then $\theta^\alpha \partial^{|\alpha|}$ factors out of $R_\theta(\partial^\alpha f)$. But this is no problem because $\theta \in S^{n-1}$. Also the directions for the Radon case have to satisfy Louis' condition V. This proves the theorem. $\square$

As a corollary we get a minor generalization of one of the results of B.F. Logan [11], P. Maass [17] and A.K. Louis [13] cited in the introduction.

COROLLARY 17. *For the x-ray transform, if ϑ is a finite set of p directions in $\mathbf{S}^{n-1}$, if f_0 and f_1 are in $L^2(\Omega)$ and if $P_\vartheta f_0 = P_\vartheta f_1$, then*

$$\|f_0 * \Phi_c - f_1 * \Phi_c\|_{H^s(\mathbf{R}^n)} \leq \sqrt{\lambda_p(c)} \|f_0 - f_1\|_{H^s_0(\Omega)}$$

In the Radon case, let ϑ be a finite set of p directions in $\mathbf{S}^{n-1}$ which satisfies condition V. If f_0 and f_1 are in $L^2(\Omega)$ and if $R_\vartheta f_0 = R_\vartheta f_1$, then

$$\|f_0 * \Phi_c - f_1 * \Phi_c\|_{H^s(\mathbf{R}^n)} \leq \sqrt{\mu_p(c)} \|f_0 - f_1\|_{H^s_0(\Omega)}$$

REMARKS

1. In the part of the proof where we use $\|\widehat{(f - g_1)} \cdot \phi_c\| \leq \|\widehat{f - g_1}\|$, there is some loss of energy. However the idea is to apply this result to functions with most of their energy in bandwidth c, in which case this loss is negligible.

2. As mentioned above, Khalfin and Klebanov [9] have achieved similar results in $\mathbf{R}^2$. Their main result for approximately equal projections states: **Theorem 0.5** [9] Given $p \geq 2$, let $\Theta_j = (\cos\left(\pi \frac{2j-1}{2j}\right), -1)$ for $j = 1, \ldots, p$ and $\Theta_j = (1, \cos\left(\pi \frac{2(j-p)-1}{2(j-p)}\right))$ for $j = p+1, \ldots, 2p$. These Θ_j determine 2n directions in Ω. Let $V_c(x) = \frac{1}{c^2} \frac{\cos(cx_1) - \cos(2cx_1)}{x_1^2} \frac{\cos(cx_2) - \cos(2cx_2)}{x_2^2}$ be the Vallée-Poussin kernel. Let f and g be probability density functions supported on the unit square $[-1, 1] \times [-1, 1] \subset \mathbf{R}^2$ (non-negative functions with L^1-norm = 1). Then given $\epsilon > 0$, if $\left|\int_{-\infty}^\infty f(x + t\Theta_j)dt - \int_{-\infty}^\infty g(x + t\Theta_j)dt\right| \leq \epsilon$, then

$$\sup_{x \in \mathbf{R}^2} |f * V_c(x) - g * V_c(x)| \leq \epsilon \left(8 + \frac{4}{\pi} \log(p)\right) + \frac{32}{(p+1)!} c^{p+2}$$

We can note that $\int_{-\infty}^\infty f(x + t\Theta_j)dt = P_{\Theta_j} f(x)$ so the result of Khalfin and Klebanov can be restated in the form

$$\|f * V_c(x) - g * V_c(x)\|_{L^\infty(\mathbf{R}^2)} \leq \left(8 + \frac{4}{\pi} \log(p)\right) \|P_\vartheta f - P_\vartheta g\|_{L^\infty(\mathbf{R})} + \frac{32}{(p+1)!} c^{p+2}$$

where L^∞ denotes the space of bounded functions with the sup norm.

Let us compare this result to our result:

$$\|f * \Phi_c - g * \Phi_c\|_{H^s(\mathbf{R}^n)} \leq \frac{1}{\lambda} \|P_\vartheta f - P_\vartheta g\|_{H^s(\vartheta, w)} + \sqrt{\lambda_p(c)} \|f - g\|_{H^s_0(\Omega)}$$

Except for the differences in using sup norms in the one case and Sobolev norms in the other and except for the difference in the filters (Vallée-Poussin vs. ideal low bandpass), we get formally the same type of estimates. However our results are valid in any $\mathbf{R}^n$ and for any finite set of p directions ϑ, while the results of Khalfin and Klebanov are valid only for $\mathbf{R}^2$ and for the special Tchebyshev directions given by the Θ_j. Also their functions must be probability density functions. However, this is not a strong restriction. We note that the Khalfin and Klebanov coefficient $\left(8 + \frac{4}{\pi}\log(p)\right)$ is analogous to our coefficient $\frac{1}{\lambda}$. If we take n equally spaced directions in $\mathbf{R}^2$, then $\frac{1}{\lambda} \leq \sqrt{p}$ so they have a better estimate than we do for this part of the inequality. If we take the bandwidth somewhat less than the number of directions, say $c = \alpha p$ where α is less than but close to 1, then their estimate for the second term $\frac{32}{(p+1)!}c^{p+2}$ is approximately equal to $\frac{\alpha}{\sqrt{2\pi(p+1)}}\left(\frac{\alpha e p}{p+1}\right)^{p+1}$ by Stirling's approximation. For this term to be small, one would need to take $\alpha < \frac{1}{e}$, whereas our corresponding term $\sqrt{\lambda_p(c)}\|f - g\|_{H_0^s(\Omega)}$ gets very small even if c is close to but less than a large p. For example, if we are going to compare L^2 functions to probability densities, then it would make sense to assume that $\|f - g\|_{H_0^s(\Omega)} < 1$. Then we can ask how $\frac{\alpha}{\sqrt{2\pi(p+1)}}\left(\frac{\alpha e p}{p+1}\right)^{p+1}$ compares to $\sqrt{\lambda_p(c)}$. As one example we take $p = 20$ and $\alpha = 0.9$ so $c = 18$. Then $\sqrt{\lambda_p(c)} < 0.019$ while $\frac{\alpha}{\sqrt{2\pi(p+1)}}\left(\frac{\alpha e p}{p+1}\right)^{p+1} > 4 \times 10^6$, while if $p = 180$ and $\alpha = 0.9$ so $c = 162$, then $\lambda_p(c) < 6.1 \times 10^{-35}$ while $\frac{\alpha}{\sqrt{2\pi(p+1)}}\left(\frac{\alpha e p}{p+1}\right)^{p+1} > 2 \times 10^{68}$. It is only when $\alpha < \frac{1}{e}$ that the estimate of Khalfin and Klebanov is useful.

3. In the corollary, let f_0 represent an object and f_1 a tomographic reconstruction with the same x-ray projections from p different directions. If p is large enough and $c < p + \frac{n}{2} - 1$ and f_0 is low bandwidth in the sense that $f_0 * \Phi_c$ is close to f_0 and if the energy of f_1 is comparable to that of f_0, then an immediate consequence of this theorem is that f_0 will be close to f_1.

4. How large must p be to make the estimate in the corollary close? In other words how small is $\lambda_p(c)$? In dimension 2, for example, if the number of directions p is 20 and if the bandwidth $c < 18$ (90% of p), then $\lambda_p(c) < 3.5 \times 10^{-4}$, while if $p = 180$ and $c = 162$ (90% of p), then $\lambda_p(c) < 6.1 \times 10^{-35}$.

5. B. F. Logan [11] has a result similar to the corollary in dimension 2 similar to this theorem: in his result the object f_0 is unfiltered and the approximation f_1 is best among ridge functions with the same p projections. But as mentioned above, the corollary (in L^2) is just an easy consequence of the definitions.

6. In dimension $n = 2$ Davison and Grünbaum [4] have constructed a singular value decomposition for the finite Radon transform R_ϑ (or equally well in this dimension for the finite x-ray transform P_ϑ). The next theorem summarizes their results for this singular value decomposition.

THEOREM 18 [Davison and Grünbaum]. [4] Let $\vartheta = \{\theta_1, \cdots, \theta_p\} \subset \mathbf{S}^1$ be a set of directions in $\mathbf{R}^2$, and let the weight $w(t)$ be given by

$$w(t) = \frac{2}{\pi}(1 - t^2)^{-\frac{1}{2}}$$

Then the finite Radon transform $R_\vartheta : L^2(\Omega) \longrightarrow \bigoplus_{j=1}^p L^2(\mathbf{R}, w)$ has a singular value decomposition with singular values λ_i such that

$$\lambda = \inf(\lambda_i) > 0$$

Furthermore, if the angles θ_j are equally spaced on $\mathbf{S}^1$ then

$$\lambda \geq \sqrt{\frac{1}{p}}$$

Proof. Let $P = R_\vartheta$. By lemma 5.1, page 91 [4] the nonzero eigenvalues γ_i of PP^* are bounded away from zero. A standard construction for singular value decompositions then gives a singular value decomposition for P with singular values $\lambda_i = \sqrt{\gamma_i}$. This proves the first part of the theorem.

From section 8 of [4] it follows that $\lambda \geq \sqrt{\frac{1}{p}}$ if p is odd and $\lambda \geq \sqrt{\frac{2}{p}}$ if p is even. Although slightly better estimates occur in the even case versus the odd case, we accept the weaker estimate independent of parity in order to simplify the statement of the theorem. □

7. The constructions in Davison and Grünbaum [4] are much more general than the one stated here. In the proof above only weights for the Gegenbauer case are considered and only for the parameter $\lambda = 1$ occurring in [4].

8. By arguments with compact operators we can show that singular value decompositions of P_ϑ and R_ϑ exist in higher dimensions than $n = 2$. However, there do not seem to be higher dimensional estimates on the singular values. Also there are results in higher dimensions for the pure Radon and x-ray transforms (Davison [5], [6] and Louis [14] for the Radon transform and Maass [17] for the x-ray transform.

4. Dense Subspaces of the Range of the Radon Transform

Our second result gives a general criterion for approximating functions in the range of the Radon transform - it characterizes dense subspaces of the range of the Radon transform. The subspaces considered here consist of linear combinations of products of spherical harmonics (in the angular direction) with functions of the radial variable.

There have been several attempts to reconstruct functions in the range of the Radon transform. The general idea is to select a space A of L^2 functions on $[-1, 1]$ and to use linear combinations of the form

$$(9) \qquad h(t, \omega) = \sum a_{lk}(t) Y_{lk}(\omega)$$

where $a_{lk}(t) \in A$ and $Y_{lk}(\omega)$ are spherical harmonics, and where h lies in the range of the Radon transform, to approximate given projection data $g \in L^2(Z)$. For example one can try to minimize the L^2 norm $\|h - g\|$ where g is given projection data and where h has the form 9 and is in the range of the Radon transform. If g differs only somewhat from the true Radon transform of an object in $L^2(\Omega)$ and if the space of functions of the form 9 which lie in the range of the Radon transform are dense in that range, then one should be able to get an L^2 close aproximation to the original object. Then the results of the first part of this paper would give estimates on the accuracy of the reconstruction, since both the original object and the reconstruction would have projections close to each other. Our interest in this problem stems from previous work using spline functions for the space A [1], [2], [3]. M. Lautsch [10] has developed a much better method in the case that A consists of spline functions. Also R. B. Marr [18] has used this idea in the case that A is the set of polynomials.

We begin with a result of A. K.Louis [12]

THEOREM 19 [Louis [12]]. *If $\nu > \frac{n}{2} - 1$, then the Radon transform is an operator $R: L^2\left(\Omega, br_{\nu-\frac{n}{2}}^{-1}\right) \to L^2\left(Z, br_{\nu-\frac{1}{2}}^{-1}\right)$. Furthermore, any $f \in L^2\left(\Omega, br_{\nu-\frac{n}{2}}^{-1}\right)$ and its Radon transform have expansions:*

$$f(s\omega) = br_{\nu-\frac{n}{2}}(s) \overbrace{\sum_{m=0}^{\infty} \sum_{l=0}^{m} T_{m,l}^{\nu,n}(s) \sum_{k=1}^{M(n,l)} d_{mlk} Y_{lk}(\omega)}^{\text{in polar coordinates}}$$

$$Rf(s,\omega) = br_{\nu-\frac{1}{2}}(s) \sum_{m=0}^{\infty} C_m^{\nu}(s) \sum_{\substack{l=0 \\ m+l \text{ even}}}^{m} \sum_{k=1}^{M(n,l)} d_{mlk} Y_{lk}(\omega)$$

where $T_{m,l}^{\nu,n}$ are polynomials of degreee m, Y_{lk} are spherical harmonics of degree l on $\mathbf{S}^{n-1}$, C_m^{ν} are Gegenbauer polynomials of degree m and d_{mlk} complex numbers. Also $M(n,l)$ is the dimension of the space of spherical harmonics of degree l on S^{n-1}.

Proof. A.K. Louis has proved in [12] that R is an operator from $L^2\left(\Omega, br_{\nu-\frac{n}{2}}^{-1}\right)$ to $L^2\left(Z, br_{\nu-\frac{1}{2}}^{-1}\right)$. The remainder of this theorem is just an adaptation of theorem 4.1 equation (4.21) of [12]. Our polynomials $T_{m,l}^{\nu,n}(s)$ are the $C(n,m,\nu,l)Q_{m,l}^{\nu,n}(s)$ of [12] where the constants $C(n,m,\nu,l)$ are defined in his theorem 3.1 equation (3.3) and where the polynomials $Q_{m,l}^{\nu,n}$, which are adapted from the Jacobi polynomials of degree m, are defined in his theorem 3.1, equation (3.2). □

COROLLARY 20. *If $\mu > -\frac{1}{2}$ and $f \in BR^{\mu}(\Omega)$ and if K is the total degree of the polynomial part of f, then there exist $d_{mlk} \in \mathbf{C}$ such that*

$$Rf(s,\omega) = br_{\mu+\frac{n-1}{2}}(s) \sum_{m=0}^{K} C_m^{\mu+\frac{n}{2}}(s) \sum_{\substack{l=0 \\ m+l \text{ even}}}^{m} \sum_{k=1}^{M(n,l)} d_{mlk} Y_{lk}(\omega).$$

The main result of this section is the following theorem.

THEOREM 21. *Let A be a dense subspace of $H_0^{\mu+\frac{n-1}{2}}([-1,1])$ with the symmetry property:*

$$f \in A \text{ implies } t \longmapsto f(-t) \in A.$$

Define the space of functions

$S_A = \{ \ g \ : \ g$ is in the range of the Radon transform and
$$g(s,\omega) = \sum_{l=0}^{K} \sum_{k=1}^{M(n,l)} f_{lk}(s) Y_{lk}(\omega), \text{ where } f_{lk} \in A, Y_{lk} \text{ are}$$
spherical harmonics and K is an integer $\geq 0\}$

Then S_A is dense in the range of the Radon transform R: $H_0^{\mu}(\Omega) \to H^{\mu+\frac{n-1}{2}}(Z)$.

Proof. First we note that it is a consequence of a result of F. Natterer that the Radon transform is an operator $H_0^\mu(\Omega) \to H^{\mu+\frac{n-1}{2}}(Z)$ (c.f. [19]).

For this proof we use the Hahn-Banach theorem: let $f = RF \in R(H_0^\mu(\Omega))$. Assume that $<f, h>_{\mu+\frac{n-1}{2}} = 0$ for all $h \in S_A$. We propose to prove that f must equal 0. If f were not 0, then there would be no loss in generality by assuming that $\|f\|_{\mu+\frac{n-1}{2}} = 1$. We assume this for contradiction.

By theorem 6 there exists a function $G \in BR^\mu(\Omega)$ such that $\|RF - RG\|_{\mu+\frac{n-1}{2}} < \frac{1}{2}$. This is to say that

$$\|f - RG\|_{\mu+\frac{n-1}{2}} < \frac{1}{2} \tag{10}$$

But the definition of the Bochner-Riesz space, the fact that the Gegenbauer polynomials span the space of polynomials and corollary 20 imply that

$$RG(s, \omega) = br_{\mu+\frac{n-1}{2}}(s) \sum_{m=0}^{K} \sum_{\substack{l=0 \\ m+l \text{ even}}}^{m} \sum_{k=1}^{M(n,l)} d_{mlk} C_m^{\mu+\frac{n}{2}}(s) Y_{lk}(\omega)$$

for some integer K. We can rearrange this sum:

$$RG(s, \omega) = \sum_{\substack{l=0 \\ l \text{ even}}}^{K} \sum_{k=1}^{M(n,l)} \epsilon_{lk}(s) Y_{lk}(\omega) + \sum_{\substack{l=1 \\ l \text{ odd}}}^{K} \sum_{k=1}^{M(n,l)} \varpi_{lk}(s) Y_{lk}(\omega) \tag{11}$$

where

$$\epsilon_{lk}(s) = br_{\mu+\frac{n-1}{2}}(s) \sum_{\substack{m=0 \\ m \text{ even}}}^{K} d_{mlk} C_m^{\mu+\frac{n}{2}}(s) \in BR^{\mu+\frac{n-1}{2}}([-1,1])$$

and

$$\varpi_{lk}(s) = br_{\mu+\frac{n-1}{2}}(s) \sum_{\substack{m=1 \\ m \text{ odd}}}^{K} d_{mlk} C_m^{\mu+\frac{n}{2}}(s) \in BR^{\mu+\frac{n-1}{2}}([-1,1])$$

Note that ϵ_{lk} is even and ϖ_{lk} is odd.

The next step is to find approximations to ϵ_{lk} and ϖ_{lk} in A which have the same parity and the same moments as ϵ_{lk} and ϖ_{lk} to order K.

Let $u \in H_o^\mu([-1,1])$, let $\epsilon > 0$ and let an integer K be given. Define

$$m_k = \int_{-1}^{1} u(s) C_k^{\mu+\frac{n}{2}}(s) \, ds,$$

the **k-th moment** of u with respect to the Gegenbauer poynomials.

Fix K and ϵ. To each $u \in H_o^\mu([-1,1])$ we associate a function $\tilde{u} \in A$ such that $\tilde{u}$ approximates u to within ϵ and such that $\tilde{u}$ has the same moments as u to order K.

We consider the linear map $T : [H_o^\mu([-1,1])]^K \to \mathbf{R}^{K \times K}$ defined by $T(g)_{jk} = \int_{-1}^{1} g_j(s) C_k^{\mu+\frac{n}{2}}(s) ds$. It is clear that this map is continuous. Also at $\left(g_j(s) = br_\mu(s) C_j^{\mu+\frac{n}{2}}(s)\right)$ the image under T is the identity matrix. This is because on $[-1,1]$, $br_\mu(s) C_j^{\mu+\frac{n}{2}}(s) = (1-s^2)^\mu C_j^{\mu+\frac{n}{2}}(s)$ and the Gegenbauer polynomials $\left\{C_j^{\mu+\frac{n}{2}}\right\}$ are orthonormal with respect to the weight $(1-s^2)^\mu$. Because a neighborhood of the identity matrix is invertible and because A is dense in $H_o^\mu([-1,1])$, the continuity of T implies that there exists $g = (g_j) \in A^K$ such that $T(g)$ is invertible. Define $a(s) = T(g)^{-1} g(s)$. Then it is easy to check that $a \in A^K$ and that $T(a) = I$.

Given $\delta > 0$, by the density, we can find $v \in A$ such that $\|u - v\|_{H_o^\mu([-1,1])} < \delta$. Let $<\cdot,\cdot>$ denote the inner product over $L^2[-1,1]$ Then define

$$\widetilde{u}(s) = v(s) + \sum_{k=0}^{K} <u-v, C_k^{\mu+\frac{n}{2}}> a_k(s)$$

It is clear that $\widetilde{u} \in A$. Also, for $j = 0, \cdots, K$ we can compute:

$$<\widetilde{u}, C_j^{\mu+\frac{n}{2}}> = <v, C_j^{\mu+\frac{n}{2}}> + \sum_{k=0}^{K} <u-v, C_k^{\mu+\frac{n}{2}}><a_k, C_j^{\mu+\frac{n}{2}}>$$
$$= <v, C_j^{\mu+\frac{n}{2}}> + <u-v, C_j^{\mu+\frac{n}{2}}> = <u, C_j^{\mu+\frac{n}{2}}> = m_k$$

In this calculation we used the fact that $<a_k, C_j^{\mu+\frac{n}{2}}> = [T(a)]_{kj} = [I]_{kj} = \delta_{jk}$. Next,

$$\|u - \widetilde{u}\|_\mu \leq \|u - v\|_\mu + \sum_{k=0}^{K} \left|<u-v, C_k^{\mu+\frac{n}{2}}>\right| \|a_k\|_\mu$$
$$\leq \|u - v\|_\mu + \sum_{k=0}^{K} \|u - v\|_\mu \left\|C_k^{\mu+\frac{n}{2}}\right\|_0 \|a_k\|_\mu$$
$$\leq const \cdot \|u - v\|_\mu$$

where the constant depends only on a finite number of norms of the Gegenbauer poynomials and on the norms of the functions a_k. Therefore, given the previously specified $\epsilon > 0$, we can choose $\delta > 0$ such that $\|u - \widetilde{u}\|_\mu < \epsilon$.

Thus we have shown that u can be approximated to within ϵ by a function $\widetilde{u} \in A$ with the same moments as u to order K. This is because the Gegenbauer polynomials of degree up to K span the poynomials of degree up to K.

If u is even, we can go one step further: use $\epsilon/2$ instead of ϵ, as above and define a new $\widetilde{u}$ as $\frac{1}{2}[\widetilde{u}(s) + \widetilde{u}(-s)]$. Clearly this function is even, is in A by the symmetry hypothesis and approximates u to within ϵ in Sobolev norm.. Also an easy calculation shows that the values of the moments to order K are the same as those for u. A similar argument can be used for odd functions. This finishes the step referred to above.

Now define

$$h(s,\omega) = \sum_{\substack{l=0 \\ l \, even}}^{K} \sum_{k=1}^{M(n,l)} \widetilde{\epsilon}_{lk}(s) Y_{lk}(\omega) + \sum_{\substack{l=1 \\ l \, odd}}^{K} \sum_{k=1}^{M(n,l)} \widetilde{\omega}_{lk}(s) Y_{lk}(\omega)$$

where the approximations $\tilde{\epsilon}_{lk}$ and $\tilde{\varpi}_{lk}$ are chosen with K as previously specified and with ϵ chosen so small that

(12) $$\|f-h\|_{\mu+\frac{n-1}{2}} < \frac{1}{2}$$

Smith, Solmon & Wagner [23] have proved a generalization of the Helgason - Ludwig consistency conditions [7], [16] for the range of the Radon transform. More precisely, as a consequence of theorem 13.4 in Smith, Solmon & Wagner [23] the following are necessary and sufficient conditions for a function to be in the range of the Radon transform on $H_0^\mu(\Omega)$:

(a) $g \in H_0^{\mu+\frac{n-1}{2}}(Z)$
(b) g is even
(c) $g(s,\omega) = 0$ if $s > 1$
(d) $\int_{-\infty}^{\infty} s^k g(s,\omega)ds$ is a homogeneous poynomial of degree $\leq k$

for all integers $k \geq 0$

We will use this result to show that h is in the range of the Radon transform. Condition (a) is obvious from the definition of h. Condition (b) is true since $\tilde{\epsilon}_{lk}$ and Y_{lk} are even for l even and since $\tilde{\varpi}_{lk}$ and Y_{lk} are odd for l odd. Condition (c) is true since $\tilde{\epsilon}_{lk}$ and $\tilde{\varpi}_{lk}$ are in A which is contained in $H_0^{\mu+\frac{n-1}{2}}([-1,1])$. Next for $k \leq K$

$$\int_{-\infty}^{\infty} s^k h(s,\omega)ds = \sum_{\substack{l=0 \\ l\,even}}^{K} \sum_{k=1}^{M(n,l)} \int_{-\infty}^{\infty} s^k \tilde{\epsilon}_{lk}(s)ds Y_{lk}(\omega) + \sum_{\substack{l=1 \\ l\,odd}}^{K} \sum_{k=1}^{M(n,l)} \int_{-\infty}^{\infty} s^k \tilde{\varpi}_{lk}(s)ds Y_{lk}(\omega)$$

$$= \sum_{\substack{l=0 \\ l\,even}}^{K} \sum_{k=1}^{M(n,l)} \int_{-\infty}^{\infty} s^k \epsilon_{lk}(s)ds Y_{lk}(\omega) + \sum_{\substack{l=1 \\ l\,odd}}^{K} \sum_{k=1}^{M(n,l)} \int_{-\infty}^{\infty} s^k \varpi_{lk}(s)ds Y_{lk}(\omega)$$

because the moments of ϵ_{lk} and ϖ_{lk} are the same as those of $\tilde{\epsilon}_{lk}$ and $\hat{\varpi}_{lk}$ for $k \leq K$. From this equation it follows that

$$\int_{-\infty}^{\infty} s^k h(s,\omega)ds = \int_{-\infty}^{\infty} s^k \left[\sum_{\substack{l=0 \\ l\,even}}^{K} \sum_{k=1}^{M(n,l)} \epsilon_{lk}(s) Y_{lk}(\omega) + \sum_{\substack{l=1 \\ l\,odd}}^{K} \sum_{k=1}^{M(n,l)} \varpi_{lk}(s) Y_{lk}(\omega) \right] ds$$

$$= \int_{-\infty}^{\infty} s^k RG(s,\omega)ds$$

(13)

Since RG is in the range of the Radon transform, the Helgason - Ludwig consistency conditions apply. In particular condition (d) shows that the right hand side of equation (13) is a homogeneous polynomial of degree $\leq k$ for $k \leq K$. This then completes the proof of condition (d) for h since for $k > K$, $\int_{-\infty}^{\infty} s^k h(s,\omega)ds = 0$.

We thus conclude that h is in S_A. We recall from the beginning of the proof that $<f,h> = 0$ when $h \in S_A$. Thus by (10) and (12) we get:

$$\|f\|^2 = <f,f> = <f-h,f> = <f-RG,f> + <RG-h,f>$$
$$\leq \|f-RG\| \cdot \|f\| + \|RG-h\| \cdot \|f\| < \tfrac{1}{2}\|f\| + \tfrac{1}{2}\|f\| = \|f\|$$

This shows that $\|f\|$ cannot equal 1, contradicting the hypothesis made at the beginning. Thus $f = 0$, completing the proof. □

References

1. W.K. Cheung, G.T. Herman and A. Markoe, *An approach to Image Reconstruction using Cubic Spline functions: its significance and applications*, Proc. of the Thirteenth Northeast Bioengineering Conference, (1987) 13-15.

2. W. K. Cheung and A. Markoe, *Image reconstruction using spline Harmonics in the range of the Radon transform to approximate the projections data: mathematical basis.*, MIPG Technical Report #MIPG158, Medical Image Processing Group, Dept. of Radiology, University of Pennsylvania, 1989.

3. W.K. Cheung, G.T. Herman and A. Markoe, *A method of Image Reconstruction using spline harmonics*, Proc. of the Twelfth Annual International Conference of the IEEE Engineering in Medicine and Biology Society, 1990, 381-382.

4. M. E. Davison and F. A. Grünbaum *Tomographic Reconstruction with Arbitrary Directions*, Comm. Pure Appl. Math. 34 (1981) 77-120.

5. M. E. Davison *A singular value decomposition for the Radon transform in n-dimensional Eucldian space*, Numer. Func. Anal. Optim. 3 (1981) 321-340.

6. M. E. Davison *The Ill-Conditioned Nature of the limited angle tomography problem*, SIAM J. Appl. Math. 43 (1983) 428-448.

7. S. Helgason, *The Radon Transform on Euclidean space, compact two-point homogeneous spaces and Grassman manifolds*, Acta Math. 113 (1965)153-180.

8. L. Hörmander, *The Analysis of Partial Differential Operators I, second ed.*, Springer-Verlag, Berlin, 1990.

9. L. A. Khalfin and L. B. Klebanov *On Some Problems of the Computer Tomography*, preprint 1993.

10. M. Lautsch, *A Spline Inversion Formula for the Radon Transform*, SIAM J. Numer. Anal., 26 (1989) 456-467.

11. B. F. Logan *The Uncertainty Principle in Reconstructing Functions from Projections*, Duke Math. J. (1975) 661-706.

12. A.K. Louis, *Orthogonal function series expansions and the null space of the Radon transform*, SIAM J. Math. Anal. 15 (1984) 621-633.

13. A. K. Louis *Nonuniqueness in Inverse Radon Problems: The Frequency Distribution of the Ghosts*, Math Z. 185 (1984) 429-440.

14. A. K. Louis *Tikhonov - Phillips regularization of the Radon Transform*, Constructive Methods for the Practical Treatment of Integral Equations, ed. G. Hammerlin and K. H. Hoffman, Birkhauser, Boston, 1985, 211- 223

15. A.K. Louis and F. Natterer, *Mathematical problems of computerized tomography*, IEEE Proc. 71(3)(1983) 379-389.

16. D. Ludwig, *The Radon transform on Euclidean spaces*, Comm. Pure Appl Math 19 (1966) 49-81.

17. P. Maass *The x-ray Transform: Singular Value Decomposition and Resolution*, Inverse problems 3 (1987) 729-741.

18. R. B. Marr, *Techniques for three-dimensional reconstruction*, Proceedings of an international workshop, Brookhaven National Laboratory, Upton, New York, July 16-19, 1974

19. F. Natterer, *The Mathematics of Computerized Tomography*, John Wiley & Sons, New York, 1986.

20. J. Radon, *Über die bestimmung von Funktionen durch ihre Integralwerte lands gewisser Mannigfaltigkeiten*, Ber. Vern. Sachs Akad. Weiss. Leibzig 69 (1917) 262-277.

21. R.T. Seeley, *Spherical Harmonics*, Amer. Math. Monthly 73 (1966) 115-121.

22. D. Slepian *Prolate Spheroidal Wave Functions, Fourier Analysis and Uncertainty - IV: Extensions to Many Dimensions; Generalized Prolate Spheroidal Wave Functions*, Bell Syst. Tech. J. 43 (1964) 3009-3058.

23. K.T. Smith, D.C. Solmon & S.J. Wagner, *Practical and mathematical aspects of the problem of reconstructing objects from radiographs*, Bull. Amer. Math. Soc. 83 (1977) 1227-1270.

24. E. Stein & G. Weiss, *Introduction to Fourier Analysis on Euclidean Spaces*, Princeton University Press, Princeton, 1975

25. H. Triebel, *Interpolation Theory, Function Spaces, Differential Operators*, North-Holland, Amsterdam, 1977

W.K. CHEUNG, 400 BUCHNER PLACE, APT 215, LACROSSE, WI 54603

DEPARTMENT OF MATHEMATICS & PHYSICS, RIDER COLLEGE, LAWRENCEVILLE, NJ 08648
E-mail address: markoe@enigma.rider.edu

On a Spatial Limited Angle Model for X-ray Computerized Tomography

ARLENE CORREA, RODNEY CRUZ AND PABLO M. SALZBERG

ABSTRACT. In this contribution we further develop a spatial limited angle model for computerized X-ray tomography (Cf. [10,11]). This model proposes a continuous extension of the Radon transform on vector spaces over finite fields.

1. Introduction

Some discrete planar models were extensively studied in the earlier days of X-ray tomography (Cf. [4] and references therein). In the case of these models, the solution of the tomographic problem leads to the inversion of a large matrix which, in general, is an ill-conditioned problem. One of the simplest techniques used in computerized tomography that avoids inverting large matrices is the back-projection technique (BPT) introduced by Kuhl and Edwards [7]. In this contribution we exhibit a technique close to filtered BPT, which is based on combinatorial properties of lines in the affine geometry $\mathcal{G} = AG(F_q, d)$. In section 2 we exhibit a fast inversion transform (Cf.(2.2)) which permits us to retrieve a density distribution on $\mathcal{G}$ by means of a corrected average of the probabilities of the set (web) of lines passing through each point. Since this transform acts on each point individually, it will allow us to reconstruct the density by means of parallel computations. This transform furnishes the heuristic for a continuous model on the 3-D torus T_3 (Cf. section 3), which is obtained by overlapping the lines of $\mathcal{G}$ with real (Euclidean) lines. However, lines on the torus radiating from one point intersect in rather complex patterns introducing errors in the reconstructions. To estimate the magnitude of these errors, as well as to choose

---

1991 *Mathematics Subject Classification.* Primary 68U10, 15A24, 05B15, 51E20; Secondary 05B25, 51A25.

Key words and phrases. Tomography, image processing, fast inversion transform, 3-d torus, incidence patterns, affine geometries, finite geometries, cyclic groups, generators.

The authors are partially supported by NIH, MBRS Program, under grant 5S-06GM08102.

the lines of the geometry that minimize them, it is necessary to understand the incidence pattern of the web of lines passing through a point. We deal with this problem in the closing section, in which we construct the basic tool for performing this task, namely, a generator for the finite cyclic group formed by the intersection points common to a set of rational lines. The results in this section extend previous results (Cf. [9]).

There are several advantages in dealing with the discrete model we are proposing. A significant one is that the model gives us a simple solution also in the case of spatial tomography. This is not the case for the analytical models currently in use (Cf. [2,3]). Moreover, it is a limited angle model, i.e., the beam of X-rays must sweep a 90° angle (a quadrant) for the planar case and an octant in the spatial model. This fact is especially important in the design of the scanning device, which could be simplified to the extent of eliminating the tunnel shape of current scanners.

2. A Fast Inversion Transform

The tomographic problem we are considering in this paper can be succinctly described in the following terms: Let Ω be a finite set endowed with a collection of 'directions' $\mathcal{L} \subset \mathcal{P}(\Omega)$, and let us assume that unknown weights $w_1, w_2, \ldots$, are assigned to the points of Ω. How can these values be obtained from the weights $w(L) = \sum_{P \in L} w(P)$ along each direction $L \in \mathcal{L}$?

Some structure must be imposed on the set of feasible directions to retrieve the individual weights. The following result, which is of a rather general nature, shows the kind of conditions to be imposed on $\mathcal{L}$.

2.1 THEOREM. *Let $\mathcal{S} = (\Omega, \mathcal{A}, \mu)$, where μ denotes an additive functional over an algebra $\mathcal{A}$ of subsets of Ω. Let $\{L_1, \ldots, L_k\} \subset \mathcal{A}$ denote a web in Ω i.e., a subset of $\mathcal{A}$ satisfying the following three conditions:*

(1) $k \geq 2$,
(2) $\mu(L_i \cap L_j) = \mu(\cap_{i=1}^{k} L_i)$, *for* $1 \leq i \neq j \leq k$, *and*
(3) $\mu(\Omega) = \mu(\cup_{i=1}^{k} L_i)$.

Then,

$$(2.1) \quad \mu(\cap_{i=1}^{k} L_i) = \frac{1}{k-1}\left(\sum_{i=1}^{k} \mu(L_i) - \mu(\Omega)\right).$$

PROOF. $\mu(\Omega) = \mu(\cup_{i=1}^{k} L_i) = \sum_{i=1}^{k} \mu(L_i) - (k-1)\mu(\cap_{i=1}^{k} L_i)$. □

Returning to the above question, theorem 2.1 shows that a sufficient set of requirements to be satisfied by $\mathcal{L}$ is the following, where $\mathcal{B}_P := \{L \in \mathcal{L} \mid P \in L\}$:

(1) $|\mathcal{B}_P| \geq 2$, for every $P \in \Omega$,
(2) $L \cap L' = \{P\}$, for any P and $L, L' \in \mathcal{B}_P, L \neq L'$, and
(3) $\bigcup \mathcal{B}_P = \Omega$, for every $P \in \Omega$.

The next result follows as a consequence of theorem 2.1 and the fact that the set $\mathcal{L}$ of lines of any affine space satisfies the three conditions in the above roster.

2.2 COROLLARY. *Let $\mathcal{G} = AG(F_q, d)$ be a d-dimensional affine geometry over the finite field F_q $(d \geq 2)$. Let Ω and $\mathcal{L}$ denote the sets of points and lines in $\mathcal{G}$, and let $\mathcal{B}_P \subset \mathcal{L}$ denote the web of lines passing through any given point $P \in \Omega$. Let also $w \colon \Omega \to R$ be a real-valued function, extended additively to any subset in $\mathcal{P}(\Omega)$. Then, for any given $P \in \Omega$,*

$$(2.2) \qquad w(P) = \frac{1}{\mid \mathcal{B}_P \mid - 1} \left(\sum_{L \in \mathcal{B}_P} w(L) - w(\Omega) \right).$$

This transform is essentially a corrected average of the weights of the lines in the web radiating from the point to be reconstructed. It is clear that the reconstruction can be performed simultaneously on each point, allowing us to program the computational work in a highly parallel fashion.

The reader is referred to [1, 5, 8] (and references therein), for similar Radon transforms on ambient spaces over finite fields.

3 The Continuous Case

Corollary 2.2 establishes the heuristic on which we base our reconstruction algorithm.

Given p prime and a $p \times p \times p$ grid G, we can endow G with a structure of affine space $\mathcal{G} = AG(Z_p, 3)$ in a canonical form: the set Ω of points are the cells (or the terns (i, j, k) labeling the positions of the cells, where (i, j, k) denotes the representative in $\{0, 1, ..., p-1\}^3$ of $(\bar{i}, \bar{j}, \bar{k}) \in Z_p^3$). The $p^2(p^2 + p + 1)$ lines in $\mathcal{L}$ are given by the sets

$$(3.1) \qquad L_{b,m} = \{b + tm \mid t \in Z_p\},$$

where $b, m \in Z_p^3$.

In our approach we assume that an image is given by a $p \times p \times p$ spatial array of non-negative values $W = [w_{ijk}]$. Conceptually, we can thing of this array as obtained by overlapping a fine 3-D grid over the real object we are scanning. Moreover, we can consider the cells of this grid as being homogeneous (i.e., endowed with a uniform density) by taking their norm small enough. These densities are precisely the entries of W, and according to the previous section, we can retrieve the w's from the weights of the lines in the geometry $\mathcal{G}$ by means of the transform given in (2.2).

However, in practical applications we work with continuous rays, as it is the case of paths described by particles. When we overlap the lines of the finite geometry $\mathcal{G}$ with euclidean lines, i.e., when we allow t in (3.1) to vary continuously and consider $\tilde{L}_{b,m} = \{b + tm \pmod{p} \mid t \in R\}$, these sets can be regarded as lines immersed in a 3-dimensional torus $T_3 = R^3/Z^3$.

Therefore, to simulate the action of a CT scanner we assume that the scanning field is $W = [w_{ijk}]$, whose entries are the unknown densities. (As mentioned above, we identify the grid G with W and consider the geometry whose space consists of the terns (i, j, k) labeling the position of the entries of the matrix.)

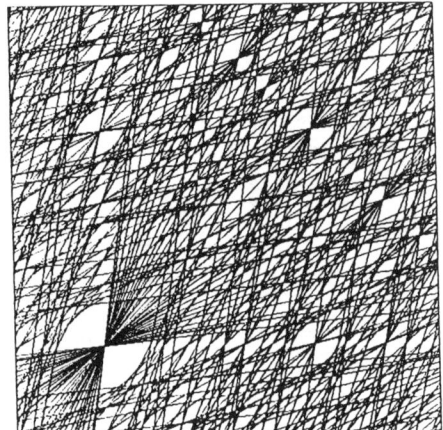 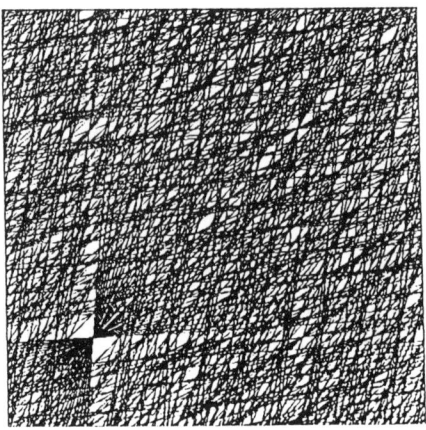

The next step is to 'irradiate' with p^2 parallel beams in each of the $p^2 + p + 1$ directions given by $\{(m_1, m_2, 1), (m_1, 1, 0), (1, 0, 0)\}$ where $\overline{m}_1, \overline{m}_2 \in Z_p$. To reconstruct the density at a given point we just consider the 'attenuation' along the web of 'rays' passing through that point. However, in contrast with the discrete case, lines in a web on the torus intersect in a rather complex pattern. For instance, Figure 1 shows the incidence pattern for 35 lines in a pencil (2-d web) uniformly distributed on a quadrant with angles in $\pi/100$ increments. The slopes have been rounded off to the nearest fraction with denominator less or equal 10. Figure 2 shows the pattern when the round off is to the nearest fraction with denominator less or equal 17.

Unfortunately, these intersections introduce errors in the reconstructions (Cf.[11]). To estimate their magnitude, as well as to choose the lines of the geometry that minimize this effect, it is necessary to understand the incidence pattern of the lines in a web. We deal with this problem in the next section, in which we exhibit a generator for the finite cyclic group formed by the intersection points common to a set of rational lines in the 3-D torus. These results extend previous ones for the planar case (Cf. [9]).

4. Incidence Pattern in the 3-D Torus

Given $x = (x_1, x_2, x_3) \in R^3$, we shall denote by $[x]$ its equivalence class in T_3. Analogously, $[A] = \bigcup \{[x] \mid x \in A\}$, where $A \subset R^3$. It is clear that $[x] \in [A]$ if and only if there exists $n \in Z^3$ such that $x + n \in A$. Thus, any element $[x] \in T_3$ will have a representative in the cube $[0, 1)^3$.

In what follows, given $m \in R^3 - \{0\}$, we shall denote the line passing through the origin with direction m as L_m.

Now, let $M \subset Q^3$ ($\mid M \mid \geq 2$) be such that any two elements of M are not collinear. We shall use the notation $m = u/v = (u_1/v_1, u_2/v_2, u_3/v_3)$ to represent the elements in M, with the implicit assumption that $gcd(u_i, v_i) = 1$.

In this section we shall be concerned with the problem of describing the elements of $\mathcal{I} = \bigcap_{m \in M}[L_m]$. The following result is an extension of the main result in [9], and can be proven by similar methods.

4.1 THEOREM. $(\mathcal{I}, +)$ is a finite cyclic subgroup of T_3. Moreover, $\mathcal{I} \subset [Q^3]$.

In what follows we shall exhibit a generator of the group $(\mathcal{I}, +)$, which will be described in terms of the coefficients of the lines.

4.2 LEMMA. Let $[\mu/\nu]$ be a generator of $\mathcal{I}$, i.e., $\mathcal{I} = \langle [\mu/\nu] \rangle$, and let $\ell = lcm\{\nu_1, \nu_2, \nu_3\}$. Then $|\mathcal{I}| = \ell$.

PROOF. First notice that $|\mathcal{I}| [\mu/\nu] = [(|\mathcal{I}| \mu)/\nu] = [0]$, which in turn yields $\nu_i \setminus |\mathcal{I}|$ for i=1,2,3. Hence, $\ell \setminus |\mathcal{I}|$. On the other hand, $(\ell \mu_i)/\nu_i \in Z$ ($i = 1, 2, 3$) implies $[\ell \mu/\nu] = [0]$, i.e., $|\mathcal{I}| \setminus \ell$. □

Notice that if for some $m \in M$ and $i \in \{1, 2, 3\}$ we have $m_i = 0$, then $\mu_i/\nu_i \in Z$, and μ_i and ν_i can be replaced by 0 and 1, respectively. In general, we shall assume $u_j = 0$ and $v_j = 1$ whenever $u_j/v_j \in Z$. Therefore, we are interested in determining μ_i/ν_i only for those subindices i such that $m_i \neq 0$ for all $m \in M$. Let us denote by I ($\subset \{1, 2, 3\}$) the set of such subindices. If $\mathcal{I}$ is not trivial, then we can select a fixed $i \in I$ and assume, without any lost in generality, that all $u/v \in M$ satisfy $u_i/v_i = 1$. Let us denote by M_i the set of such vectors.

In the sequel we shall describe, under some mild restrictions, a generator of $\mathcal{I}$ in terms of the components of those $m \in M_i$.

Now, let us assume $|\mathcal{I}| > 1$. Given a generator $[\mu/\nu]$ of $\mathcal{I}$, and $m \in M_i$, let $t_m \in Q$ be such that $t_m m = \mu/\nu + n$ for some $n \in Z^3$. Also, denote $t'_m := t_m \nu_i$. Since $m \in M_i$ (i.e., $m_i = u_i/v_i = 1$) then it is clear that

(4.1) $$t'_m \equiv \mu_i \pmod{\nu_i}.$$

Furthermore, $t_m m - t_{\tilde{m}} \tilde{m} \in Z^3$ hold for all $m, \tilde{m} \in M_i$. This expression can be rewritten as the following system of congruences:

(4.2) $$t'_m - t'_{\tilde{m}} \equiv 0 \pmod{\nu_i}, \text{ and}$$

$$t'_m \frac{u_j}{v_j} - t'_{\tilde{m}} \frac{\tilde{u}_j}{\tilde{v}_j} \equiv 0 \pmod{\nu_i}, \text{ for } m, \tilde{m} \in M_i \text{ and } j \neq i.$$

After some computations (4.2) yields:

(4.3) $$t'_m (u_j \tilde{v}_j - \tilde{u}_j v_j) = (h\tilde{u}_j + c_j \tilde{v}_j) \nu_i v_j,$$

for $j \neq i$ and some $h, c_j \in Z$.

At this point, let us introduce some notation in order to simplify the increasing complexity of the expressions. Given $m, \tilde{m} \in M_i$, let us denote
(4.4)
$$r_j(m, \tilde{m}) := u_j \tilde{v}_j - \tilde{u}_j v_j, \text{ and } s_j(m, \tilde{m}) := gcd(v_j, r_j(m, \tilde{m})) = gcd(v_j, \tilde{v}_j).$$

For the sake of brevity, we shall avoid using $(m, \tilde{m})$ in the notations of r_j and s_j when there is no risk of confusion.

In what follows we shall consider $m \in M_i$ as arbitrary but fixed.

Thus, (4.3) can be rewritten shortly as $t'_m r_j = (h\tilde{u}_j + c_j \tilde{v}_j)\nu_i v_j$, which implies, after dividing both terms by v_j, that $(v_j/s_j)\backslash t'_m$. Therefore,

$$(4.5) \qquad t_1 := lcm\ \{\frac{v_j}{s_j(m,\tilde{m})} \mid \tilde{m} \in M_i,\ j \neq i\},$$

is a factor of t'_m. In addition, (4.3) yields:

$$h\tilde{u}_j \equiv \frac{t'_m s_j}{\nu_i v_j} \frac{r_j}{s_j} \pmod{\tilde{v}_j},\ j \neq i.$$

Since h does not depend on j and $gcd(\tilde{u}_j, \tilde{v}_j) = 1$ for $j = 1, 2, 3$, the *Chinese Remainder Theorem* implies (Cf. [12], Theorem 5.4.3.):

(where as usual, $\{\ ,\ \}$ denotes l.c.m, and $(\ ,\ )$ denotes g.c.d.):

$$(4.6) \qquad \frac{t'_m}{\{\frac{v_j}{s_j}, \frac{v_{j'}}{s_{j'}}\}} \frac{d_{jj'}}{\nu_i} \equiv 0 \pmod{(\tilde{v}_j, \tilde{v}_{j'})}, \text{ where } \tilde{m} \in M_i,\ j, j' \neq i \text{ and}$$

$$(4.7) \qquad d_{jj'} := \tilde{u}_j \{\frac{v_j}{s_j}, \frac{v_{j'}}{s_{j'}}\} \frac{s_{j'}}{v_{j'}} \frac{r_{j'}}{s_{j'}} - \tilde{u}_{j'} \{\frac{v_j}{s_j}, \frac{v_{j'}}{s_{j'}}\} \frac{s_j}{v_j} \frac{r_j}{s_j}.$$

We can summarize the preceding discussion as follows:

4.3 LEMMA. *If $[\mu/\nu]$ is a generator for $\mathcal{I}$, then (4.6) holds.*

In the sequel, we shall use this lemma to find expressions for t'_m and ν_i in terms of the components of the directions in M_i. These expressions will furnish a generator of the group.

By expressing $(\tilde{v}_j, \tilde{v}_{j'}) = (d_{jj'}, (\tilde{v}_j, \tilde{v}_{j'}))\frac{(\tilde{v}_j, \tilde{v}_{j'})}{(d_{jj'}, (\tilde{v}_j, \tilde{v}_{j'}))}$, we conclude from (4.6)

that $f_{jj'} := \frac{(\tilde{v}_j, \tilde{v}_{j'})}{(d_{jj'}, (\tilde{v}_j, \tilde{v}_{j'}))}$ must be a factor of $\frac{t'_m}{\{\frac{v_j}{s_j}, \frac{v_{j'}}{s_{j'}}\}}$, i.e., $f_{jj'}\{\frac{v_j}{s_j}, \frac{v_{j'}}{s_{j'}}\} \backslash t'_m$,

and therefore, the integer

$$(4.8) \qquad t_2 := lcm\ \{f_{jj'}\{\frac{v_j}{s_j}, \frac{v_{j'}}{s_{j'}}\} \mid \tilde{m} \in M_i,\ j, j' \neq i\},$$

is also a factor of t'_m. The preceding discussion suggests us to take, as an estimator of t'_m, the expression:

$$(4.9) \qquad t^*_m := \{t_1, t_2\},$$

where t_1 and t_2 have been defined in (4.5) and (4.8), respectively. Notice that we can not establish that $(d_{jj'}, (\tilde{v}_j, \tilde{v}_{j'}))$ divides $d_{jj'}/\nu_i$ unless $(\nu_i, (d_{jj'}, (\tilde{v}_j, \tilde{v}_{j'}))) = 1$. Thus, t'_m could have a factor of $(d_{jj'}, (\tilde{v}_j, \tilde{v}_{j'}))$ not included in t^*_m.

Now, replacing (4.1) in (4.3) yields $\mu_i r_j \equiv 0 \pmod{\nu_i s_j}$ for $\tilde{m} \in M_i$, and $j \neq i$, which imply (since $(\mu_i, \nu_i) = 1$) that $\nu_i \setminus (r_j/s_j)$. Therefore, we define:

$$(4.10) \qquad \nu_i^* = \gcd \left\{ \frac{r_j(m, \tilde{m})}{s_j(m, \tilde{m})} \mid m, \tilde{m} \in M_i, \; j \neq i \right\}.$$

4.4 THEOREM. *$\mathcal{I}$ is a subgroup of $\langle [\frac{t_m^*}{\nu_i^*} m] \rangle$.*
Furthermore, if $\gcd(\nu_i^*, d_{jj'}, \tilde{v}_j, \tilde{v}_{j'}) = 1$ for all $\tilde{m} \in M_i$, and $j, j' \neq i$, then $[\frac{t_m^*}{\nu_i^*} m]$ generates $\mathcal{I}$, where $d_{jj'}$, t_m^* and ν_i^* were defined in (4.7),(4.9) and (4.10), respectively.

PROOF. Since $t_m^* \setminus t_m'$ and $\nu_i \setminus \nu_i^*$, then $t_m' = k t_m^*$ and $\nu_i^* = \kappa \nu_i$ for some $k, \kappa \in \mathbb{Z}$. from which we obtain:

$$(4.11) \qquad \frac{t_m^*}{\nu_i^*} = \frac{t_m'}{k \kappa \nu_i}.$$

Therefore, $n[(t_m^*/\nu_i^*)m]$ generates $\mathcal{I}$ for some $n \in \mathbb{Z}$, which proves the first assertion.

On the other hand, for any $\tilde{m} \in M_i$ and $j \neq i$, we obtain from the definition of ν_i^* : $r_j = c_j s_j \nu_i^*$, which in turn yields

$$\frac{t_m^*}{v_j} \frac{r_j}{\nu_i^*} = \frac{t_m^*}{v_j} c_j s_j.$$

Since $(\tilde{u}_j, \tilde{v}_j) = 1$, the Chinese Remainder Theorem states the existence of $h, h_j \in \mathbb{Z}$ such that:

$$(4.12) \qquad h \tilde{u}_j + h_j \tilde{v}_j = c_j t_m^* \frac{s_j}{v_j}, \; j \neq i,$$

(or equivalently, the existence of a solution h for the system

$$(4.12') \qquad h \tilde{u}_j \equiv c_j t_m^* \frac{s_j}{v_j} \pmod{\tilde{v}_j}, \; j \neq i,)$$

if and only if

$$\tilde{u}_j t_m^* c_{j'} \frac{s_{j'}}{v_{j'}} - \tilde{u}_{j'} t_m^* c_j \frac{s_j}{v_j} \equiv 0 \pmod{(\tilde{v}_j, \tilde{v}_{j'})}, \text{ for } j, j' \neq i.$$

After replacing $c_j = r_j/(s_j \nu_i^*)$ in the preceding expressions and rearranging some terms, we obtain:

$$\frac{t_m^*}{\{\frac{v_j}{s_j}, \frac{v_{j'}}{s_{j'}}\}} \frac{d_{jj'}}{\nu_i^*} \equiv 0 \pmod{(\tilde{v}_j, \tilde{v}_{j'})}, \text{ for } j, j' \neq i.$$

It is easy now to prove that these congruences hold. Indeed, they are a straightforward consequence of Lemma 4.3, the definition of t_m^* and the hypothesis of this theorem. Therefore (4.12') holds and, after rearranging some terms we obtain: $t_m^*(u_j/v_j) - t_{\tilde{m}}^*(\tilde{u}_j/\tilde{v}_j) \equiv 0 \pmod{\nu_i^*}$, where $t_{\tilde{m}}^* \equiv t_m^* \pmod{\nu_i^*}$ for $m, \tilde{m} \in M_i$ and $j, j' \neq i$, i.e. $(t_m^*/\nu_i^*)m - (t_{\tilde{m}}^*/\nu_i^*)\tilde{m} \equiv 0 \pmod{1}$, for $m, \tilde{m} \in M_i$, and $j \neq i$, which implies $(t_m^*/\nu_i^*)m \in \mathcal{I}$.

By (4.11), $order((t_m^*/\nu_i^*)m) \geq order(t_m m) = |\mathcal{I}|$. □

This theorem extends a previous result (Cf. [9], Theorem 3) for the planar case.

EXAMPLE.

Let us consider the pencil of lines

$$\{t(1, \frac{1}{3}, \frac{3}{4}) + (\frac{1}{2}, \frac{4}{7}, \frac{2}{3}), \; t(1, \frac{3}{4}, \frac{1}{3}) + (\frac{1}{2}, \frac{4}{7}, \frac{2}{3})\}.$$

After translation of this pencil to the origin we shall consider the set of directions $M = \{(1, \frac{1}{3}, \frac{3}{4}), (1, \frac{3}{4}, \frac{1}{3})\}$. Since these vectors have no null component, it follows that $I = \{1, 2, 3\}$. Let us take, for instance, $i = 1$ (in this case $M_1 = M$), and let $m = (1, \frac{1}{3}, \frac{3}{4})$. Therefore,

$$t_m^* = lcm\{\frac{3}{(3,4)}, \frac{4}{(3,4)}\} = 12, \text{ and}$$

$$\nu_1^* = gcd\{\frac{4}{(3,4)} - \frac{9}{(3,4)}, \frac{9}{(3,4)} - \frac{4}{(3,4)}\} = 5.$$

Since $(\nu_i^*, (\tilde{v}_2, \tilde{v}_3)) = gcd(5, 3, 4) = 1$, according to Theorem 4.4, $[(t_m^*/\nu_i^*)m] = [\frac{12}{5}(1, \frac{1}{3}, \frac{3}{4})] = [(\frac{2}{5}, \frac{4}{5}, \frac{4}{5})]$ is a generator for $\mathcal{I}$, i.e.,

$$\mathcal{I} = \{[(\frac{2}{5}, \frac{4}{5}, \frac{4}{5})], [(\frac{4}{5}, \frac{3}{5}, \frac{3}{5})], [(\frac{1}{5}, \frac{2}{5}, \frac{2}{5})], [(\frac{3}{5}, \frac{1}{5}, \frac{1}{5})], [(0, 0, 0)]\}.$$

Therefore, the intersection points of the pencil are given by $\mathcal{I} + [(\frac{1}{2}, \frac{4}{7}, \frac{2}{3})]$. □

The importance of Theorem 4.4 becomes clear when we analyze the behavior of lines on the 3-d torus T_3. Each toroidal line consists of flat bundles of equidistant parallel segments distributed on planes which, in turn, are parallel and equidistant in the space. Moreover, if we identify the 3-d torus T_3 with the unit cube, then it is easy to see that the number of intersections of a line with direction $m = (m_1, m_2, m_3)$, where $gcd(m_1, m_2, m_3) = 1$, with each face of the cube is given by m_1, m_2, and m_3, respectively (opposite faces have the same number of intersections). As a rule of thumb, for larger values of these integers we obtain more dense bundles. As a consequence, the number and multiplicity of (the number of lines passing through) the intersections of the lines in a web tends to increase. Furthermore, these intersections form patterns which exhibit very interesting fractal type properties (Cf. figure 1 and 2 for a pencil of lines on the plane). Unfortunately, these patterns tend to hide (becomes fuzzy) when we increase the number of lines.

Theorem 4.4 allows us to determine analytically the locations of the intersection points of the lines in a web, as well as their multiplicities, which is essential for the selection of an adequate geometry.

The search for efficient algorithms in performing this task is still in progress.

References

1. E. Bolker, *The finite Radon transform*, Integral Geometry, Contemp. Math. **63** (1987), 27 –50.
2. R. A. Brooks and G. Di Chiro, *Theory of image reconstruction in computed tomography*, Radiology **117** (1975), 561 –572.
3. _____, *Principles of computer assisted tomography (CAT) in radiographic and radioisotopic imaging*, Physics in Medicine and Biology **21** (1976), 689 – 732.
4. R. A. Gordon, *A tutorial on ART (Algebraic Reconstruction Techniques)*, IEEE Trans. Nuclear Science **21** (1974), 78 – 93.
5. E. L. Grinberg, *The Admissibility Theorem for the Hyperplane Transform over a Finite Field*, J. Combinatorial Th., Series A **53** (1990), no. 2, 316 – 320.
6. M. Hall, Jr., *Combinatorial theory*, (2nd. ed.) Wiley-Interscience Series In Discrete Mathematics, John Wiley & Sons, New York, 1986.
7. D. E. Kuhl and R. Q. Edwards, *Reorganizing data from transverse section scans of the brain using digital processing*, Radiology **91** (1968), 975 – 983.
8. J. P. S. Kung, *Reconstructing finite radon transforms*, Nuclear Physics B (Proc. Suppl.) **5A** (1988), 44 –49.
9. P. M. Salzberg and R. Figueroa, *Pencil of lines in the 2-D torus*, Ars Combinatoria (to appear).
10. P. M. Salzberg, *Tomography in projective spaces: a heuristic for limited angle reconstructive models*, SIAM J. Matrix Anal. Appl. **9, No. 3** (1988), 393 – 398.
11. _____, *An application of finite field theory to computerized tomography: a spatial limited angle model*, Finite fields, coding theory, and advances in communications and computing, Gary L. Mullen and Peter Jay-Shyong Shiue (eds), Marcel Dekker, Inc, New York, 1992, pp. 395–402.
12. H. N. Shapiro, *Introduction to the theory of numbers*, Wiley Interscience, John Wiley & Sons, New York, 1983.

DEPARTMENT OF MATHEMATICS, UNIVERSITY OF PUERTO RICO, P.O.BOX 23355, RIO PIEDRAS CAMPUS, PUERTO RICO 00913.

E-mail address: p_salzberg@ upr1.upr.clu.edu

The Backpropagation Method in Inverse Acoustics

GIOVANNI F. CROSTA

ABSTRACT. Determining the shape of a sound soft obstacle from knowledge of both the incident and scattered far fields is one of the simplest problems of inverse scattering, which may be put in variational form and stated as the minimization of a suitable norm. The solution method presented herewith relies on the properties of complete families of linearly independent solutions of Helmholtz equation. Said properties provide a unifying view over approximate direct and inverse problem solvers. To begin with, two known direct solvers are examined, which determine the scattered far field by projection onto some subspaces followed by forward propagation: Waterman's T-matrix [J. Acoust. Soc. Amer., **45** (1969), pp. 1417 – 29] and another least squares method [see e.g., D S JONES, X Q MAO, Inverse Problems, **5** (1989), pp. 731–48]. Some error relations for the Waterman scheme are provided and convergence for the coefficients yielded by the least squares method is stated. Then, obstacle reconstruction by approximate back propagation (ABP) is described in detail. This procedure minimizes the *boundary defect*, where the approximate scattered field on the obstacle boundary is a linear combination of outgoing spherical wave functions. The coefficients in the combination are obtained by the two stages of estimation and backpropagation. Namely, the far field coefficients are estimated from scattering amplitude data, then are transformed by a matrix, the ABP operator. Two properties distinguish the ABP method from existing ones, also based on the approximation of the scattered field: *i*) no penalty term is needed in the objective function; *ii*) if the obstacle is known, the minimum attainable values of the boundary defect in various circumstances can be estimated and computed. The ABP algorithm and the related computer code are outlined. Several reconstruction problems are considered. Their solution is not a pure "numerical experiment" because the performance of ABP can be assessed by some independently computable estimates. The relevant numerical and graphical results are provided.

1991 MSC. *Primary*: 35J05, 81U20, 81U40, *Secondary*: 76Q05.
The author thanks the Seminar Organizers for accepting his contribution, Prof. Margaret Cheney and the Referee for their constructive criticism and precious advice. Thanks also to Prof. Alexander G. Ramm for some remarks. This research has been mainly funded by the Italian Ministry of University and Scientific Research (*MURST 60%*, 1992). The financial support by the American Mathematical Society is also gratefully acknowledged. This paper is in final form and no version of it will be submitted for publication elsewhere.

1. Introduction

The problem addressed herewith is the identification of the shape of an impenetrable acoustic scatterer in the resonance region from suitable information. Since it is one of the simplest problems in the realm of inverse scattering, it has been extensively considered before, both from the analytic and the numerical points of view. A survey of prior methods and results is found in [4, 16].

It often happens that the investigation of an inverse problem brings about improved understanding of some methods used to solve the related direct problem. Indeed, this paper centers on the interplay between approximate forward and inverse solvers, where the link is provided by the families of metaharmonic functions [19] in $\mathbf{R}^3$, related to the homogeneous Helmholtz equation

$$(1.1) \qquad (\nabla^2 + k^2) v = 0$$

in exterior domains.

Among these families are outgoing spherical waves, their real parts and the normal derivatives on the (Lyapunov) surface Γ of any bounded domain containing the origin. Conditions are available, under which a family is linearly independent and complete. Unless some additional, restrictive hypotheses are introduced about Γ, these families are not a Schauder basis in $L^2(\Gamma)$. Nonetheless, some of them provide an essential tool for discretizing and solving direct problems in the least squares sense [2; 15, Ch. 4]: the guideline is to establish a relation between sets (in fact, vectors) of expansion coefficients of the incident and scattered fields by means of suitable matrices, the entries of which are inner products of said functions.

As these matrices can describe (forward) propagation of the scattered field from the obstacle boundary to the far zone, it seems natural to use them for performing a key step in data inversion i.e., applying a far field – to – boundary field map. This is the distinctive feature of the recently introduced "approximate back propagation" (ABP) method, a preliminary description of which is given in [5]. The purpose of this paper is to state the known properties of the ABP method, provide some indicators, by which its performance is predicted and demonstrate its numerical capability in inverting the (simulated) scattering amplitude data.

SECTION 2 deals with two schemes for the approximate solution of the direct problem: they determine some expansion coefficients of the scattered field v, which complies with EQ. 1.1, with a Dirichlet boundary condition

(1.2) $$(v + w)|_\Gamma = 0$$

on Γ, where w is known, and with Sommerfelds' s radiation condition "at infinity". These schemes respectively are Waterman' s **T** matrix [20] and the least squares method used e.g., by [8]. Both rely on projecting the known and unknown fields onto finite dimensional subspaces of order L spanned by some complete families. Waterman' s scheme is shown to entail two approximation steps. Denote by $\mathbf{f}^{(L)}$ the first $(L+2)\frac{L+1}{2}+1$ exact far field coefficients and by $\mathbf{f}^{(W,L)}$ their Waterman approximates, then the error vector $\mathbf{f}^{(L)} - \mathbf{f}^{(W,L)}$ consists of two contributions, coming from the scattered field and from the forward propagated incident field, respectively. The other method starts with determining the expansion coefficients, $\mathbf{c}^{(L)}$, for the scattered field on Γ which appear in the linear combination of outgoing waves and comply with the Dirichlet BC on Γ in the least squares sense i.e., minimize the boundary defect $B^{(L)}$, a squared norm in $L^2(\Gamma)$; then an affine transformation is applied to propagate $\mathbf{c}^{(L)}$ forward and yield another approximation, $\mathbf{p}^{(L)}$, to $\mathbf{f}^{(L)}$. The $\mathbf{p}^{(L)}$ are obtained under less restrictive conditions than the $\mathbf{f}^{(W,L)}$ above. An estimate for the error $\mathbf{f}^{(L)} - \mathbf{p}^{(L)}$ is given. Moreover the first $\lambda_0 + 1$ entries of $\mathbf{p}^{(L)}$, where λ_0 is arbitrarily large, fixed, converge uniformly to their counterparts in $\mathbf{f}^{(L)}$, as $L \to \infty$. These results find application to the ABP method.

SECTION 3 deals with the inverse obstacle problem and its least squares solution based on a backward propagator. The incident plane wave is known, as well as the scattering amplitude. Some prior information is available about the obstacle: it is star shaped with respect to the origin and has an axis of symmetry. The unknown is the vector of shape parameters, $\vec{\psi}$, appearing in a linear combination of e.g., trigonometric functions. The ABP method consists of two steps: *i)* the determination, once for all, of far field coefficients, say $\tilde{\mathbf{f}}^{(L)}$, from scattering amplitude data, followed by *ii)* the iterative identification of $\vec{\psi}$, which minimizes $B^{(L)}$. The vector $\tilde{\mathbf{f}}^{(L)}$ cannot appear as such in the approximate representation of the boundary scattered field in $B^{(L)}$: a matrix $\mathbf{W}^{(L)}$, the ABP operator, is defined such that, $\mathbf{W}^{(L)} \cdot \tilde{\mathbf{f}}^{(L)}$ is "close" to $\mathbf{c}^{(L)}$. One factor of $\mathbf{W}^{(L)}$ is the inverse of Waterman's **T** matrix. All quantities in $B^{(L)}$, except $\tilde{\mathbf{f}}^{(L)}$, depend on $\vec{\psi}$. The properties of $\mathbf{W}^{(L)}$, hence of $B^{(L)}$ and of the ABP method in general, are all affected by the properties of the involved complete families. This is why the minimum attainable value of $B^{(L)}$ and other performance indices can, in some circumstances, be determined and computed before carrying out any iterative identification. The value of $B^{(L)}$ at $\mathbf{W}^{(L)}$. $\mathbf{f}^{(W,L)}$ is determined as the solution to a particular minimization problem.

According to the classification in Ch. 5 of [4], the ABP method relies on "the approximation of the scattered field" and implements non linear, least squares. It differs from methods in the same class e.g., AKR [1] and JM [8], because the boundary expansion coefficients (counterpart of $\mathbf{c}^{(L)}$) are no longer independent unknowns: they are yielded by the $\vec{\psi}$-dependent far – to – boundary field map, $\mathbf{W}^{(L)}$. As a consequence the penalty term based on the far field error, which other methods need, disappears from the objective function. Finally, the above mentioned performance estimates are made possible.

SECTION 4 describes the algorithm concisely and presents several new numerical and graphical results. Obstacles can be only identified from full aperture data. The backpropagation and minimization stages can be kept separate: this simplifies the code and speeds up computation. The examples have been selected with the twofold purpose of highlighting the features of the method and making the computational results easily readable. Every result, except the one yielded by adding noise to $\tilde{\mathbf{f}}^{(L)}$, is interpreted by means of the analytical tools developed in the preceeding SECTIONS. Because of the relationship between $\mathbf{W}^{(L)}$ and the Waterman scheme, the inversion of $\mathbf{f}^{(W,L)}$ data must yield the best results (which is the case) and is not sufficient, alone, to validate the ABP method. To this purpose, the scattering amplitude is computed from the least squares scheme of SECT. 2. Results remain acceptable as long as the assumptions in SECT. 3 are satisfied.

2. T – Matrix Schemes

The purpose of this SECTION is to introduce some linearly independent, complete families of functions, summarize some of their properties and apply them to two different schemes, which approximately solve the direct scattering problem.

2.1. Complete Families.
Consider the index triple $\{l, m, p\}$, where $0 \leq m \leq l \leq \infty$ and $p = 0, 1$. Outgoing spherical waves are the functions $v_{l,m,p}$ defined by

$$(2.1) \quad v_{l,m,p} = h_l^{(1)}(kr) P_l^m(\cos\theta) [(1-p)\cos m\phi + p \sin m\phi] g_{l,m},$$

where k is wavenumber, $\{r, \theta, \phi\}$ are the spherical coordinates of a point $\mathbf{r} \in \mathbf{R}^3$, $h_l^{(1)}(.)$ is the l-th order spherical Hankel function of the 1st kind,

$P_l^m(.)$ a Legendre associated function and $g_{l,m}$ its normalization factor. These functions solve the homogeneous Helmholtz equation in any exterior domain $\{ r \mid r > R > 0 \}$ in $\mathbf{R}^3$ and satisfy Sommerfeld's radiation condition. One of their relevant properties is stated by the following LEMMA.

LEMMA 2.1 (after THM. 14 of [13]).
I) *If the twice continuously differentiable function v satisfies*

$$(2.2) \qquad (\nabla^2 + k^2) v = 0 , \quad r > R$$

then, $\forall\, r > R$, *the series*

$$(2.3) \qquad v = \sum_{l=0}^{\infty} \sum_{m=0}^{l} \sum_{p=0}^{1} f_{l,m,p}\, v_{l,m,p} ,$$

where $f_{l,m,p}$ *stand for the (complex valued)* **far field expansion coefficients**, *converges uniformly in every closed subregion of* $r > R$.
II) *Every series of the form (2.3), which converges uniformly in every said subregion represents there a solution to* EQ. 2.2.

From now on the multi-index λ will replace the triple $\{ l, m, p \}$ and the set it spans will be denoted by Λ.

Consider a bounded domain V in $\mathbf{R}^3$ enclosed by the surface $\partial V \equiv G$, which shall be of Lyapunov class: the normal vector $\hat{n}(x)$ to G at x shall exist $\forall\, x \in G$ and there shall exist constants $\alpha, \gamma > 0$ such that the angle $\beta(x, y)$ between $\hat{n}(x)$ and $\hat{n}(y)$ satisfies $\beta(x, y) \leq \gamma |x - y|^{\alpha}$, $\forall\, x, y \in G$ (see e.g., p 51 of [4]).

DEFINITION 2.1. (e.g., p 146 ff of [15]) Let G and $\{ w_\lambda \mid \lambda \in \Lambda, w_\lambda \in L^2(G) \}$ be a linearly independent family. This family is said to be **complete** in $L^2(G)$ provided $\forall\, \epsilon > 0$, $\forall\, h \in L^2(G)$ there exist an approximation order $M(\epsilon)$ and a set of coefficients $\{ c_\lambda^{(M(\epsilon))}(h), \lambda \in \Lambda(M(\epsilon)) \}$, which depend both on h and on $M(\epsilon)$ such that,

$$(2.4) \qquad \left\| h - \sum_{\lambda \in \Lambda(M(\epsilon))} c_\lambda^{(M(\epsilon))}(h)\, w_\lambda \right\|^2_{L^2(G)} < \epsilon$$

From now on **complete** will be shorthand for "linearly independent and complete".

LEMMA 2.2. (e.g., [19, 15]). *Let G be Lyapunov and let $\partial_n (.)|_G$ denote outward normal differentiation on G, then both $\{ v_\lambda \mid \lambda \in \Lambda \}$ of EQ. 2.1 and $\{ \partial_n v_\lambda|_G \mid \lambda \in \Lambda \}$ are complete, linearly independent families in $L^2(G)$.*

Under suitable conditions, **real wave functions**, defined by $u_\lambda :=$ $= \mathrm{Re}[v_\lambda]$, and their normal derivatives can also exhibit the completeness property.

LEMMA 2.3 [10, 15]. *Denote the spectra of the interior Dirichlet and Neumann negative Laplacians by $\sigma(-\Delta_D)$, resp. $\sigma(-\Delta_N)$. The family of* **real waves** $\{ u_\lambda \mid \lambda \in \Lambda \}$ *is complete in $L^2(G)$ if and only if $k^2 \notin \sigma(-\Delta_D)$. Similarly the family of their normal derivatives $\{ \partial_n u_\lambda|_G \mid \lambda \in \Lambda \}$ is complete in $L^2(G)$ if and only if $k^2 \notin \sigma(-\Delta_N)$.*

REMARK 2.1. The completeness of the above families does not imply that they are either a Schauder or a Riesz basis in $L^2(G)$. A basis $\{ w_\lambda \}$ is **Schauder** if it allows a unique representation of any $h \in L^2(G)$ by a converging series $\sum_\lambda \xi_\lambda w_\lambda$. A **Riesz basis** is isomorphic to an orthonormal basis. It can be shown [see e.g., Ch. 4 of 15] that

$\{ v_\lambda \mid \lambda \in \Lambda \}$ *is a Riesz basis in $L^2(S_r)$, the (open) sphere of radius $r \geq R$ centered at the origin.*

Notwithstanding the limitation set by the previous REMARK, it makes sense to introduce the linear subspaces spanned by a finite number of functions in a family. Let L (≥ 0) stand for the **approximation order**: the indices m and l span the interval $0 \leq m \leq l \leq L$. To this case the notation $\lambda \in \Lambda(L)$ applies.

Said subspaces are denoted as follows, where the families are numbered 1 to 4 for the ease of reference:

(2.5) $X_1^{(L)} := \mathrm{span}\{ v_\lambda \mid \lambda \in \Lambda(L) \}$; $X_2^{(L)} := \mathrm{span}\{ \partial_n v_\lambda \mid \lambda \in \Lambda(L) \}$;

(2.6) $X_3^{(L)} := \mathrm{span}\{ u_\lambda \mid \lambda \in \Lambda(L) \}$; $X_4^{(L)} := \mathrm{span}\{ \partial_n u_\lambda \mid \lambda \in \Lambda(L) \}$;

They imply the orthogonal decomposition

(2.7) $$L^2(G) = X_i^{(L)} \oplus X_i^{\perp}, \text{ where } i = 1, 2, 3 \text{ or } 4.$$

The same properties apply when instead of G the boundary $\partial\Omega \equiv \Gamma$ of the obstacle Ω is considered, provided Γ is also of Lyapunov class. From now on every statement will refer to Γ. In particular, if the origin is properly chosen (see SECT. 3.1.1), R will stand for the radius of the sphere circumscribed to Ω. Denote arrays by bold square brackets, [ ] and inner products in $L^2(\Gamma)$ by $\langle . | . \rangle$. Norms $\| \cdot \|$ without a subscript also refer to $L^2(\Gamma)$. Multi-indices λ, μ satisfy $\lambda, \mu \in \Lambda(L)$. Some finite dimensional matrices of inner products in $L^2(\Gamma)$ are introduced next.

DEFINITION 2.2.

(2.8) $\mathbf{L}^{(L)} := -\frac{ik}{4\pi} [\langle v_\lambda | \partial_n v_\mu \rangle]; \quad \mathfrak{R}\mathbf{L}^{(L)} := -\frac{ik}{4\pi} [\langle u_\lambda | \partial_n v_\mu \rangle];$

(2.9) $\mathbf{M}^{(L)} := -\frac{ik}{4\pi} [\langle \partial_n u_\lambda | \partial_n u_\mu \rangle];$

(2.10) $\mathbf{P}^{(L)} := [\langle v_\lambda | v_\mu \rangle]; \quad \mathfrak{R}\mathbf{P}^{(L)} := [\langle v_\lambda | u_\mu \rangle];$

(2.11) $\mathbf{Q}^{(L)} := [\langle \partial_n u_\lambda | v_\mu \rangle]; \quad \mathfrak{R}\mathbf{Q}^{(L)} := [\langle \partial_n u_\lambda | u_\mu \rangle].$

$\mathbf{P}^{(L)}$ and $\mathbf{M}^{(L)}$ (up to a multiplicative constant) are the order L Gramians for families # 1 and 4 respectively. The entries of $\mathfrak{R}\mathbf{Q}^{(L)}$ are real valued. Although in general those of $\mathfrak{R}\mathbf{L}^{(L)}$ and $\mathfrak{R}\mathbf{P}^{(L)}$ are not, the prefix $\mathfrak{R}$ here serves as the reminder of a dual pairing between a spherical and a real wave function. A remark about the meaning of the superscript $^{(L)}$: with the above matrices it simply designates the size of the array (see below for the actual value), with their inverses and with vectors obtained by solving algebraic systems containing any of said matrices, the superscript will imply that the entries, not just their size, depend on L.

The known invertibility results for the above matrices are now listed. The matrices obtained by letting $L \to \infty$ show no superscript.

LEMMA 2.4.

I) $\forall L$, (finite), $\exists [\mathbf{L}^{(L)}]^{-1}$.

II) $\forall L$, (finite), $\exists [\mathbf{P}^{(L)}]^{-1}$.

III) If $k^2 \notin \sigma(-\Delta_N)$ then $\forall L$, (finite), $\exists [\mathbf{M}^{(L)}]^{-1}$.

IV) *Provided all involved families are also Schauder bases and the following restrictions apply to k^2, all corresponding infinite dimensional matrices can be inverted:*

k^2 is arbitrary	then	$\exists\ [\mathbf{L}]^{-1}$ and $[\mathbf{P}]^{-1}$
$k^2 \notin \sigma(-\Delta_D)$	then	$\exists\ [\Re\mathbf{L}]^{-1}$ and $[\Re\mathbf{P}]^{-1}$
$k^2 \notin \sigma(-\Delta_N)$	then	$\exists\ [\mathbf{M}]^{-1}$ and $[\mathbf{Q}]^{-1}$
$k^2 \notin \{\sigma(-\Delta_D) \cup \sigma(-\Delta_N)\}$	then	$\exists\ [\Re\mathbf{Q}]^{-1}$.

Statement I is LEMMA A.5 in [10]. Statements II and III follow immediately from the completeness of $\{v_\lambda\}$ and resp., $\{\partial_n u_\lambda\}$. Statement IV is the COROLLARY to LEMMA A.3 in [10].

REMARK 2.2. When L is finite, even if k^2 is constrained as in statement IV above, the invertibility of $\Re\mathbf{L}^{(L)}$, $\Re\mathbf{P}^{(L)}$, $\mathbf{Q}^{(L)}$ and $\Re\mathbf{Q}^{(L)}$ cannot be established in general. In fact examples of obstacles can be produced [6], where $\Re\mathbf{Q}^{(L)}$ is **not** invertible.

2.2. The Waterman or $X_4^{(L)}$ Scheme. Assume a unit amplitude plane wave

$$(2.12) \qquad u = \exp[\,i\,\mathbf{k} \cdot \mathbf{r}\,]$$

impinges upon an obstacle Ω, the boundary of which, Γ, is sufficiently smooth (see SECT. 2.1). Denote the exterior domain $\mathbf{R}^3 \setminus (\Omega \cup \partial\Omega)$ by Ω^c. According to LEMMA 2.1, the scattered field v can be represented by EQ. 2.3, at least outside the sphere circumscribed to Ω. Moreover the plane wave can be represented everywhere in $\mathbf{R}^3$ as a superposition of real waves [12, p 55], [13, LEMMA 36]

$$(2.13) \qquad u = \sum_{\mu \in \Lambda} a_\mu u_\mu.$$

If Ω is a body of revolution around the z axis, only the colatitude incidence angle, θ_{inc}, matters, whereas the azimuth incidence angle, ϕ_{inc}, can be set to 0; therefore all relevant base functions have even parity ($p = 0$ in EQ. 2.1) and $\text{card}[\Lambda(L)] = N + 1$, where $N := (L+2)\dfrac{L+1}{2}$. In particular the expansion coefficients in EQ. 2.13 only depend on l, m and θ_{inc} and read

$$(2.14) \qquad a_{l,m} = i^l \sqrt{(2l+1)\epsilon_m \frac{(l-m)!}{(l+m)!}}\ P_l^m(\cos\theta_{inc}),$$

where $\epsilon_0 = 1$, $\epsilon_m = 2$, $m \neq 0$.

For subsequent application, u of EQ. 2.13 is split into the following finite sum and remainder

$$(2.15) \quad u = \sum_{\mu \in \Lambda(L)} a_\mu u_\mu + \sum_{\mu \notin \Lambda(L)} a_\mu u_\mu := u_a^{(L)} + u_{rem}^{(L+1)}.$$

The notation reminds that $u_a^{(L)}$ is **not** the projection of u onto $X_3^{(L)}$, neither is $u_{rem}^{(L+1)}$ its orthogonal complement, unless Γ is the surface of a sphere.

Consider the exterior problem for the homogeneous Helmholtz equation, subject to the Dirichlet boundary condition

$$(2.16) \quad (v + u)|_\Gamma = 0$$

and to Sommerfeld's radiation condition i.e., $r(\partial_r v - ikv) \to 0$ as $r \to \infty$, with $k = |\mathbf{k}|$. If the known procedures of potential theory are applied (see Appendix), then the expansion coefficients f_λ in EQ. 2.3 and, resp. a_μ of EQ. 2.14 can be expressed by inner products in $L^2(\Gamma)$

$$(2.17) \quad f_\lambda = -\frac{ik}{4\pi} \langle u_\lambda | \partial_n (u+v) \rangle, \quad \lambda \in \Lambda$$

$$(2.18) \quad a_\mu = \frac{ik}{4\pi} \langle v_\mu | \partial_n (u+v) \rangle, \quad \mu \in \Lambda.$$

Here the incident wave u and its normal derivative on the obstacle surface, $\partial_n u|_\Gamma$, are known, whereas the normal derivative of the scattered field, $\partial_n v|_\Gamma$, is unknown. Therefore the f_λ's are also unknown. One may obtain $\partial_n v|_\Gamma$ exactly or approximately from EQ. 2.18, then substitute it into EQ. 2.17 and determine f_λ.

Several implementations of this basic procedure exist. One of them is the $X_4^{(L)}$- or Waterman [20] scheme of order L: it determines the card$[\Lambda(L)]$ entries of the vector $\mathbf{f}^{(W,L)} := [f_\lambda^{(W,L)}]$, which approximate the corresponding f_λ's, from knowledge of finitely many coefficients a_μ i.e., from the vector $\mathbf{a}^{(L)} := [a_\mu]$, again with $\mu \in \Lambda(L)$. The procedure relies on approximating the normal derivative of the total field $h = \partial_n (v + u)|_\Gamma$.

In the next few paragraphs the intermediate steps will be outlined as well as the corresponding error relations. To begin with, the normal derivative of the total field is assumed to be known and a minimization problem in $X_4^{(L)}$ is considered (THM. 2.1). Its solution leads to some far field coefficients, $f^{(4,L)}$, which are related to the exact ones by THM. 2.2.I. Next h is considered as the unknown to be determined from the inversion of EQ. 2.18. This time the approximation to h is computable from $\mathbf{a}^{(L)}$ and the appropriate matrices of inner products. The link between $\mathbf{a}^{(L)}$ and $\mathbf{f}^{(W,L)}$ is established by means of Waterman's $\mathbf{T}$ matrix. This scheme is shown herewith to imply two approximation steps, both of which contribute to the error relation of THM. 2.2.II.

THEOREM 2.1. *Let Γ be of Lyapunov class and the BC of EQ. 2.16 hold; assume that, as a result, $h := \partial_n(v+u)|_\Gamma \in L^2(\Gamma)$; choose the incident wavenumber k such that, $k^2 \notin \sigma(-\Delta_N)$ and fix the order L. If h is known, then*

I) *there exists a unique solution $\vec{\alpha}^{(L)} := [\alpha_\mu^{(L)}]$, $\mu \in \Lambda(L)$, to the approximation problem:*

$$(2.19) \qquad B_4^{(L)} := \| h - \sum_{\mu \in \Lambda(L)} \alpha_\mu^{(L)} \partial_n u_\mu \|^2_{L^2(\Gamma)} = \min .$$

II) *The minimum value of the objective function is*

$$(2.20) \qquad \min B_4^{(L)} = \| h^{\perp}_4 \|^2_{L^2(\Gamma)} ,$$

where $h^{\perp}_4$ is the orthogonal complement of h to $X_4^{(L)}$ of 2.6.

III)

$$(2.21) \qquad \lim_{L \to \infty} \| h^{\perp}_4 \| = 0 .$$

Proof. Denote $\sum_{\mu \in \Lambda(L)} \alpha_\mu^{(L)} \partial_n u_\mu$ by $h_4^{(L)}$ ($\in X_4^{(L)}$, hence the name of this scheme).

I) From LEMMA 2.4.III, $\exists \, [\mathbf{M}^{(L)}]^{-1}$, hence the minimizing vector is found from solving the algebraic system of normal equations

$$(2.22) \qquad \mathbf{M}^{(L)} \cdot \vec{\alpha}^{(L)} = -[\langle \partial_n u_\lambda | h \rangle] .$$

II) The statement is implied by the projection theorem in Hilbert spaces.

III) The property is a consequence of completeness of family # 4 under the stated hypotheses. □

REMARK 2.3. The following may occur as $L \to \infty$.

a) $\mathbf{M}^{(L)}$ is asymptotically not invertible (recall that a sufficient condition is listed in LEMMA 2.4), hence $\lim_{L \to \infty} \vec{\alpha}^{(L)}$ does not exist.

b) $\mathbf{M}^{(L)}$ is asymptotically invertible without family # 4 being a Schauder basis. Then $\exists \lim_{L \to \infty} \vec{\alpha}^{(L)}$, however no convergence property can be established for $\vec{\alpha}^{(L)}$.

In either case 2.21 holds.

Now let $\dagger$ denote Hermitean conjugation and T plain transposition. Introduce the two vectors of approximate far field coefficients, whenever they make sense

$$(2.23) \qquad \mathbf{f}^{(4,L)} := - \Re\mathbf{Q}^{T(L)} \cdot \vec{\alpha}^{(L)}$$

and

$$(2.24) \qquad \mathbf{f}^{(W,L)} := - \Re\mathbf{Q}^{T(L)} \cdot [\mathbf{Q}^{\dagger(L)}]^{-1} \cdot \mathbf{a}^{(L)},$$

let $\mathbf{f}^{(L)}$ stand for the vector of exact far field coefficients of size $\mathrm{card}[\Lambda(L)]$ and define the error vector

$$(2.25) \qquad \mathbf{r}_4^{(L)} := [\,\langle\, v_\lambda \,|\, h_4^{\perp} \,\rangle\,] \,.$$

Whenever it exists, the matrix $-\Re\mathbf{Q}^{T(L)} \cdot [\mathbf{Q}^{\dagger(L)}]^{-1}$ is the transition or $\mathbf{T}^{(L)}$ matrix. The pertaining error relations are provided next.

THEOREM 2.2.

I) *Under the same hypotheses on* Γ , *h and k as in* THM. 2.1, **the error made in replacing** $\mathbf{f}^{(L)}$ **by** $\mathbf{f}^{(4,L)}$ **is**

$$(2.26) \qquad \mathbf{f}^{(L)} - \mathbf{f}^{(4,L)} = - \frac{ik}{4\pi} [\,\langle\, u_\lambda \,|\, h_4^{\perp} \,\rangle\,] \,.$$

It satisfies

$$(2.27) \qquad \lim_{L \to \infty} |f_\lambda - f_\lambda^{(4,L)}| = 0$$

uniformly in $0 \leq \lambda \leq \lambda_0$, where $\lambda_0 \in \Lambda(L)$ is arbitrarily large, fixed.

II) *In addition assume* $\exists\, [Q^{(L)}]^{-1}$, *then the error made in replacing* $f^{(L)}$ *by* $f^{(W,L)}$ *consists of two contributions*

$$(2.28) \quad f^{(L)} - f^{(W,L)} = -\frac{ik}{4\pi}\left([\langle u_\lambda | h\frac{1}{4}\rangle] + T^{(L)} \cdot r\frac{(L)}{4}\right).$$

Proof.

I) Decompose h by the sum $h^{(L)}_{\frac{1}{4}} + h\frac{1}{4}$, apply the definitions of f_λ (EQ. 2.17) and $f_\lambda^{(4,L)}$ and subtract to obtain EQ. 2.26. Now choose L sufficiently large and fix $\lambda_0 \in \Lambda(L)$. For every λ in the interval $0 \leq \lambda \leq \lambda_0$ each entry of the vector in EQ. 2.26 depends on λ only through u_λ and on L only through $h\frac{1}{4}$. Since $\| u_\lambda \|_{L^2(\Gamma)}$ can be uniformly bounded $\forall\, \lambda$ and EQ. 2.21 holds, index-wise convergence in the specified interval, EQ. 2.27, is established.

II) Substitute the above sum for h in the ket of a_μ (EQ. 2.18) and obtain

$$(2.29) \quad a_\mu = \frac{ik}{4\pi} \langle v_\mu | \sum_{\lambda \in \Lambda(L)} \alpha_\lambda^{(L)} \partial_n u_\lambda + h\frac{1}{4} \rangle, \mu \in \Lambda$$

i.e., the affine algebraic system w. r. to $\vec{\alpha}^{(L)}$ of THM. 2.1

$$(2.30) \quad \frac{ik}{4\pi} Q^{\dagger(L)} \cdot \vec{\alpha}^{(L)} = a^{(L)} - \frac{ik}{4\pi}[\langle v_\mu | h\frac{1}{4}\rangle].$$

Neglect the affine term in EQ. 2.30 (this is the second approximation step) and obtain a linear system for the new unknown $\vec{\beta}^{(L)}$

$$(2.31) \quad \frac{ik}{4\pi} Q^{\dagger(L)} \cdot \vec{\beta}^{(L)} = a^{(L)}.$$

The vector $f^{(W,L)}$ of EQ. 2.24 results from replacing h in EQ. 2.17 by the sum $\sum_{\lambda \in \Lambda(L)} \beta_\mu^{(L)} \partial_n u_\mu$: namely

$$(2.32) \quad f^{(W,L)} = -\frac{ik}{4\pi}[\langle u_\lambda | \sum_{\lambda \in \Lambda(L)} \partial_n u_\mu \beta_\mu^{(L)} \rangle] =$$

$$= -\frac{ik}{4\pi} \Re Q^{T(L)} \cdot \vec{\beta}^{(L)} = -\Re Q^{T(L)} \cdot [Q^{\dagger(L)}]^{-1} \cdot a^{(L)},$$

where EQ. 2.11 has been recalled.

Comparison between EQNS. 2.30 and 2.31 yields

(2.33) $$\vec{\beta}^{(L)} = \vec{\alpha}^{(L)} + [Q^{\dagger(L)}]^{-1} \cdot r_4^{(L)},$$

hence

(2.34) $$f_\lambda - f_\lambda^{(W,L)} = -\frac{ik}{4\pi} \langle u_\lambda \mid h - h_4^{(L)} \rangle - \frac{ik}{4\pi} (T^{(L)} \cdot r_4^{(L)})_\lambda,$$

which is EQ. 2.28 written component-wise. □

REMARK 2.4. *i*) The error appearing in EQ. 2.26 is related to the scattered field, whereas the error in EQ. 2.28 carries a forward propagated contribution from the incident field, due to $r_4^{(L)}$.

ii) The 1st summand on the r.h.s of EQ. 2.28 vanishes asymptotically (see 2.27). On the other hand it is still an open problem to find suitable conditions on **k** and Γ s.t., the 2nd term vanishes, without the (non trivial) requirement that any of the involved complete families be also Riesz bases.

iii) The vector $f^{(4,L)}$ has been introduced with the sole purpose of attaining the above error relations. It never appears in any application. The interesting quantity is $f^{(W,L)}$, the determination of which rests on the datum $a^{(L)}$ and on other computable arrays.

The algorithm, which implements the $X_4^{(L)}$ scheme and computes $f^{(W,L)}$ is well known [20, 11] and can be summarized as follows.

1 Fix an approximation order L, apply EQ. 2.14 to obtain $a^{(L)}$, the first card$[\Lambda(L)]$ entries of the vector **a**.
2 Specify the obstacle (see SECT. 3.1.1 below for shape parameterization). Compute the appropriate inner products of base functions in $L^2(\Gamma)$ and form the matrices of order L, $\Re Q^{(L)}$ and $Q^{(L)}$ of EQ. 2.11. For axially symmetric obstacles both matrices are block diagonal.
3 Invert $Q^{(L)}$, usually by conditioning and orthogonalization. This step may fail if $k^2 \in \sigma(-\Delta_N)$.
4 If Step 3 succeeds, apply EQ. 2.24 to obtain $f^{(W,L)}$.

Alternatives to the $X_4^{(L)}$ scheme exist and come e.g., from projecting $\partial_n v \mid_\Gamma$ alone either onto $X_4^{(L)}$ or onto $X_1^{(L)}$. The next SUBSECTION is devoted to one of these schemes.

2.3. The $X_1^{(L)}$ (Affine – Least Squares) Scheme. Consider the same exterior boundary value problem as in SUBSECT. 2.2. Another way of approximately determining the far field coefficients relies on the next LEMMA 2.5 and DEF. 2.4.

DEFINITION 2.3. The vector of **boundary coefficients** of order L, $\mathbf{c}^{(L)} :=$
$= [c^{(L)}_\lambda]$, $\lambda \in \Lambda(L)$, provided it exists, appears in the approximation to the the boundary scattered field $v^{(L)}_1 |_\Gamma$

$$(2.35) \qquad v^{(L)}_1 |_\Gamma = \left(\sum_{\lambda \in \Lambda(L)} c^{(L)}_\lambda v_\lambda \right) |_\Gamma$$

and shall minimize the **boundary defect**

$$(2.36) \qquad B^{(L)}(\mathbf{c}^{(L)}) := \| v^{(L)}_1 + u \|^2_{L^2(\Gamma)}.$$

The definition is appropriate, because it leads to a well posed problem.

LEMMA 2.5.
I) *The problem of determining the boundary coefficients of a given order L has a unique solution, obtained from the algebraic system*

$$(2.37) \qquad \mathbf{P}^{(L)} \cdot \mathbf{c}^{(L)} = -\mathbf{g}^{(L)} := -[\langle v_\lambda | u \rangle] \, , \, \lambda \in \Lambda(L).$$

II) *The value of the corresponding minimum boundary defect (with by now obvious notation) is*

$$(2.38) \qquad B^{(L)}(-[\mathbf{P}^{(L)}]^{-1} \cdot \mathbf{g}^{(L)}) = \| u^\perp_1 \|^2_{L^2(\Gamma)}.$$

III) *The asymptotic behaviour of the relevant quantities is expressed by*

$$(2.39) \qquad \lim_{L \to \infty} \| u^\perp_1 \| = 0$$

and

$$(2.40) \qquad \lim_{L \to \infty} | c^{(L)}_\lambda - f_\lambda | = 0$$

uniformly in $0 \leq \lambda \leq \lambda_0$, λ_0 as in THM. 2.2.

For the proof, which relies on LEMMA 2.4.II and on the regularity of the fundamental solution, reference is made to [2], p. 169 ff. of [15] and [5].

Although EQ. 2.40 suggests that $\mathbf{c}^{(L)}$ may be used as such in stead of $\{f_\lambda\}$, there is another procedure, which deserves attention: it has been applied e.g., by [8] in connection to an inversion problem. Herewith its relation to the complete family framework is established.

DEFINITION 2.4. *The* $X_1^{(L)}$ *forward propagator is the affine transformation acting on* $c^{(L)}$

$$(2.41) \qquad p^{(L)} := \Re L^{(L)} \cdot c^{(L)} + b^{(L)},$$

where $b^{(L)} := -\frac{ik}{4\pi} [\langle u_\lambda | \partial_n u \rangle]$.

EQ. 2.41 is obtained if the unknown normal derivative $\partial_n v|_\Gamma$ is approximated by differentiating the sum in EQ. 2.35 term-wise i.e.,

$$(2.42) \qquad p_\lambda^{(L)} = -\frac{ik}{4\pi} \langle u_\lambda | \partial_n (u + v_1^{(L)})|_\Gamma \rangle,$$

whereas no approximation affects $\partial_n u|_\Gamma$, because Γ and u are known. Therefore the difference betwen exact and $X_1^{(L)}$-approximated coefficients is

$$(2.43) \qquad f_\lambda - p_\lambda^{(L)} = -\frac{ik}{4\pi} \langle u_\lambda | \partial_n (v_1^\perp)|_\Gamma \rangle.$$

The basic steps of the affine – least squares algorithm for an axially symmetric obstacle are the following.
1 Fix an approximation order L. From knowledge of u, compute the inner products and form the vector $g^{(L)}$ of EQ. 2.37.
2 Form the Gramian $P^{(L)}$, which is both Hermitean conjugate and block diagonal.
3 Solve the linear algebraic system EQ. 2.37 for $c^{(L)}$ e.g., by a Kholetskij method. Unlike $Q^{(L)}$ in the $X_4^{(L)}$ scheme, the inversion of $P^{(L)}$ poses no restriction on k.
4 Form the matrix $\Re L^{(L)}$ of EQ. 2.8 and the vector $b^{(L)}$ in DEF. 2.4, then apply EQ. 2.41 to obtain the forward propagated coefficients $p^{(L)}$.

REMARK 2.5.

i) The index – wise convergence of $p_\lambda^{(L)}$ to f_λ is controlled by the asymptotic behaviour of $\partial_n (v_1^\perp)|_\Gamma$, not to be confused with $(\partial_n v)_1^\perp$, because projection and normal differentiation do not commute. Namely

$$(2.44) \qquad |f_\lambda - p_\lambda^{(L)}| \leq \frac{k}{4\pi} \| u_\lambda \| \, \| \partial_n (v_1^\perp)|_\Gamma \|.$$

Indeed *uniform convergence of $p_\lambda^{(L)}$ in the range $0 \leq \lambda \leq \lambda_0$ holds, provided the obstacle is sufficiently smooth.* The proof is carried out in close analogy to that on p. 169 ff. of [15]. It relies on the boundedness of the map

$$(2.45) \quad \mathcal{B}_g : \mathcal{C}^{1,\alpha}(\Gamma) \longrightarrow \mathcal{C}^{0,\alpha}(\Gamma)$$

$$u_1^\perp \longmapsto \partial_{n_x} \left(\int_\Gamma u_1^\perp \partial_{n_y} g(x-y) dy \right) \Big|_\Gamma = \partial_n (v_1^\perp) \Big|_\Gamma ,$$

where $g(.,.)$ is the Green function for the Dirichlet boundary value problem. Further details are not reported herewith for reasons of space. The main consequence is the existence of a class of obstacles and a set $\{\mathbf{k}\}$ such that, for some sufficiently large L the right hand side of INEQ. 2.44 is "small" for the first few λ's, those which are involved in computation. See § 4.2.3 below for some related numerical results.

ii) As it can be deduced from EQNS. 2.16, 2.37 and 2.42, the $X_1^{(L)}$ scheme relies on the following finite dimensional counterpart of the Dirichlet – to – Neumann map, $\mathcal{M}^{(L)}$

$$(2.46) \quad \mathcal{M}^{(L)} : L^2(\Gamma) \longrightarrow X_2^{(L)}$$

$$v|_\Gamma \longmapsto \partial_n (v_1^{(L)}) \Big|_\Gamma =$$

$$= - \sum_{\mu \in \Lambda(L)} ([\mathbf{P}^{(L)}]^{-1} \cdot [\langle v_\lambda | u \rangle])_\mu \, \partial_n v_\mu ,$$

where $v|_\Gamma$ is known. The rightmost linear combination is **not** the projection of $\partial_n v|_\Gamma$ onto $X_2^{(L)}$, because the coefficients $\mathbf{c}^{(L)}$ come from minimization in $X_1^{(L)}$ (recall EQNS. 2.35 and 2.36).

3. Obstacle Identification

3.1. Outline of the Algorithm.

3.1.1. **Data and Prior Information**. The data for an inverse problem may consist of the incident wave e.g., u of EQ. 2.12 and the **scattering amplitude** $F(\hat{\mathbf{x}}, \mathbf{k})$, which appears in the asymptotic representation of the scattered field

$$(3.1) \quad v = \frac{e^{ikr}}{r} F(\hat{\mathbf{x}}, \mathbf{k}) + O(r^{-2}) \text{ as } r \to \infty ,$$

with $\hat{\mathbf{x}} \in S^2$, the surface of the unit sphere. In realistic situations the values of $F(\hat{\mathbf{x}}, \mathbf{k})$ may be known for one or a few incident wave vectors $\mathbf{k}$ at some regularly spaced grid points, say $\{\hat{x}_j \mid 1 \leq j \leq J\}$ on the whole of S^2. Estimation from a limited solid angle, which leads to the so called **limited aperture reconstruction** [4, p. 134], is not considered herewith. In fact it is not allowed by the current implementation of the ABP method.

Prior information about the obstacle plays a basic role: as already pointed out, the domain Ω is bounded, open, simply connected, star – shaped with respect to the origin and axially symmetric. Hence its surface is described by the function $s(\theta)$, $s \in C^{1,\alpha}\{[0, \pi]\}$, $\alpha > 0$. By further restriction, $s(\theta)$ is parameterized: a dimension I is chosen and the following law is applied

$$(3.2) \qquad \frac{1}{s^2}(\theta) = \sum_{i=0}^{I} \psi_i \Psi_i(\theta) ,$$

where $\Psi_i(\theta)$ are trigonometric functions

$$(3.3) \{\Psi_i(\theta) , 0 \leq i \leq I\} = \{1, \cos\theta, \sin\theta, \cos 2\theta, \sin 2\theta, \ldots\} .$$

The unknown in the obstacle identification problem is $\{\psi_i\} \equiv \vec{\psi}$, the vector of **shape parameters**, which shall comply with several constraints. Namely an admissible set may be defined by

$$(3.4) \qquad \Psi_{ad} :=$$
$$= \{\vec{\psi} \mid \vec{\psi} \in \mathbb{R}^{I+1}; s \in C^2([0,\pi]); 0 < s_L \leq s \leq s_H, \forall \theta \in [0,\pi]\} ,$$

where s_L and s_H are the lower and upper bounds respectively. Since the surface must be of class C^2, the parameters are not all independent: they are related by some linear equations, which are not presented for reasons of space.

3.1.2. Basic Steps. The ABP identification algorithm consists of the following.

1 Fix an approximation order L and obtain estimates $\tilde{f}^{(L)}$ of the far field coefficients from the available scattering amplitude data at $\{\hat{x}_j\}$.

2 From the current, say n-th with $n \geq 0$, admissible estimate $\vec{\psi}^{(n)} \in \Psi_{ad}$ of the parameters, which describe the shape $\Gamma^{(n)}$

  2.1 determine the entries of a matrix, $W^{(L)}$, the **approximate back propagator** (ABP) of order L ,

  2.2 multiply $\tilde{f}^{(L)}$ by $W^{(L)}$ and obtain the coefficients $\tilde{c}^{(L)}$

  2.3 evaluate the boundary defect

$$(3.5) \qquad B^{(L)}(\vec{\psi}^{(n)}) := \| \sum_{\lambda \in \Lambda(L)} \tilde{c}^{(L)}_\lambda v_\lambda + u \|^2_{L^2(\Gamma^{(n)})}$$

2.4 minimize it with respect to $\vec{\psi}$, taking all constraints into account: the newly determined shape parameters are the **update** $\vec{\psi}^{(n+1)}$.

2.5 If no stopping condition is met, return to step 2.1.

Step 1 is carried out once, whereas step 2 is carried out iteratively.

The algorithm is therefore based on the constrained minimization of an objective function (see EQ. 3.5). Several methods based on similar principles exist by now. The distinctive features of ABP are presented in § 3.2 below.

3.1.3. Existence and Uniqueness of Minimizers.

The existence of at least one minimizer follows from the continuity of $B^{(L)}$ w. r. to $\vec{\psi}$ and the finite dimension of the bounded set Ψ_{ad}. There is a relevant uniqueness result [4, p 107], [16, p 100], which applies to infinite dimensional problems.

LEMMA 3.1. *Let Γ_1, Γ_2 be two obstacles, which satisfy $\Gamma_1, \Gamma_2 \subset S_R$, $kR < \pi$; let their scattering amplitude functions coincide for one incident wave with wave number k. Then $\Gamma_1 = \Gamma_2$.*

Of course the finiteness of L and of the sampling point number, J, as well as numerical roundoff errors, may impair uniqueness and make e.g., the computed minimizer depend on the initial vector $\vec{\psi}^{(0)}$.

3.1.4. Relationship with the Domain Derivative.

Step 2 requires the gradient and Hessian of $B^{(L)}$ with respect to $\vec{\psi}$ i.e., the determination of a domain derivative. Very briefly, in a typical shape optimization problem (see e.g., [18]) the boundary condition is either a constant or a function of the surface coordinates. This leads to the simultaneous solution of the primal (the original PDE) and adjoint state equations. In obstacle identification, on the other hand, the boundary value $u|_\Gamma$ and the base functions depend on the absolute coordinates $\{ r, \theta, \phi \}$, hence the framework, as it could be shown, is substantially simpler.

The notion of back propagation must be now explained.

3.2. The Approximate Back Propagator (ABP).

3.2.1. Definition and Properties.
Fix L, assume the obstacle is known through the reference parameters $\vec{\psi}_{ref} \in \Psi_{ad}$ and choose k such that, two conditions are fulfilled

$$(3.6) \qquad i)\ k^2 \notin \sigma(-\Delta_N)\ ;\qquad ii)\ \exists\ [\Re Q^{(L)}]^{-1}.$$

By recalling DEF. 2.2 the following matrix is introduced.

DEFINITION 3.1. (The approximate back propagator of order L)

$$(3.7) \qquad \mathbf{W}^{(L)}(\vec{\psi}_{ref}) := [\mathbf{P}^{(L)}]^{-1} \cdot \Re \mathbf{P}^{(L)} \cdot \mathbf{Q}^{\dagger(L)} \cdot [\Re \mathbf{Q}^{T(L)}]^{-1}.$$

From its structure, $\mathbf{W}^{(L)}$ is expected to connect the far field coefficients yielded by the $X_4^{(L)}$ scheme (§ 2.2) to the coefficients, which minimize a boundary defect (§ 2.3). This is made precise by the next statement, which is repeated from [5].

THEOREM 3.1.
I) *Recall the decomposition of u (EQ. 2.15) and introduce the error vector*

$$(3.8) \qquad \mathbf{w}^{(L+1)} = [\langle v_\lambda | u_{rem}^{(L+1)} \rangle].$$

Then there is an affine relationship between $\mathbf{f}^{(W,L)}$ (EQ. 2.24) and $\mathbf{c}^{(L)}$ (DEF. 2.3)

$$(3.9) \qquad \mathbf{c}^{(L)} = \mathbf{W}^{(L)} \cdot \mathbf{f}^{(W,L)} - [\mathbf{P}^{(L)}]^{-1} \cdot \mathbf{w}^{(L+1)}.$$

II) *Name $\mathbf{W}^{(L)} \cdot \mathbf{f}^{(W,L)}$ the vector of approximately back propagated coefficients. The corresponding value of the boundary defect is*

$$(3.10) \qquad B^{(L)}(\vec{\psi}_{ref}; \mathbf{W}^{(L)} \cdot \mathbf{f}^{(W,L)}) =$$
$$= \| u_1^\perp \|^2_{L^2(\Gamma)} + \| (u_{rem}^{(L+1)})_1^{(L)} \|^2_{L^2(\Gamma)}$$

where the rightmost squared norm comes from the projection of $u_{rem}^{(L+1)}$ onto $X_1^{(L)}$.

III) *If $k^2 \notin \sigma(-\Delta_D)$ then $\lim_{L \to \infty} |\langle v_\lambda | u_{rem}^{(L+1)} \rangle| = 0$, $\forall$ fixed λ.*

The key steps to prove I are: start with the vector $\mathbf{g}^{(L)}$ on the right hand side of EQ. 2.37, represent u according to EQ. 2.15, recall EQNS. 2.10 and replace the first summand $[\langle v_\lambda | u_a^{(L)} \rangle]$ by the product $\mathfrak{R}P^{(L)} \cdot a^{(L)}$. The other summand $[\langle v_\lambda | u_{rem}^{(L+1)} \rangle]$ is left unchanged. Since $\mathfrak{R}Q^{(L)}$ is assumed to be invertible, EQ. 2.24 can be solved for $a^{(L)}$. The result is

(3.11) $\quad P^{(L)} \cdot c^{(L)} = \mathfrak{R}P^{(L)} \cdot Q^{\dagger(L)} \cdot [\mathfrak{R}Q^{T(L)}]^{-1} \cdot f^{(W,L)} - w^{(L+1)}$,

from which EQ. 3.9 follows by virtue of LEMMA 2.4.II.

In order to prove II, start with the product $P^{(L)} \cdot W^{(L)} \cdot f^{(W,L)}$, apply the available definitions and obtain the identity

(3.12) $\quad\quad\quad P^{(L)} \cdot W^{(L)} \cdot f^{(W,L)} = -\mathfrak{R}P^{(L)} \cdot a^{(L)}$,

which can be read as the system of normal equations obtained from the minimization problem

(3.13) $\quad\quad\quad \min \left\| \sum_{\lambda \in \Lambda(L)} b_\lambda^{(L)} v_\lambda + u_a^{(L)} \right\|^2_{L^2(\Gamma)}$,

the solution to which is by definition $b^{(L)} = W^{(L)} \cdot f^{(W,L)}$. The sum $\sum_{\lambda \in \Lambda(L)} b_\lambda^{(L)} v_\lambda$ is the opposite of the projection of $u_a^{(L)}$ onto $X_1^{(L)}$ i.e., $-(u_a^{(L)})_1^{(L)}$. By suitably decomposing u and cancelling terms out, the squared norm of EQ. 3.13 becomes the right hand side of EQ. 3.10. □

REMARK 3.1. EQ. 3.10 is the consequence of a two step approximation process: disregard of the affine term, $w^{(L+1)}$, followed by projection onto a finite dimensional subspace, $X_1^{(L)}$. The analogy to the procedure and result of THM. 2.2 is thus very close.

As a corollary to both THMS. 2.2 and 3.1, $B^{(L)}$ can be evaluated when $W^{(L)}$ acts on $f^{(L)}$ i.e., on the first $\text{card}[\Lambda(L)]$ exact far field coefficients.

COROLLARY 3.1. *Recall (2.25) and let ζ stand for the function*

(3.14) $\quad \zeta := -\dfrac{ik}{4\pi} \sum_{\mu \in \Lambda(L)} \{ ([T^{(L)}]^{-1} \cdot [\langle u_\lambda | h_4^{\perp} \rangle])_\mu u_\mu + r_{4,\mu}^{(L)} u_\mu \}$.

Then the boundary defect evaluated at $W^{(L)} \cdot f^{(L)}$ reads

(3.15) $\quad B^{(L)}(\vec{\psi}_{ref}; W^{(L)} \cdot f^{(L)}) = \|u_1^{\perp}\|^2_{L^2(\Gamma)} + \|(u_{rem}^{(L+1)} + \zeta)_1^{(L)}\|^2_{L^2(\Gamma)}$.

The result is obtained by combining EQ. 2.28 with EQ. 3.10. Unlike EQ. 3.10, the right hand side of EQ. 3.15 depends on $\mathbf{T}^{(L)}$ and on $h_{\frac{1}{4}}$. At this stage the right hand side could be estimated from above for a given obstacle. No attempt in this direction is made herewith.

3.2.2. Justification of ABP.
The practical significance of the ABP method and its computational effectiveness can be assessed by means of the indicators specified next.

ASSUMPTION 3.1. *There exist a class of obstacles in Ψ_{ad}, an incident wavevector $\mathbf{k}$, an order L_0 and two non negative functions, $c_1(L)$, $c_2(L)$ such that, $\forall\ L \geq L_0$ the following occur simultaneously.*

I) *the value $c_1(L_0)$ is "large" and $c_1(L)$ increases fast enough,*

II) $c_2(L)$ *decreases fast enough,*

III)

$$(3.16) \qquad (0 \leq)\ c_2(L) < c_1(L)\ ,$$

IV) *the defect evaluated at the exact far field coefficients, $B_{exa}^{(L)}$, and the defect in EQ. 3.15, now denoted by $B_{ABP}^{(L)}$, respectively satisfy*

$$(3.17) \qquad B_{exa}^{(L)} := \Big\| \sum_{\lambda \in \Lambda(L)} f_\lambda\, v_\lambda + u \Big\|^2_{L^2(\Gamma)} = c_1(L)\ ;$$

$$B_{ABP}^{(L)} := \Big\| \sum_{\lambda \in \Lambda(L)} (\mathbf{W}^{(L)} \cdot \mathbf{f}^{(L)})_\lambda\, v_\lambda + u \Big\|^2_{L^2(\Gamma)} = c_2(L)\ .$$

Since $\mathbf{f}^{(L)}$ is never available, condition IV must be restated in terms of quantities computable e.g., by the scheme of SECT. 2.3, the order of which is now denoted by M. Let the forward solver yield the coefficients $\{p_\lambda^{(M)}\}$, where $\lambda \in \Lambda(M)$. From REM. 2.5.*i*, the solver exhibits convergence in the range $0 \leq \lambda \leq \lambda_0$ as $M \to \infty$. Let M_0 denote the order, which satisfies $\mathrm{card}[\Lambda(M_0)] = \lambda_0 + 1$. The alternative to IV becomes the following.

v) *Choose $M > M_0 > L > L_0$. Assume EQS. 3.17 hold even if f_λ is replaced by $p_\lambda^{(M)}$ of EQ. 2.41 and $\mathbf{f}^{(L)}$ by the first $\mathrm{card}[\Lambda(L)]$ entries of $\mathbf{p}^{(M)}$.*

In other words, the partial sums in $B_{exa}^{(L)}$ shall form a diverging sequence, hence the family $\{v_\lambda\}$ is not a Schauder basis in $L^2(\Gamma)$. Yet, propagating $\mathbf{f}^{(L)}$ or $\mathbf{p}^{(M)}$ backwards by $\mathbf{W}^{(L)}$ shall return a "small" value of $B_{ABP}^{(L)}$, thus improving accuracy as L increases.

The numerical verification of INEQ. 3.16 and EQS. 3.17 provides a heuristic guideline for selecting some examples and predicting whether ABP will succeed or fail, as it will be described in § 4.2.3.

3.2.3. Distinctive Features of ABP.

From the above properties, a comparison with existing identification methods can be outlined.

i) There is *no separate penalty term* in the objective function, which is usually based on the discrepancy between the known and computed scattering amplitude values (see [1], [8] and the other references listed in Ch. 5 of [4]).

ii) The only unknowns are the *shape parameters*. Namely, other methods consider far field coefficients as additional unknowns. A functional relationship between them and the boundary coefficients never seems to have been taken into account by other Authors.

iii) If the reference obstacle is known, which occurs when the scattering amplitude results from the simulation of a direct scattering process, the *minimum* achievable value of the *boundary defect* can be determined (EQ. 3.10) or estimated (EQ. 3.15) before carrying out any numerical iteration.

The ABP operator here incorporates the known linear (up to an error term, recall EQ. 3.9) constraints between sets of coefficients. As a consequence, the only constraints to be treated separately during an iteration are those on the shape parameters, implied by the definition of Ψ_{ad} of EQ. 3.4.

4. Numerical Implementation

4.1. The Computer Code.

A synopsis of the interaction between direct and inverse problem solvers is provided by Fig 4.1. The two top rows show the data flow for the solution of the direct problem by either the $X_4^{(M)}$ or $X_1^{(M)}$ schemes. The bottom row describes shape reconstruction from far field data.

4.1.1. Solution of the Direct Problem.

Since no experimental data from scattered fields are available, all numerical examples to be described rely on computed far field coefficients and scattering amplitudes. For simplicity only one incident wavevector, **k**, is considered. Either scheme, $X_1^{(M)}$ or $X_4^{(M)}$, is used, where M is the approximation order, in accordance to SECT. 3.2.2. The following quantities control a direct problem solver: M, I, $\vec{\Psi}_{ref}$ and J, the number of grid points on S^2 (see the beginning of § 3.1.1). The solid angle $[0, \pi) \times [0, 2\pi)$ is replaced by $J = n_p^2$ Gaussian quadrature points. The coefficients $\mathbf{p}^{(M)}$ of EQ. 2.41 yield the far field $\tilde{v}(\mathbf{p}^{(M)})$ on S^2 through the known relationship

$$\text{(4.1)} \qquad \tilde{v}(\mathbf{p}^{(M)}) = \sum_{\lambda \in \Lambda(M)} p_\lambda^{(M)} \tilde{v}_\lambda ,$$

where

$$\text{(4.2)} \quad \tilde{v}_\lambda = \sqrt{2} \left(\frac{k}{\pi}\right)^{3/2} (-i)^l g_{l,m} P_l^m(\cos\theta) \cos m\phi , \quad \lambda \in \Lambda(M), \; r=1.$$

Similarly, $\mathbf{f}^{(W,M)}$ of EQ. 2.24 yields $\tilde{v}(\mathbf{f}^{(W,M)})$.

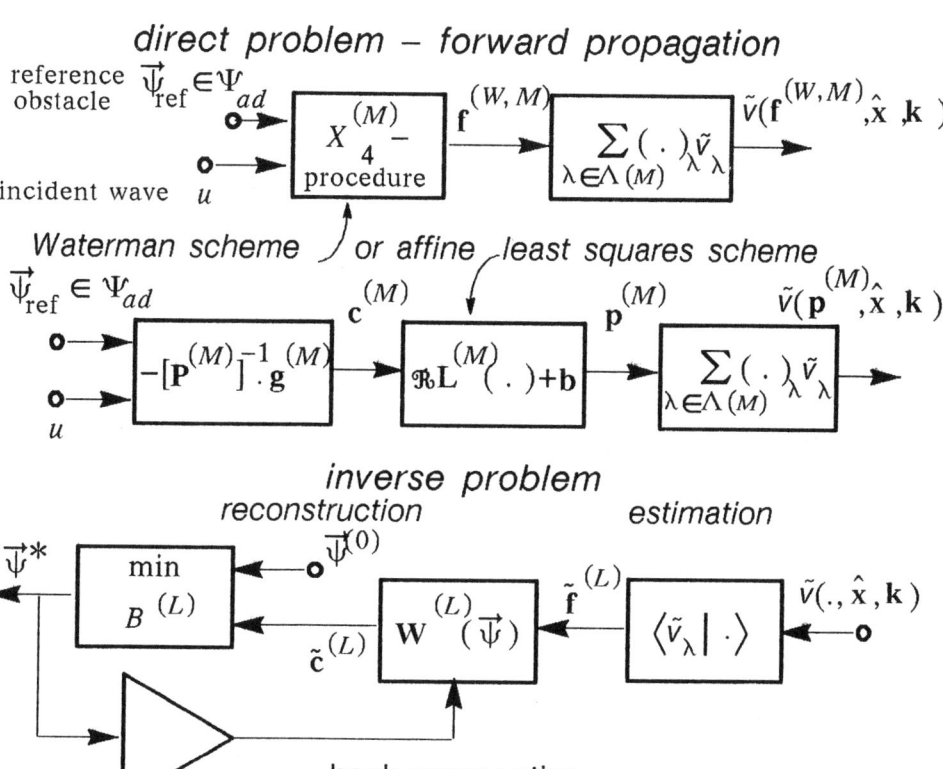

FIGURE 4.1
Synopsis of data flow for the direct and inverse problems.
Scattering amplitude data for the numerical examples below come from the $X_1^{(M)}$ (affine, least squares) scheme only.

4.1.2. Estimation of $\tilde{f}^{(L)}$.
Given **k** and L, step 1 of the algorithm requires to reverse EQ. 4.1 by approximately evaluating some inner products in $L^2(S^2)$. Of course the orders M and L may differ; moreover integration may be carried out over a different grid of n_o^2 points.

4.1.3. Minimization of $B^{(L)}$.
The objective function to be iteratively minimized with respect to $\vec{\psi} \in \Psi_{ad}$ is $B^{(L)}(\vec{\psi}; \mathbf{W}^{(L)}(\vec{\psi}) \cdot \tilde{f}^{(L)})$, where the base functions and the Jacobian in all surface integrals, including those in the entries of $\mathbf{W}^{(L)}$, depend on $\vec{\psi}$. The computed minimizer i.e., the vector at which iterations stop for some reason, will be denoted by $\vec{\psi}^*$.

Since a discrete gradient rule shall be applied, the derivatives with respect to $\vec{\psi}$ of all of these quantities would be needed. In fact iterative identification in step 2 is split into two phases to avoid the differentiation of $\mathbf{W}^{(L)}$.

The vector $\mathbf{W}^{(L)}(\vec{\psi}^{(n)}) \cdot \tilde{f}^{(L)}$ is inserted into $B^{(L)}$; the gradient and Hessian of the latter are determined as if $\{v_\lambda\}$, u and Γ in EQ. 3.5 were the only functions of $\vec{\psi}^{(n)}$. This simplifies the code substantially. Since there is no guarantee however that the updated parameters $\vec{\psi}^{(n+1)}$ yield the appropriate $\mathbf{W}^{(L)}$ for the next step, the inequality

$$(4.3) \quad B^{(L)}(\vec{\psi}^{(n+1)}; \mathbf{W}^{(L)}(\vec{\psi}^{(n+1)}) \cdot \tilde{f}^{(L)}) < \\ < B^{(L)}(\vec{\psi}^{(n)}; \mathbf{W}^{(L)}(\vec{\psi}^{(n)}) \cdot \tilde{f}^{(L)})$$

must be evaluated *a posteriori*. If it is not, the update is scaled down by means of a line search routine, which is also iterative.

4.1.4. Stopping Tests vs. Numerical Consistency.
There are two stopping tests in the algorithm i.e., the maximum allowed numbers of main iterations (steps 2.1 to 2.4 in § 3.1.2) and nested line search iterations.

Usually line search fails when the available numerical "model" is inconsistent with the function to be actually minimized. Beyond obvious roundoff errors, other sources of inconsistency are errors in the data $\tilde{f}^{(L)}$ and the limited accuracy set by L. Numerical minimization of $B^{(L)}$ is meaningless below the value set by EQ. 3.10, which could be computed if $\vec{\psi}_{ref}$ were known. Nonetheless, even if this vector is unknown, computation shall become inconsistent in its neigbourhood. This feature shows in most of the examples, where the small value of L is the only error cause.

4.2. Numerical Examples.

4.2.1. Test Shapes. Some of the reference shapes are listed in TAB. 4.1 together with their relevant radii and parameters. For oblate spheroids, ϵ is eccentricity. All of them comply with the uniqueness condition set by LEMMA 3.1, hence examples are restricted to only one incident wavevector such that $k = 1$. Oblate spheroids have been chosen, in order to show how the ABP method performs as only one control parameter, eccentricity, is varied. The other shapes have been selected because of their similarity with published examples: see again Ch. 5 of [4] and references therein.

TABLE 4.1
Test Shapes and Their Trigonometric Parameterization

Shape	l_{min}	$r(0)$	$r(\pi/2)$	$\vec{\psi}_{ref}$
oblate spheroid ($\epsilon^2 = 4/5$)	3	.44721	1	{ 3, 0, 0, 2 }
oblate spheroid ($\epsilon^2 = 8/9$)	3	.333333	1	{ 5, 0, 0, 4 }
S – bullet	5	.577	.75	{ 2, 0, 0, 0, 0, 1 }
P – peanut	7	1.0	.49	{ 2, 0, 0, –1.6, 0, 0, 0, .6 }
G – cell	11	.777	1.4	{ 1.4, 0, –.04, +.85, 0, 0, 0, –.3, 0, 0, 0, –.3 }

4.2.2. General Properties. TAB. 4.2 summarizes the relevant properties of each example. The reconstruction results will be discussed in § 4.2.4. The orders M and L have been defined in § 4.1.1 and 4.1.2 resp. as well as the numbers of grid points after n_p and n_o. The value $B_{min}^{(M)}$ is obtained from applying EQ. 2.38. The extra term in EQ. 3.10 turns out to add a negligible contribution in all cases. The quotient $\left| \frac{P_{000}}{P_{0MM}} \right|$ relates the first and last diagonal entries of the 0-th block in $\mathbf{P}^{(M)}$ and is an estimate of the reciprocal condition number of $\mathbf{P}^{(M)}$. Oblate spheroids are designated by their eccentricity squared. Moreover $\hat{q} := \frac{\hat{x} + \hat{z}}{\sqrt{2}}$. Rational numbers are given in floating point format (.mantissa **signed exponent**).

TABLE 4.2
Reconstruction Results

Shape	k	M	n_p	$B^{(M)}_{min}$	$\left\|\dfrac{P_{000}}{P_{0MM}}\right\|$	I_{inv}	L	n_o	N_{it}	$B^{(L)}(\vec{\psi}^*)$	FIG.
$\epsilon^2=4/5$	$\hat{q}$	12	63	.387−1	.25−30	7	4	15	6	.120+0	4.2
						7	5	15	7	.108+0	4.3
$\epsilon^2=8/9$	$\hat{q}$			.185+0	.27−33	7	4	15	4	.257+0	4.4
						7	5	15	7	.246+0	4.5
						7	6	15	9	.775+1	4.6
S−bullet	$\hat{z}$	12	63	.225−1	.10−27	11	4	15	10	.588−1	4.7
						11	5	15	15	.243+0	4.8
P−peanut	$\hat{z}$	12	63	.270−1	.33−29	11	4	15	5	.728−1	4.10
						11	5	15	6	.683+0	4.12
						11	6	15	8	.360+2	like 4.6
G−cell	$\hat{z}$	9	63	.399+0	.286−17	11	4	15	8	.420+0	like 4.13
						11	5	15	7	.330+0	4.13

TABLE 4.3
Numerical Assessment of the $X_1^{(L)}$ Scheme: an Example
Shape: P−peanut; $\mathbf{k} = \hat{z}$, $n_p = 63$

M	m	l	$\mathrm{Re}[p^{(M)}_{m,l}]$	$\mathrm{Im}[p^{(M)}_{m,l}]$	m	l	$\mathrm{Re}[p^{(M)}_{m,l}]$	$\mathrm{Im}[p^{(M)}_{m,l}]$
9	0	0	−.453881+00	−.437046+00	0	1	.321796+00	−.644392−01
12	0	0	−.457111+00	−.437885+00	0	1	.323543+00	−.649501−01
15	0	0	−.458153+00	−.437552+00	0	1	.327485+00	−.663813−01

M	m	l	$\mathrm{Re}[p^{(M)}_{m,l}]$	$\mathrm{Im}[p^{(M)}_{m,l}]$	m	l	$\mathrm{Re}[p^{(M)}_{m,l}]$	$\mathrm{Im}[p^{(M)}_{m,l}]$
9	0	2	−.244537−01	−.161468−02	0	3	.538358−02	−.119899−02
12	0	2	−.247662−01	−.175842−02	0	3	.529813−02	−.118799−02
15	0	2	−.250729−01	−.179961−02	0	3	.537174−02	−.121514−02

M	m	l	$\mathrm{Re}[p^{(M)}_{m,l}]$	$\mathrm{Im}[p^{(M)}_{m,l}]$
9	0	4	−.634013−04	.218344−03
12	0	4	−.358098−04	.251576−03
15	0	4	−.305589−04	.252894−03

4.2.3. Numerical Assessment of the $X_1^{(L)}$ Scheme and Verification of ASSUMPTION 3.1. For each shape listed in TAB. 4.1 it is important to verify whether the computed far field coefficients exhibit the expected convergence property already at a relatively low (≤ 15), value of M. By choosing the P-peanut, letting $M = 9, 12, 15$, $\mathbf{k} = \hat{\mathbf{z}}$ and $n_p = 63$, $\mathbf{p}^{(M)}$ is computed according to EQ. 2.41. The dominant entries, which correspond to $m = 0$, $0 \leq l \leq 4$ are listed in TAB. 4.3 do not show any erratic trend. Similar properties are found for the coefficients of the other obstacles.

In order to verify conditions I, II, III and V in ASSUMPT. 3.1, let e.g., $L_0 = 4$, $M_0 = 9$, $M = 15$. The other control parameters must be the same as in TAB. 4.2, except the number of grid points, which is kept to n_p^2. For a given shape, $B_{\text{exa}}^{(L)}$ shall increase, whereas $B_{\text{ABP}}^{(L)}$ shall decrease at least when L goes from 4 to 5. Moreover INEQ. 3.16 i.e., $B_{\text{exa}}^{(L)} > B_{\text{ABP}}^{(L)}$, shall hold at each L. With reference to TAB. 4.4, these properties are satisfied by the "$\epsilon^2 = 4/5$ − spheroid" and the S-bullet, which shall therefore yield the best results. Reconstruction of the P-peanut shall be better at $L = 5$ than at $L = = 6$. Poor results are expected from the other spheroid and from the G-cell, for which ASSUMPT. 3.1.II is not verified.

TABLE 4.4
Numerical Verification of ASSUMPTION 3.1

$L_0 = 4$; $L = 4, 5$ and 6; $M_0 = 9$; $M = 15$. For a given shape, $B_{\text{exa}}^{(L)}$ shall increase, whereas $B_{\text{ABP}}^{(L)}$ shall decrease as L increases.

Shape	k	M	n_p	$B_{\text{exa}}^{(4)}$	$B_{\text{exa}}^{(5)}$	$B_{\text{exa}}^{(6)}$	$B_{\text{ABP}}^{(4)}$	$B_{\text{ABP}}^{(5)}$	$B_{\text{ABP}}^{(6)}$
$\epsilon^2 = 4/5$	$\hat{\mathbf{q}}$	15	63	.275+1	.427+1	.950+1	.149+0	.801−1	.793−1
$\epsilon^2 = 8/9$	$\hat{\mathbf{q}}$	15	63	.183+2	.526+2	.217+3	.303+0	.203+0	.205+0
S-bullet	$\hat{\mathbf{z}}$	15	63	.429+0	.457+0	.561+0	.131+0	.114+0	.868−1
P-peanut	$\hat{\mathbf{z}}$	12	63	.876+0	.196+1	.430+1	.159+0	.790−1	.860−1
G-cell	$\hat{\mathbf{z}}$	15	63	.929+1	.235+2	.248+2	.154+1	.199+1	.191+1

4.2.4. Reconstruction Results. Again with reference to TAB. 4.2, the chosen parameterization dimension is l_{inv} (plainly l in the FIGURES), which is sometimes greater than the minimum l_{min} required by $\vec{\psi}_{\text{ref}}$; the number of iterations is N_{it}. FIGURES 4.2 to 4.8 and 4.10 to 4.13 show cross sections of shapes. The reference shape is drawn by a thick solid line, the initial guess $\vec{\psi}^{(0)}$ (the unit sphere) by a thin solid line and the reconstruction by a thick dashed line. For ease of comparison, some numerical values from TAB. 4.2 are repeated inside the drawings, together with the reference frame and the incident wavevector.

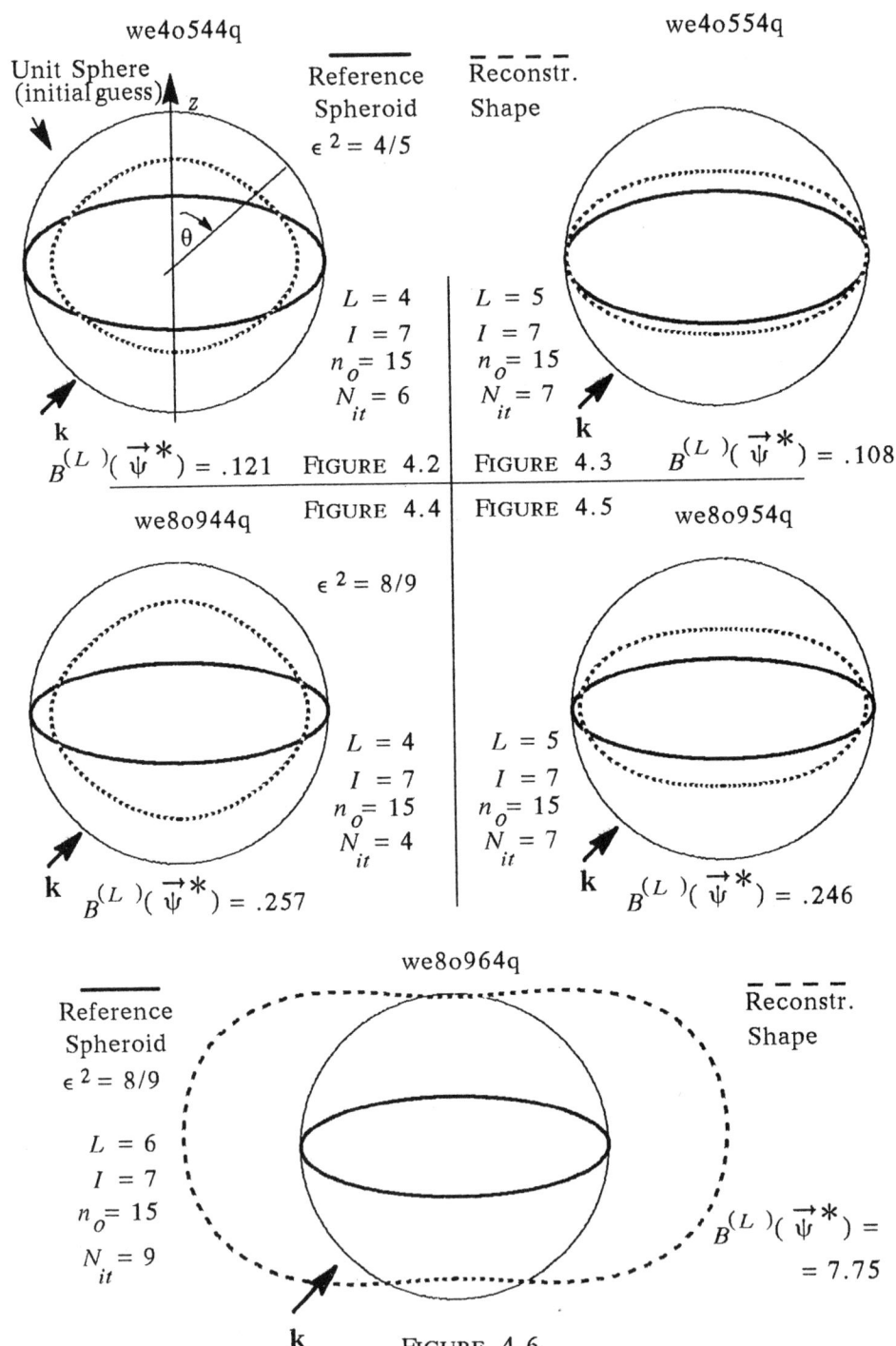

FIGURE 4.2 FIGURE 4.3 FIGURE 4.4 FIGURE 4.5 FIGURE 4.6

A relatively small value of $B^{(M)}_{min}$ and a large reciprocal condition number are required for ABP reconstruction to perform well. This shall occur with the $\epsilon^2 = 4/5$ as compared to the other spheroid in TAB. 4.2. The S-bullet and the P-peanut shall also be better reconstructed than the G-cell, the size of which yields a larger boundary defect, notwithstanding the smaller condition number.

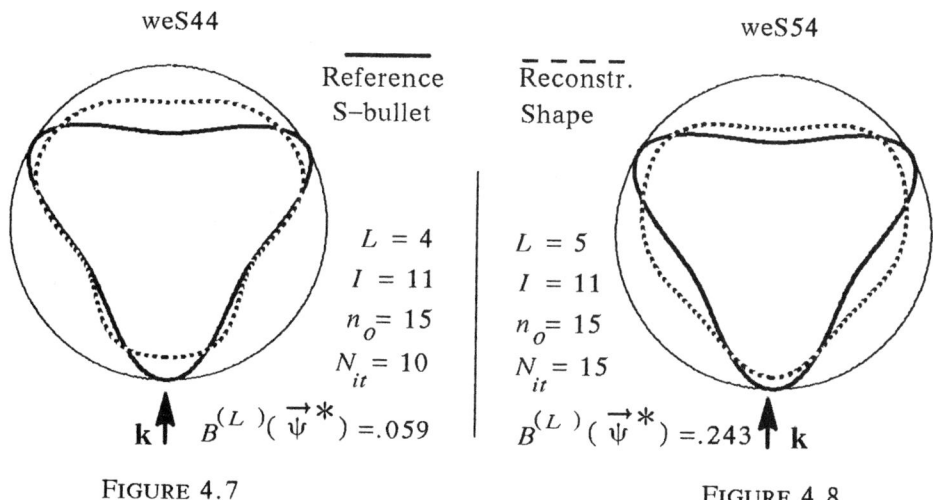

FIGURE 4.7   FIGURE 4.8

The above criteria shall be combined with the remarks in § 4.2.3 to predict the results in the ideal case. The estimation process of § 4.1.2, which relates $\tilde{v}(\mathbf{p}^{(M)})$ to $\tilde{\mathbf{f}}$, is also expected to further deteriorate the results. A typical relationship between $\mathbf{p}^{(M)}$ and $\tilde{\mathbf{f}}$ is presented in TAB. 4.5 and by the relative error bar chart of FIG. 4.9. When $m = 0$, estimation errors are acceptable up to $l = 4$. Also note that some values of $p^{(M)}_{m,l}$, $m \neq 0$, which shall be in the range of 10^{-30} are overestimated by several orders of magnitude (last line of TAB. 4.5).

FIGURES 4.7, 4.8 and more remarkably 4.13 show that reconstructions of the S-bullet and, resp. the G-cell are inaccurate in the shadow portion (North pole). The same occurs to the P-peanut, when 30% pseudo random noise is added to the estimated coefficients (FIG. 4.11). Results of course improve if there are two incident wavevectors. Although interesting, this subject is not elaborated herewith, because the purpose of this SECTION is to show the properties and limitations of ABP as they emerge from § 3.2.

TABLE 4.5
Estimation of the Far Field Coefficients
Shape: P-peanut; $\mathbf{k} = \hat{\mathbf{z}}$, $M = 15$, $n_p = 63$, $n_o = 15$

$\mathbf{p}^{(M)}$: coefficients computed by direct problem solver;

$\tilde{\mathbf{f}}$: coefficients estimated from inner products (file: *eP*)

m	l	$\text{Re}[p^{(M)}_{m,l}]$	$\text{Im}[p^{(M)}_{m,l}]$	$\text{Re}[\tilde{f}^{(M)}_{m,l}]$	$\text{Im}[\tilde{f}^{(M)}_{m,l}]$
0	0	-.458153+00	-.437552+00	-.457111+00	-.437885+00
0	1	+.327485+00	-.663813-01	+.323543+00	-.649501-01
0	2	-.250729-01	-.179961-02	-.247662-01	-.175842-02
0	3	+.537174-02	-.121514-02	+.529813-02	-.118799-02
0	4	-.305589-04	+.252894-03	-.358102-04	+.251577-03
0	5	-.114611-04	+.997759-06	-.480301-05	-.311150-06
0	6	+.125029-05	+.139571-05	+.906245-06	+.143026-05
0	7	-.212421-06	+.407371-07	-.388520-05	+.831400-06
0	8	+.478894-08	+.101865-08	-.121307-04	-.160722-05
0	9	-.505232-09	+.107915-09	-.158304-03	+.328336-04
0	10	+.469515-11	-.458851-11	-.390571-03	-.181758-03
0	11	-.248225-12	+.692860-13	-.295032-02	+.601804-03
0	12	-.332990-14	-.862566-14	-.621592-02	-.423765-02
...					
12	12	+.486057-34	-.291008-30	+.136123+00	+.124774+00

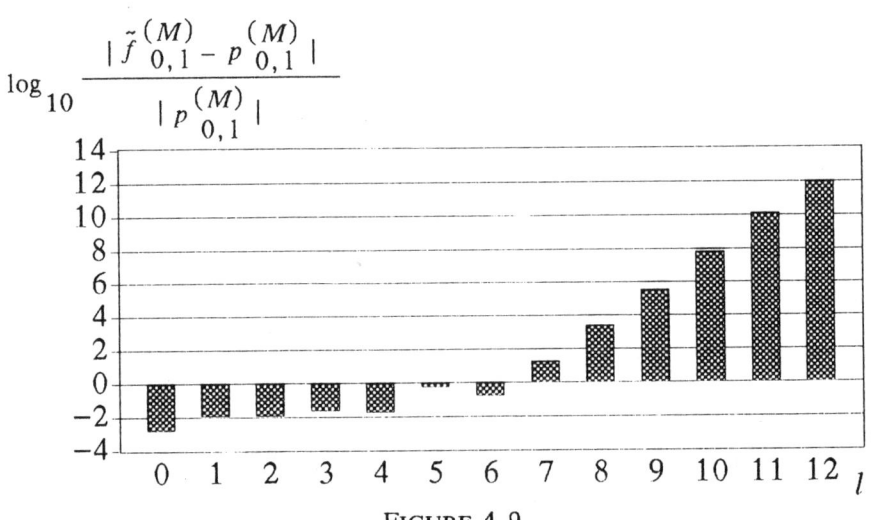

FIGURE 4.9

Log_{10} bar chart of the relative error made in estimating the far field coefficients from inner products.

REMARKS. Description has been deliberately limited to simulations closer to realistic conditions and expected to yield the poorest results. Far field data have come from an $X_1^{(M)}$-scheme and the estimation of $\tilde{\mathbf{f}}$ has been performed on a coarser grid ($n_o < n_p$), in order to minimize cross talk between the forward and the inverse solver. The data from the $X_4^{(M)}$ scheme consistently yield slightly better results, because of the structural analogy between the forward ($\mathbf{T}^{(M)}$) and backward ($\mathbf{W}^{(L)}$) propagators.

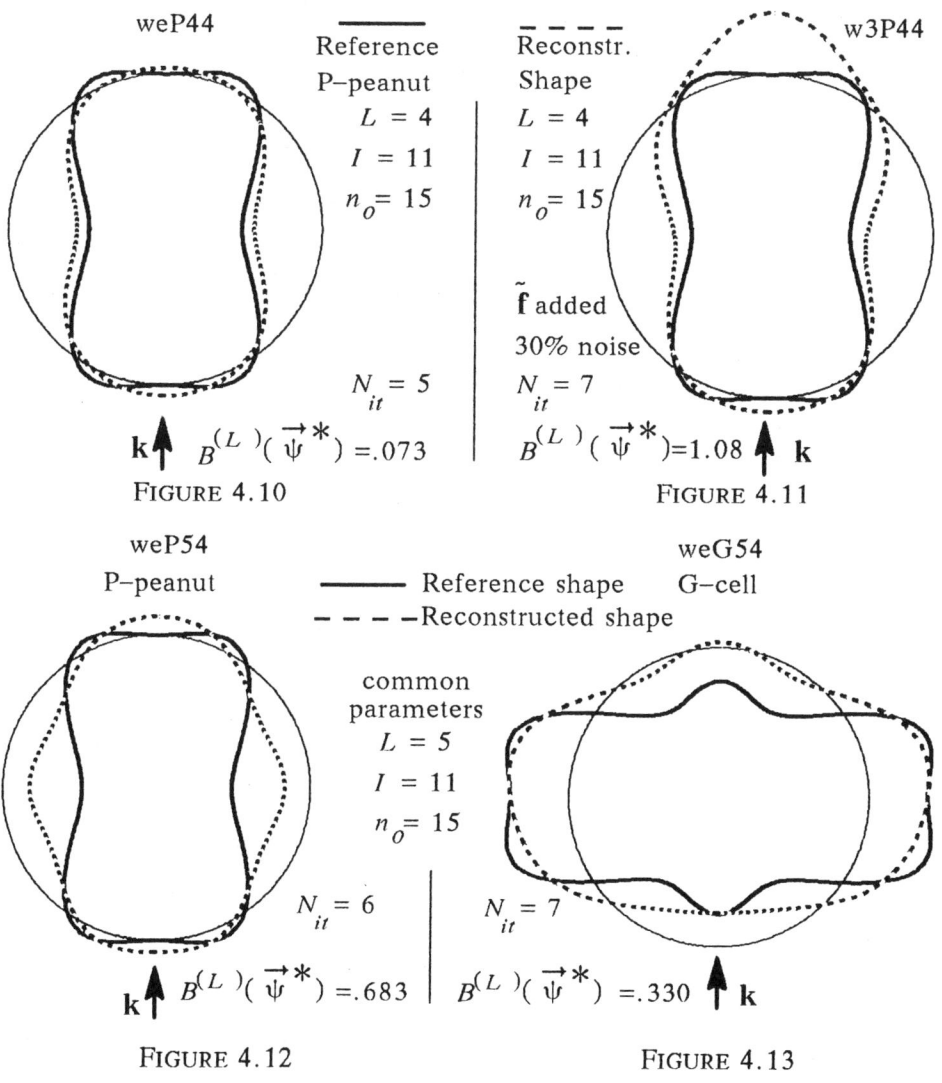

FIGURE 4.10

FIGURE 4.11

FIGURE 4.12

FIGURE 4.13

Computation has been carried by an IBM RT PC 6151/115 run by AIX version 2.2.1 operating system and the FORTRAN 77 version 1.1.1 level

1245. It must be pointed out that different hardware and software versions for machines of the same class may yield slightly different numerical results.

Conclusion

The properties of complete families in $L^2(\Gamma)$ and the variational approach, which translates into a least squares approximation in linear subspaces, together provide a unifying view over approximation schemes affecting both the direct and the inverse scattering problems. In this context, the ABP method arises as an immediate application. Moreover the error, which characterizes each scheme can be expressed and in some cases estimated. Some properties of ABP have been outlined. In accordance with the results of § 3.2, several numerical examples have been designed and solved. Conversely, given a reference shape, some means to predict the performance of ABP have been outlined.

The identification of obstacles exhibiting a Neumann BC has not been covered so far: it could be carried out by suitably modifying the ABP operator.

Of course the validation, not only of ABP but of the whole approach based on complete families will benefit from the merger with methods set in different frameworks e.g., the direct solvers based on the Nystroem scheme [4, p. 68], [14, Ch. 18] or Kleinman's et al. [9] procedure and the inverse solvers based on approximations of the incident field, the Herglotz function method in particular [4, § 5.5].

Finally, the stability [7, see also 17] of the solutions to infinite and finite dimensional problems: it is a property which deserves an investigation plan of its own, as far as the ABP method is concerned. The result of FIG. 4.11 could e.g., be interpreted accordingly.

Appendix

In order to derive EQ. 2.17, denote by $\Phi(x-y) = (1/D)\exp[ikD]$, $D := |x-y|$, the fundamental solution to EQ. 1.1. By Green's identity, the scattered field v is the solution to the following integral equation

$$(\text{A.1}) \quad v(x) = \frac{1}{4\pi} \int_\Gamma \Phi(x-y)\, \partial_n(u+v)\, d\Gamma(y), \quad x \in \Omega^c.$$

Outside the sphere circumscribed to Ω, v is to be represented according to EQ. 2.3. Recall the known expansion of $\Phi(x, y)$

$$(\text{A.2}) \quad \Phi(x-y) = ik \sum_{\lambda \in \Lambda} v_\lambda(k\, r_>)\, u_\lambda(k\, r_<)$$

by products of base functions, where $|r_>|$ and $|r_<|$ are respectively the greater and lesser of $|x|$, $|y|$. Insert this expansion into EQ. A.1, choose x on the surface of a sphere centered at the origin and circumscribed to the obstacle: hence $r_> = x$, $r_< = y$ and the v_λ ' s are orthogonal. By equating the coefficients of like multiindices, EQ. 2.17 follows.

In order to derive EQ. 2.18, assume now $x \in \Omega$ and recall Helmholtz formula (see e.g., §§ 3.2 and 3.9 of [3])

$$(A.3) \quad 0 = u(x) - \frac{1}{4\pi}\int_\Gamma \Phi(x-y)\,\partial_n(u+v)\,d\Gamma(y), x \in \Omega.$$

In particular, choose x on the surface of a sphere inscribed in the obstacle: here $r_> = y$, $r_< = x$ and the u_λ ' s are orthogonal. Substitute the representation EQ. 2.13 for u and equate the coefficients of like multiindices. EQ. 2.18 follows.

The above procedures are based on SECT. 1 of [20].

REFERENCES

1. T S ANGELL, R E KLEINMAN, G F ROACH, An Inverse Transmission Problem for the Helmholtz Equation, Inverse Problems **3** (1987), 149–80

2. R G BARANTSEV, V V KOZACHEK, Issledovanie Matrizy Rasseyaniya na Ob'ektach Slozhnoi Formy (Investigation of the Scattering Matrix for Bodies of Complicated Form), Vestnik Leningr. Univers., # 7 (1968), 71 – 77

3. D COLTON, R KRESS, *Integral Equation Methods in Scattering Theory*, Wiley: New York, 1983

4. D COLTON, R KRESS, *Inverse Acoustic and Electromagnetic Scattering Theory*, Springer: Berlin, 1992

5. G CROSTA, A Shape Optimization Problem in Inverse Acoustics, to appear in J Lagnese, D L Russel, L White, Eds., IMA Volumes in Mathematics and Its Applications: *Control and Optimal Design of Distributed Parameter Systems*, Springer: New York, 1994

6. A G DALLAS, The Waterman Algorithm for Approximation of the Transition Matrix in Scattering by Obstacles, talk delivered at the XXII General Assembly of the International Union of Radio Science, Tel Aviv, Aug. 24–Sep. 2, 1987

7. V ISAKOV, Stability Estimates for Obstacles in Inverse Scattering, J. Computational and Applied Math. **42** (1992), 79 – 88

8. D S JONES, X Q MAO, A Method for Solving the Inverse Problem in Soft Acoustic Scattering, Inverse Problems **5** (1989), 731–48

9. R E KLEINMAN, G F ROACH, L S SCHUETZ, J SHIRRON, An Iterative Solution to Acoustic Scattering by Rigid Objects, Journal of the Acoust. Soc. Amer. **84** (1988), 385 – 91

10. R E KLEINMAN, G F ROACH, S E G STROEM, The Null Field Method and Modified Green Functions, Proc. Royal Soc. of London A **394** (1984), 121–36

11. G KRISTENSSON, P C WATERMAN, The T Matrix for Acoustic and Electromagnetic Scattering by Circular Disks, Journal of the Acoust. Soc. Amer. **72** (1982) 1612 – 25

12. W F MAGNUS, F OBERHETTINGER, *Formulas and Theorems for the Special Functions of Mathematical Physics*, Chelsea Publishing: New York, 1949

13. C MUELLER, *Foundations of the Mathematical Theory of Electromagnetic Waves*, Springer: Berlin, 1969

14. W H PRESS, S A TEUKOLSKY, W T VETTERLING, B P FLANNERY, *Numerical Recipes in C: The Art of Scientific Computing, Second Edition*, Cambridge University Press: Cambridge (UK), 1992

15. A G RAMM, *Scattering by Obstacles*, Reidel: Dordrecht, 1986

16. A G RAMM, *Multidimensional Inverse Scattering Problems*, Longman: Harlow, 1992

17. A G RAMM, Stability Estimates in Inverse Scattering, Acta Appl. Math. **28**, #1 (1992), 1 – 42

18. J SIMON, Differentiation with Respect to the Domain in Boundary Value Problems, Numer. Funct. Anal. and Optimiz. **2** (1980) 649 –87

19. I N VEKUA, O Polnote Sistemy Metagarmoniceskikh Funktsii (On the Completeness of Systems of Meta-Harmonic Functions), Doklady Ak. Nauk SSSR **90**, # 5 (1953), 715 – 18

20. P C WATERMAN, New Formulation of Acoustic Scattering, Journal of the Acoust. Soc. Amer. **45** (1969), 1417 – 29

DIPARTIMENTO DI SCIENZE DELL' INFORMAZIONE, UNIVERSITA' DEGLI STUDI DI MILANO, 39, via Comelico, I-20135 MILAN (IT);
e_mail: crosta@imiucca.csi.unimi.it ; FAX: +39 (2) 55 00 63 73 .

Lectures in Applied Mathematics
Volume 30, 1994

Some Nonlinear Aspects of the Radon Transform

LEON EHRENPREIS

ABSTRACT. We study three nonlinear problems in integral geometry. In the first two problems we start with functions defined on a manifold M and we integrate them over the intersection of M with suitable linear varieties. In the third problem the functions are defined on R^n and the integrals are over nonlinear varieties.

1. Introduction

In integral geometry we start with a manifold M equipped with a positive measure dx_M (or simply dx of no confusion is possible). We also have submanifolds $\{L\}$ each equipped with a measure. We are interested in studying functions f on M in terms of their integrals (Radon transform)

$$(1) \qquad \mathbf{R}f(L) = \int_L f$$

Radon's original treatment dealt with $M = R^n$ and $\{L\}$ the set of hyperplanes with the Euclidean measure. Many generalizations have been made in the literature. In particular $\{L\}$ can be a (suitable subset) of the planes in R^n of dimension $< n - 1$. We consider this the linear theory. For the nonlinear theory we study "curved" M or L.

The most powerful tool for dealing with the linear theory is the Fourier transform on R^n. The present paper deals with various nonlinear problems which can be studied using analogs of Fourier analysis which are adjusted to the problem.

We can introduce a Fourier-like analysis to study this problem when the geometry defined by $\{L\}$ has a *spread* structure. This means that $\{L\}$ can be "organized" to be a disjoint union of spreads S_g. Each S_g consists of $\{L(g,s)\}$ where

---

1991 *Mathematics Subject Classification.* Primary 44A12; Secondary 42B99.
Work supported by NSF Grant No. 33-1807-231

© 1994 American Mathematical Society
0075-8485/94 $1.00 + $.25 per page

(a) $\bigcup_s L(g,s) = M$.

(b) $L(g, s_1)$ and $L(g, s_2)$ are disjoint for $s_1 \neq s_2$.

If the L are hypersurfaces in M then under some mild conditions for each g there is a function $S_g(x)$ on M whose level sets are the *leaves* $L(g,s)$ of S_g. If the L have codimension k then we want the $L(g,s)$ to be the intersections of the level sets of $S_g^1, \ldots, S_g^k$. In this paper we shall assume $k = 1$. There are only technical differences in passing to general k.

Of course, there are many functions $S_g(x)$ whose level sets are the leaves of the spread S_g. Each $S_g(x)$ can be thought of as defining a "local structure" at each spread. But for a good theory we need a more global structure. This means that we want a function $e(x, y)$ depending on the parameter y such that

(c) For each g there is a set $\{y\} = Y_g$ for which $e(x, y)$ is constant on the leaves of S_g.

Using the function $e(x, y)$ we can define a sort of Fourier transform

$$\hat{f}(y) = \int_M f(x) e(x, y) \, dx_M \tag{2}$$

For $y \in Y_g$ the integration can be performed first on the leaves of the spread S_g and then in the "orthogonal direction." To make this sensible we assume the *Fubini property*

(d) For any g the measure dx_M splits in the form

$$dx_M = ds_g \, dl(g, s) \tag{3}$$

Here $dl(g, s)$ is the given measure on $L(g, s)$ and ds_g is a measure in the spread parameter.

Given the Fubini property we can write, for $y \in Y_g$,

$$\hat{f}(y) = \int e(x, y) \, ds_g \int_{L(g,s)} f(x). \tag{4}$$
$$= \int (\mathbf{R} f)(g, s) e(x, y) \, ds_g$$

for $y \in Y_g$. Equation (4) can be regarded as a general *projection-slice theorem*. Thus the left side of (4) is the "slice" meaning the restriction of $\hat{f}$ to Y_g while the right side involves $\mathbf{R}f(g, s)$ which can be thought of as a sort of projection of f on functions depending only on s_g that is, on the leaves of S_g.

In the classical case $M = R^n$, $\{L\}$ is the set of hyperplanes in R^n, and the spreads are the parallel families of hyperplanes. $e(x, y) = \exp(ix \cdot y)$ and (4) is the standard projection-slice theorem.

In order for the Fourier transform (2) to be useful we require

(e) The map $f \to \hat{f}$ is injective on functions of compact support on M.

(f) If h is any function of s_g then the map

(5)
$$h \to \int h(s_g) e(x,y)\, ds_g = \hat{h}(y)$$

for $y \in Y_g$, is injective.

In this paper we shall present several examples of integral transforms with spread structures and related Fourier kernels $e(x,y)$. In the first example M is an algebraic variety and we produce an integral transform with injectivity. In the second example M is the homogeneous space of a group and we can make a fairly exhaustive study of the Radon transform. In both these examples the L are linear. For our third example $M = R^n$, but the L are nonlinear.

This paper represents an outline of techniques. Full details are presented in the author's book [**RT**] which contains a complete bibliography.

2. Radon transform on algebraic varieties.

Suppose that f is a function on some smooth submanifold M of R^n of dimension k. M is endowed with a given positive measure denoted by dx_M. f is identified with the measure $f dx_M$ on R^n which we sometimes write as $f\delta(M)$. If the L meet M nicely then formula (1) is meaningful. It seems reasonable that we do not need all hyperplanes but rather a submanifold Γ of dimension $k-1$ of the space of all L and the translates of these $L_0 \in \Gamma$. A spread is the set of translates of a fixed L_0.

PROBLEM 1. Find pairs (M, Γ) for which $f \to \mathbf{R}f(L_0, s)$ is injective on a suitable space of functions or distributions on M when L_0 varies in Γ and s represents the amount of translation of L_0. Such (M, Γ) is called a *Radon pair*.

Once we have such a pair (M, Γ) we can ask the usual questions that one asks for the ordinary Radon transform, such as, range characterization, inversion formula.

Although we have no method for constructing "all" Radon pairs (M, Γ), we do have a technique which allows us to construct some pairs.

Let $\vec{p}(x) = (p_1(x), \ldots, p_l(x))$ where the p_j are homogeneous polynomials of degree $m_j > 1$. A function h on R^n is called $\vec{p}$ *harmonic* if

(6)
$$\partial p_j(h) = 0 \quad \text{for all } j$$

Here ∂p_j is the differential operator obtained from p_j by replacing each x_k by $\partial/\partial x_k$. In particular, if $l = 1$ and $p(x) = \sum x_k^2$ then p harmonicity is usual harmonicity.

In [**RT**] we demonstrate the following result:

THEOREM 1. *Let M be defined by*

(7)
$$\vec{p}(x) = \vec{Y}(x)$$

where Y_j is a polynomial of degree $< m_j$. If q is any polynomial in R^n then there *is a unique harmonic polynomial h with*

(8) $$q = h \quad \text{on } M.$$

COROLLARY 2. *For M as in Theorem 1 the restrictions of harmonic functions to M are dense in the space of all C^∞ functions on M.*

Remark 1. The space $C^\infty(M)$ can be replaced by suitable function spaces on M which are defined by growth conditions which are larger than exponential.

COROLLARY 3. *If g is a smooth function of compact support on M then*

(9) $$\int_M gh = 0 \quad \text{all harmonic } h$$

implies $g = 0$.

We have found candidates for M. How about candidates for Γ?

Let V^c be the complex affine algebraic variety defined by

(10) $$V^c: \quad p_j(x) = 0 \quad \text{all } j.$$

Note that V is a cone.

It is shown in [**FT**] that harmonic functions can be expressed as suitable Fourier integrals over V^c. In case the polynomial ideal generated by the p_j is equal to its radical (i.e. consists of all polynomials vanishing on V^c) and V^c is a cone over a nonsingular base Γ^c (more generally over a base with "reasonable singularities") then it is shown in [**RT**] that a basis for harmonics is the set of Fourier transforms of the form

(11) $$h(x) = \widehat{\frac{\partial^l}{\partial \hat{\eta}^l} \delta_0}$$

Here $\partial/\partial\hat{\eta}$ is the derivative along a generator $\hat{\eta}$ of V^c.

Now for the crucial observation: For any direction $\hat{\eta}$ the Fourier transform h given by (11) is constant in directions orthogonal to $\hat{\eta}$. Put in different terms, the nondegenerate quadratic form used to define the Fourier transform enables us to think of $\hat{\eta}$ as a covector and h is constant on the hyperplanes defined by this covector.

In order to avoid complications arising from the complex structure of V^c, we shall assume that V^c is the complexification of a real cone V over a nonsingular real algebraic variety Γ whose complexification is the complex base Γ^c of V^c.

Let $\hat{\eta}$ be a fixed direction in V. Then the linear combinations (over l) of the h defined by (11) are all constant in the codirection defined by $\hat{\eta}$. Corollary 2 asserts that the linear combinations of such polynomials are dense in suitable function spaces on M.

This is an analytic statement; the Radon transform is a geometric construct. Let $L_{\hat{\eta}}$ be the hyperplane through the origin whose normal is $\hat{\eta}$. Call $\delta(L_{\hat{\eta}})$ the distribution representing integration over $L_{\hat{\eta}}$. Then $\delta(L_{\hat{\eta}})$ as well as its translates are constant in the direction of $\hat{\eta}^{\perp}$. Moreover, it is easily seen that the linear combinations of the translates of $\delta(L_{\hat{\eta}})$ are dense, in spaces of large (in the sense of Remark 1) distributions which are constant in the covector defined by $\hat{\eta}$. This means that

The closure of the linear combinations of
  (a) *The translates of* $\delta(L_{\hat{\eta}})$
  (b) $\left\{ \widehat{\dfrac{\partial^l}{\partial \hat{\eta}^l}} \delta_0 \right\}$
are the same.

In this assertion the words "the same" mean "the same as distributions in R^n." We want to apply the distributions in (a), (b) to measures of the form $f(x)\,dx_M$ which means $f\delta(M)$.

We can put this in other terms. Suppose for simplicity that f is a C^∞ function of compact support on M. We extend f to $\tilde{f} \in \mathcal{D}(R^n)$. Then we can think of

(12) $$(\mathbf{R}f)(L) = (\mathbf{R}\tilde{f})(L\delta(M))$$

where $L\delta(M)$ means the product of $\delta(L)$ with δM. It is standard that this product is well defined and has suitable continuity properties so long as M and L intersect properly.

We have thus proven

THEOREM 4. *Suppose that M intersects properly with the translates of the hyperplanes defined by the codirections $\hat{\eta}$ of V. Then (M, Γ) is a Radon pair.*

Remark 2. For any covector $\hat{\eta} \in \Gamma$ we can regard the set of translates of $L_{\hat{\eta}}$ as a spread. Corollary 2 asserts that the linear combinations of the spread polynomials are dense in suitable spaces on M. The proof of Theorem 4 explains how to pass from spread polynomials to the δ functions of the translates of the $L_{\hat{\eta}}$.

Remark 3. Theorem 4 can also be thought of in terms of the *Fourier transform on submanifolds of* R^n. The restriction to M of the Fourier transform of a measure on V defines the Fourier transform from V to M. The proof of Theorem 4 shows that the range of the Fourier transform is dense in suitable function spaces. The uniqueness statement in Theorem 1 is equivalent to the injectivity for this Fourier transform when restricted to measures supported at the origin on V. The Fourier transform is not injective on more general measures. Moreover even when we can establish injectivity it seems difficult to find an inverse.

3. Manifolds related to Lie groups.

Theorem 4 is relevant to the injectivity of the Radon transform. Because of the difficulties mentioned in Remark 3, we do not know of any general method of determining the range. In case there is a group structure we have more tools at our disposal. We illustrate how things work for the Lorentz group $G = SO(1,2)$ in 3 dimensions.

For M we choose the positive sheet of the hyperboloid $t^2 - x^2 - y^2 = 1$. p is the Minkowski length $p = t^2 - x^2 - y^2$ so p harmonicity means solution of the wave equation. V is the light cone and Γ is the unit circle

(13) $$\Gamma\colon t^2 = x^2 + y^2, t = 1.$$

From a group theoretic point of view $M = G/K$ where K is the circle subgroup of G and for covectors corresponding to $\hat{\eta} \in V$ the Radon transform becomes the horocyclic Radon transform on G/K.

We mentioned above that the horocyclic Radon transform lies within the framework of the Fourier transform from V to M. This seems difficult to analyze directly. It appears to be much easier to analyze the Fourier transform from V to V because V has an uncomplicated harmonic analysis since V is the direct product of a compact group (the circle) and the scalar group which is $R^\times$, the multiplicative group of reals.

Thus we come to a major ingredient of our work, called *intertwining*. We use the fact that harmonics are solutions of the wave equation in R^3 to shift the contours of integration from M to V. In this way we can use the inversion of the Fourier transform from $\hat{V}$ to V to invert the Fourier transform from $\hat{V}$ to M. ($\hat{V}$ and V are both light cones; V lives in the original space and $\hat{V}$ lives in the dual space.)

We are led to two problems:

(P1) Invert the Fourier transform $\hat{V}$ to V.

(P2) Intertwine the Fourier transform from $\hat{V}$ to M with the Fourier transform from $\hat{V}$ to V.

Let us go through the steps in our construction. We start with a function $f \in \mathcal{D}(M)$ which we want to represent as the Fourier transform of some measure $\hat{f}_{\hat{V}}$ on $\hat{V}$. It seems reasonable that $\hat{f}_{\hat{V}}$ should be "close" to the Fourier transform of f, namely

(14) $$\hat{f}(\hat{x}) = \int_M f(x) e^{ix\cdot\hat{x}}\, dx_M$$

when restricted to $\hat{V}$.

For $\hat{x} \in \hat{V}$ the exponential $e^{ix\cdot\hat{x}}$ is a solution of the wave equation. Let $F(x)$ be the solution of the wave equation

(15) $$\Box F = 0$$

with Cauchy data on M suitably expressed in terms of f.

We can integrate by parts

(16) $$0 = \int_{M \uplus V^+} F \Box e^{ix\cdot\hat{x}} = \int_M f(x) e^{ix\cdot\hat{x}}\, dx_M - \int_{V^+} \tilde{f}\tilde{e}\, dx_V$$

where $\tilde{f}$ and $\tilde{e}$ are simply expressible in terms of F and exp. $M \uplus V^+$ refers to the region between M and V^+.

(16) gives an expression for $\hat{f}|_{\hat{V}}$ (which is the first term on the right side of (16)) in terms of a Fourier-like transform from V^+ to $\hat{V}$. Unfortunately the expression of F and hence $\tilde{f}$ in terms of f is somewhat complicated. These expressions could be computed in the present case using the fundamental solution for $\square$. We do not know how to carry out such computations in higher rank groups without using the Plancherel formula. We shall, therefore, use a simpler procedure. In fact, our method leads to a new proof of the Plancherel formula.

We can evaluate the term $\int_{V^+}$ on $\hat{V}$ in terms of the mysterious function $\tilde{f}$ because $\tilde{e}$ is essentially $\exp(ix \cdot \hat{x})$. Before explaining how this is done, let us see how to continue.

We know that

$$\hat{f}(\hat{x}) = \int_{V^+} \tilde{f}(x)\tilde{e}(x \cdot \hat{x})\, dx_V \quad \text{on } \hat{V}. \tag{17}$$

As we mentioned at the beginning of this computation, we expect that the Fourier transform F_v of $\hat{f}\,dx_V$ when restricted to M should be close to f. Since F_v is a solution of the wave equation, this could be accomplished if $\tilde{F}_v|_{V^+}$ is essentially $\tilde{f}$. We do not know $\tilde{f}$ but we know that its Fourier transform from V^+ to $\hat{V}$ is $\hat{f}$.

Since $\tilde{F}_v|_{V^+}$ is the (inverse) Fourier transform from $\hat{V}$ to V^+ of $\hat{f}$ it can be computed in terms of $\hat{f}$. Thus $\hat{\tilde{F}}_v$ which is the Fourier transform from V^+ to $\hat{V}$ of $\tilde{F}_v|_{V^+}$ can be computed in terms of $\hat{f}$.

It turns out that $\hat{\tilde{F}}_v$ is not exactly equal to $\hat{f}$ on $\hat{V}$. It differs from $\hat{f}$ by a beta function which is closely related to Harish-Chandra's c function for $M = G/K$. This means that it is not $\hat{f}|_{\hat{V}}$ whose Fourier transform on M is f but rather some function f_v on $\hat{V}$ which is expressible in terms of $\hat{f}|_{\hat{V}}$ and a c function.

Let us recapitulate the steps in the above construction.

(i) We start with $f \in \mathcal{D}(M)$ which produces $\hat{f}$ on $\hat{V}$.

(ii) We construct f_v from $\hat{f}|_{\hat{V}}$ and form the Fourier transform $\hat{f}_v$ of f_v.

To verify that $\hat{f}_v = f$ on M we want to check that $\tilde{\hat{f}}_v = \tilde{f}$ on V^+. This is the same as saying that $\hat{\tilde{\hat{f}}}_v = \hat{f}$ on $\hat{V}$.

(iii) We compute $\tilde{f}_v|_{V^+}$ in terms of f_v hence we compute $\hat{\tilde{\hat{f}}}_v|_{\hat{V}}$ in terms of f_v.

(iv) We now adjust f_v so that $\hat{\tilde{\hat{f}}}_v|_{\hat{V}} = \hat{f}|_{\hat{V}}$ and we are done (see figure).

Now let me explain some of the steps in more detail. The integration by parts in (16) is fairly standard except that we have to choose a suitable coordinate

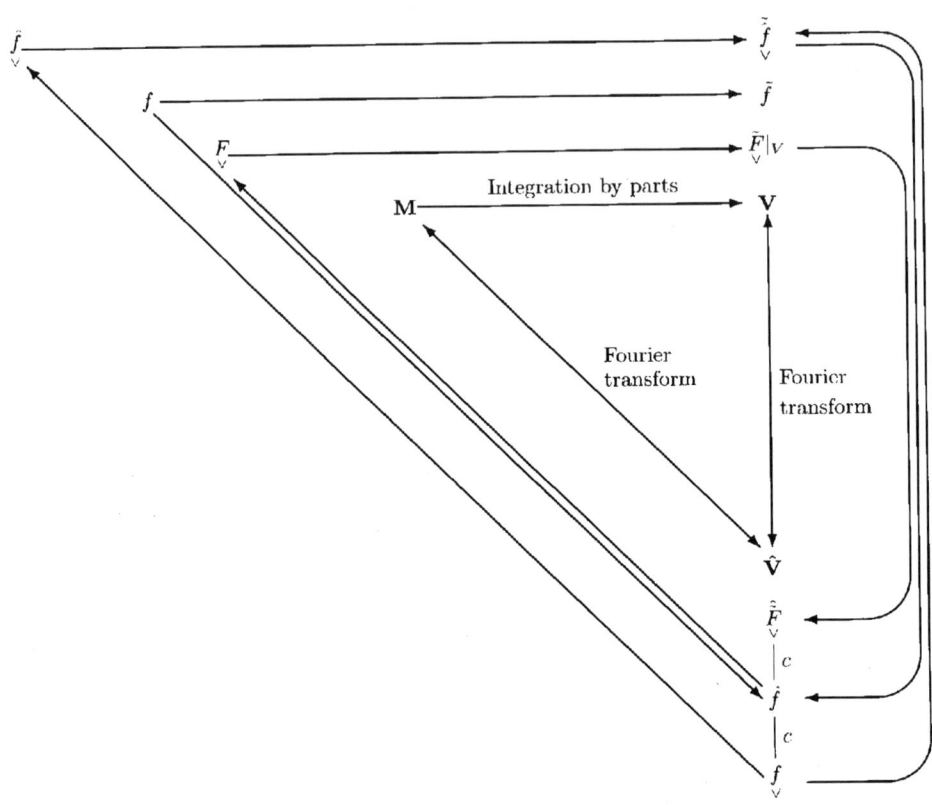

system near V^+. Also we have to be somewhat careful in dealing with the origin which is a singular point of V.

To compute the Fourier transform from V^+ to $\hat{V}$ it is best to first decompose $\tilde{f}$, and hence $\hat{\tilde{f}}$, under the action of K which is the rotation group around the t axis. We may therefore assume that $\tilde{f}$ is of the form

(18) $$\tilde{f}(r,\theta) = \tilde{f}_j(r) e^{ij\theta}$$

for a fixed j. Next we observe that, for $x \in V$, $\hat{x} \in \hat{V}$

(19) $$x \cdot \hat{x} = r\hat{r}[1 + \cos(\theta + \hat{\theta})]$$

because

(20) $$x = (r, r\cos\theta, r\sin\theta)$$

with a similar expression for $\hat{x}$.

Finally we decompose $\tilde{f}_j(r)$ under Mellin transform in r.

Thus the computations of the Fourier transforms from V^+ to $\hat{V}$ and from $\hat{V}$ to V^+ come down to the computations of integrals of the form

(21) $$\iint r^{is} e^{ir\hat{r}(1+\cos\theta)} e^{ij\theta}\, dr\, d\theta$$

Of course the integral (21) does not converge directly; it must be defined using a suitable analytic continuation. It can be expressed in terms of Bessel functions. These Bessel functions explain the deviation of $\hat{\tilde{F}}_\vee$ from $\hat{f}$ and hence the deviation of $f_\vee$ from $\hat{f}$.

The details of this argument appear in [**RT**].

Once having understood the Fourier transform from $\hat{V}$ to M we are in a position to treat the horocyclic Radon transform on M in much the same way it is treated on R^n. The Fourier transform of $\delta(\hat{\eta})$ (the δ function of the line in $\hat{V}$ with direction $\hat{\eta}$) is $\delta(\hat{\eta}^\perp)$ which is the δ function of the hyperplane through the origin corresponding to the covector $\hat{\eta}$. The Radon transform of f on the spread of hyperplanes parallel to $\hat{\eta}^\perp$ is

(22) $$\mathbf{R}f(\hat{\eta}^\perp,\ ) = \delta(\hat{\eta}) * f\ .$$

Taking the Fourier transform of (22) in the spread parameter (i.e. the parameter in $(\hat{\eta}^\perp)^\perp$) yields the usual projection-slice theorem

(23) $$[\mathbf{R}f(\eta^\perp,\ )]\hat{}\, = \hat{f}|_{\hat{\eta}}$$

Suppose that $f \in \mathcal{D}(M)$. Then $\hat{f}$ is an entire function of exponential type on all of C^n. Thus the $\hat{f}|_{\hat{\eta}}$ are, for fixed $\hat{\eta}$, entire functions of fixed exponential type. Moreover the $\hat{f}|_{\hat{\eta}}$ satisfy natural compatibility conditions at the origin which correspond to Helgason-like moment conditions on f.

However, unlike the situation in R^n, the holomorphicity and moment conditions do not suffice to characterize the range of **R** on $\mathcal{D}(M)$. There is an additional condition which comes from the Weyl group of G.

To understand this Weyl invariance, let us return to our above discussion of the Fourier transform from M to $\hat{V}$, which leads to a complete characterization of the space $\widehat{\mathcal{D}(M)}|_{\hat{V}}$. For we showed how, given a $\hat{g} \in \hat{\mathcal{D}}(\hat{V})$ we could find (if it exists) a $g \in \mathcal{D}(M)$ whose Fourier transform restricts to $\hat{g}$ on $\hat{V}$. g is given as the Fourier transform on M of a suitable $\check{\hat{g}}$ on $\hat{V}$. But the Fourier transform of this g will not equal $\hat{g}$ on $\hat{V}$ unless $\hat{g}$ is invariant under a suitable action of the Weyl group.

What is the origin of this Weyl invariance?

In studying the Fourier transform from M to $\hat{V}$ we extended a function f on M to a solution F of the wave equation $\Box F = 0$. The passage from f to F is not unique because two Cauchy data on M define a solution to the wave equation. Thus functions on M represent only "half" the solution of the wave equation.

Conversely a solution of the wave equation in the closure of the interior of V^+ is completely determined by its restriction to V^+.

The Weyl invariance picks out the "half" of the solutions which corresponds to functions on M.

We wish to give a precise statement of the characterization of the horocyclic Radon transform on $\mathcal{D}(M)$. The spreads are defined by the covectors $\hat{\eta}$ so they can be parameterized by the points in the real unit circle. Moreover rotations around the time axis operate on M. Thus functions on M can be decomposed under the action of this rotation group. This gives a Fourier series representation of $f \in \mathcal{D}(M)$ as sum of $f_m \in \mathcal{D}(M)$ each of which transforms according to a character of this rotation group.

By our above remarks the horocyclic Radon transform of f can be written in the form $F(\hat{\eta}, s)$ where s represents the amount of translation of $\delta(\hat{\eta}^\perp)$ [compare (22)]. Moreover $F(\hat{\eta}, s)$ is constant in directions parallel to $\hat{\eta}^\perp$.

THEOREM 5. *A function $F(\hat{\eta}, s)$ is the Radon transform of $f \in \mathcal{D}(G/K)$ if and only if F satisfies*
  (i) *Paley-Wiener conditions.*
  (ii) *Moment conditions.*
  (iii) *Weyl invariance.*

Let me describe these conditions precisely.
  (i) By (23) the Fourier transform $\hat{F}(\hat{\eta}, \hat{r})$ of $F(\hat{\eta}, s)$ for fixed $\hat{\eta}$ is $\hat{f}|_{\hat{\eta}}$. Thus it must be a usual Paley-Wiener function on the complex line defined by $\hat{\eta}$. In terms of the usual parameter $\hat{r}$ we must have exponential decrease as $\operatorname{Im} \hat{r} \to +\infty$. (This results from the fact that G/K lies in the region defined by $t \geq 1$.)

(ii) The moment conditions mean that the $\hat{F}(\hat{\eta}, \hat{r})$ fit together on the light cone to form a smooth function at the origin,
(iii) The Weyl invariance is best stated in terms of the F_m which are the horocyclic Radon transforms of the f_m. Thus $\hat{F}_m$ transforms according to a suitable character of the rotation group.

Call $\check{\hat{F}}_m(\hat{u})$ the Mellin transform of $\hat{F}_m$ on $\hat{r} > 0$. Then

$$(24) \qquad \check{\hat{F}}_m(1-\hat{u})(i)^{1-\hat{u}}\Gamma(\hat{u}+m) = \check{\hat{F}}_m(\hat{u})(i)^{\hat{u}}\Gamma(1-\hat{u}+m)$$

Remark 4. Helgason has obtained a characterization of the horocyclic transform of $\mathcal{D}$. His description is somewhat different from ours, and we do not know how to compare the two descriptions directly.

4. The case of nonlinear L.

In the above examples M was nonlinear but the varieties L on which we integrated were linear. We now reverse things and set $M = R^n$ but L nonlinear.

Let P be a homogeneous polynomial of degree m. The spread corresponding to P is the set of varieties

$$(25) \qquad L(p, s) = \{P(x) = s\}$$

that is, the level sets of P.

There is a Fourier transform associated to these spreads. Let p be a vector with $\binom{n+m-1}{m}$ components, these components being the monomials of degree m on R^n. Let $\hat{p}$ be a vector with the same number of components; the components of $\hat{p}$ are complex numbers. Thus $\hat{p} \cdot p$ represents the most general homogeneous polynomial of degree m.

For functions f, e.g. in $\mathcal{D}(R^n)$, we define the nonlinear Fourier transform of degree m by

$$(26) \qquad F(\hat{p}, \hat{x}) = \int f(x) e^{i\hat{p} \cdot p + i\hat{x} \cdot x} \, dx.$$

The relation of the nonlinear Fourier transform to the nonlinear Radon transform is again a projection-slice theorem. For, choose $\hat{p}_0$ so that $\hat{p}_0 \cdot p = P$. Then we can write (26) in a form analogous to (4), namely

$$(27) \qquad \begin{aligned} F(\lambda \hat{p}_0, 0) &= \int f(x) e^{i\lambda P(x)} \, dx \\ &= \int e^{i\lambda s} \, ds \int_{P(x)=s} f(x) \, dx. \end{aligned}$$

It should be noted that the measure we use on the sets $\{P(x) = s\}$ is not the Euclidean measure but rather the Euclidean measure divided by $|\operatorname{grad} P|$ in order to achieve the Fubini property.

Equation (27) states that the information given by the nonlinear Fourier transform on the line $\{(\lambda \hat{p}_0, 0)\}$ is equivalent to the information given by the Radon transform on the spread $\{\hat{p}_0 \cdot p = s\}$. This means that the Radon transform gives information about F on the $\hat{p}$ axis. On the other hand $F(0, \hat{x}) = \hat{f}(\hat{x})$ so f is determined by F on the $\hat{x}$ axis. How do we interplay the integral geometry $F(\hat{p}, 0)$ with the ordinary Fourier transform $F(0, \hat{x})$?

The nonlinear Fourier transform satisfies certain partial differential equations. Rather then deal with the complicated general situation let us illustrate the simplest case $m = n = 2$.

$$(28) \qquad p = (x_1^2, x_1 x_2, x_2^2)$$

It is clear that F satisfies the partial differential equation

$$(29) \qquad \frac{\partial^2 F}{\partial \hat{p}_1 \partial \hat{p}_2} = \frac{\partial^2 F}{\partial \hat{p}_2^2} \qquad \text{(Plücker equation)}.$$

$$(30) \qquad \frac{\partial F}{\partial \hat{p}_1} = -i \frac{\partial^2 F}{\partial \hat{x}_1^2}$$

$$\frac{\partial F}{\partial \hat{p}_2} = -i \frac{\partial^2 F}{\partial \hat{x}_1 \partial \hat{x}_2}$$

$$\frac{\partial F}{\partial \hat{p}_3} = -i \frac{\partial^2 F}{\partial \hat{x}_2^2} \qquad \text{(Heat equations)}.$$

Note that (29) is essentially the three-dimensional wave equation. Thus the geometric (Radon) information which, by (27), is given in terms of $F(\hat{p}, 0)$, is not independent. In fact, if we know $F(\hat{p}, 0)$ on a set of determination for the wave equation (and some differential conditions) then we know $F(\hat{p}, 0)$ everywhere.

We can now solve the heat equations (if we know some more differential conditions and suitable Gevrey regularity). In this way we determine $F(\hat{p}, \hat{x})$ hence $F(0, \hat{x}) = \hat{f}(\hat{x})$ hence $f(x)$.

We conclude that it is enough to know F and suitable derivates on a set of determination for the wave equation on the $\hat{p}$ axis (geometric information) to determine f.

A detailed study of the relationship between the nonlinear Fourier transform and the nonlinear Radon transform is presented in Chapter V of [**RT**]. It leads to a rather complete analysis of the nonlinear Radon transform.

Remark 5. In the usual Radon transform both M and the leaves L are linear. In Sections 2 and 3 M is nonlinear but the L are linear. In Section 4 M is linear but the L are not. It is reasonable to study cases in which neither M nor the L are linear. We have not studied such examples and we hope the problem will appeal to the reader.

References

[RT] Leon Ehrenpreis, *The Radon Transform*, to appear.
[FT] _____, *Fourier Transform in Several Complex Variables*, Wiley-Interscience, New York, 1972.

DEPARTMENT OF MATHEMATICS, TEMPLE UNIVERSITY, PHILADELPHIA, PA 19122
E-mail address: leon@math.temple.edu

Spherical Tomography and Spherical Integral Geometry

Simon Gindikin

Jim Reeds

Larry Shepp

ABSTRACT

Spherical integral geometry gives (in particular) a general and unified way to study spherical tomography, i.e. reconstructing a density, f, on the surface, S, of the ordinary sphere from its integrals over certain circles on S. We discuss the concrete practical problem of reconstructing $f = f(\mathbf{x})$, $\mathbf{x} \in S$, where $f(\mathbf{x})$ is the number of dipoles in a crystal which are oriented in each direction $\mathbf{x} \in S$. Nuclear magnetic resonance measurements give the integrals of f along any circle on S which is perpendicular to any one of a fixed set of n vectors, where $n \approx 100$, limited by practicality. Surprisingly, it is much better to choose these n vectors to lie uniformly in one **fixed** plane rather than to attempt to choose them uniformly on S. This was first observed via simulations, but a theoretical basis and an explanation of this observation is obtained via spherical integral geometry.

1. Spherical integral geometry

Let S^2 be the 2-dimensional sphere in $\mathbb{R}^2$:

$$(x_1)^2 + (x_2)^2 + (x_3)^2 = 1$$

and $f(x)$ be a C^∞ function on S^2. Let the *spherical Radon transform* $\widehat{f}(\xi)$ of f be the integral of f on plane sections

(1.1) $$\langle \xi, x \rangle = \xi_1 x_1 + \xi_2 x_2 + \xi_3 x_3 + \xi_0 = 0, \ \ \xi \in \mathbb{R}^4 \setminus \{0\}$$

so that

(1.2) $$\widehat{f}(\xi) = \int_{S^2} f(x)\delta(\langle \xi, x \rangle)\omega(x_1, x_2, x_3)$$

where

(1.3) $$\omega(x_1, x_2, x_3) = x_1 dx_2 \wedge dx_3 - x_2 dx_1 \wedge dx_3 + x_3 dx_1 \wedge dx_2 \ .$$

We can interpret $\widehat{f}$ as the usual 3-dimensional Radon transform of the distribution $f(x)\delta(x_1^2 + x_2^2 + x_3^2 - 1)$. We have

(1.4) $$\widehat{f}(\lambda \xi) = |\lambda|^{-1}\widehat{f}(\xi), \ \ \lambda \in \mathbb{R} \setminus \{0\} \ .$$

MR *Subject Classification.* Primary 92C55; Secondary 44A12.

© 1994 American Mathematical Society
0075-8485/94 $1.00 + $.25 per page

$$(1.5) \qquad \Box \widehat{f} = \frac{\partial^2 \widehat{f}}{\partial \xi_0^2} - \frac{\partial^2 \widehat{f}}{\partial \xi_1^2} - \frac{\partial^2 \widehat{f}}{\partial \xi_2^2} - \frac{\partial^2 \widehat{f}}{\partial \xi_3^2}.$$

If we consider only sections with $\xi_0 = 0$ (great circles), we obtain the classical Funk-Minkowski transform. In general, using stereographic projection, the family of all sections on S^2 transforms into the 3-parameter family of all circles and lines on $\mathbb{R}^2$. Thus $\widehat{f}$ depends essentially on 3 variables via (1.4) so that the problem of inversion of the operator $f \mapsto \widehat{f}$ is over-determined and the inversion formula is nonunique. To describe different inversion formulas we will use an analog of the kappa operator, $\varkappa$, [G-G-S, G] which allows one to describe inversion formulas in over-determined problems of integral geometry. Earlier, all known examples of the operator $\varkappa$ involved local problems in integral geometry; here, for the first time we treat an example of a nonlocal problem.

Let us consider the differential 2-form on $\mathbb{R}_\xi^4$ for fixed $x \in S^2$

$$(1.6) \qquad \begin{aligned} \varkappa \widehat{f} = \ & \frac{1}{16\pi^2 \langle \xi, x \rangle^2} \Big[(\widehat{f}(\xi) + \langle \xi, x \rangle \widehat{f}_0'(\xi)) \omega(\xi_1, \xi_2, \xi_3) \\ & + (x_1 \widehat{f}(x) + \langle \xi, x \rangle \widehat{f}_1'(\xi)) \omega(\xi_0, \xi_2, \xi_3) \\ & - (x_2 \widehat{f}(x) + \langle \xi, x \rangle \widehat{f}_2'(\xi)) \omega(\xi_0, \xi_1, \xi_3) \\ & + (x_3 \widehat{f}(x) + \langle \xi, x \rangle \widehat{f}_3'(\xi)) \omega(\xi_0, \xi_1, \xi_2) \Big] \end{aligned}$$

where

$$\widehat{f}_j'(\xi) = \frac{\partial \widehat{f}(\xi)}{\partial \xi_j}.$$

This form has singularities on the hyperplane $\langle x, \xi \rangle = 0$ in $\mathbb{R}_\xi^4$. The principal fact is that the form $\varkappa \widehat{f}$ is closed which is proved by directly verifying that both $g_1(\xi) = \widehat{f}(\xi)$ and $g_2(\xi) = \langle \xi, x \rangle^{-2}$, $x \in S^2$ are solutions to the wave equation $\Box g = 0$ with $\Box$ as in (1.5). The form $\varkappa \widehat{f}$ depends only on f along the line connecting ξ and 0, so if we restrict $\varkappa \widehat{f}$ to any 3-dimensional surface in $\mathbb{R}_\xi^4$ which intersects any line through 0 in one point we obtain a form which does not depend on the choice of this surface. For example if $\xi_0 \neq 0$ we can put $\xi_0 = 1$. But the more symmetric form (1.6) has several advantages.

Now let us explain how to use $\varkappa \widehat{f}$ for the construction of concrete inversion formulas. We will integrate $\varkappa \widehat{f}$ on different 2-dimensional cycles γ; under some natural conditions on γ the result of the integration will give $f(x)$. We can intuitively expect that this integral is proportional to $f(x)$ for the following reasons: It is clear that this integral is a linear functional on f which is invariant if we replace the cycle γ by any $\tilde{\gamma}$ in the same homology class. So the integral is a kind of residue of $\varkappa \widehat{f}$ on the submanifold $\langle \xi, x \rangle = 0$. Since the only point involved in all choices of γ is x itself, the support of this function should involve only x, i.e., the integral must be proportional to $f(x)$. Then the constant of proportionality is given by any special case. Rigorously one shows that for special choice of γ the integral reduces to the Radon inversion formula and so to $f(x)$. We will give examples of such cycles below. Of course a problem of regularization of the integral remains, since there is a singularity on the hyperplane $\langle x, \xi \rangle = 0$. This is exactly the singularity for the Radon transform on $\mathbb{R}^2$ and we can use the same methods of regularization. We also need to take singularities into account when we deform γ.

Next we consider some examples.

Example 1. We begin with $\gamma = \{\xi_3 = 0\}$, i.e. we consider only sections by planes parallel to the x_3-axis. Because of the restriction $\xi_3 = 0$ on γ we obtain

$$f(x) = \int_\gamma \varkappa \widehat{f},$$

(1.7) $\qquad \varkappa f \big|_\gamma = \dfrac{1}{16\pi^2} \dfrac{1}{\langle x, \xi \rangle^2} [x_3 \widehat{f}(\xi_0, \xi_1, \xi_2, 0) + \langle \xi, x \rangle \widehat{f}'_3(\xi_0, \xi_1, \xi_2, 0)] \omega(\xi_0, \xi_1, \xi_2) .$

So we can not reconstruct $f(x)$ if we know only $\widehat{f}(\xi_0, \xi_1, \xi_2, 0)$, but we can if we know also $\widehat{f}'_3|_\gamma$ (Cauchy data on γ). We can then use for example the following regularization of $\langle x, \xi \rangle^{-2}$, as in the usual 2-dimensional Radon inversion formula. Let

$$\xi_0 = -p, \quad \xi_1 = \cos \phi, \quad \xi_2 = \sin \phi, \quad \xi_3 = 0$$

$$\widehat{f}(p, \phi) \triangleq \widehat{f}(-p, \cos \phi, \sin \phi, 0), \quad \widehat{f}'_3(p, \phi) \triangleq \widehat{f}'_3(-p, \cos \phi, \sin \phi, 0) .$$

Then

(1.8) $\qquad f(x) = \dfrac{1}{16\pi^2} \displaystyle\int_0^\pi d\phi \int_{-\infty}^\infty dp \dfrac{x_3 \widehat{f}'_p(p, \phi) + \widehat{f}'_3(p, \phi)}{p - x_1 \cos \phi - x_2 \sin \phi},$

where we take the principal value of the integral on p. See [G-S] or [J] for theory, [S-L] for practice.

If the function $f(x)$ satisfies the symmetry condition

(1.9) $\qquad f(x_1, x_2, x_3) = f(x_1, x_2, -x_3)$

then $\widehat{f}'_3(\xi_0, \xi_1, \xi_2, 0) \equiv 0$ and we can reconstruct $f(x)$ knowing only $\widehat{f}(\xi_1, \xi_2, \xi_3, 0)$.

We obtain a formula, similar to the usual 2-dimensional Radon inversion formula, which can be obtained as follows: If we consider $f(x)$, $x \in S^2$, as a function of x_1, x_2 then $\widehat{f}(\xi_0, \xi_1, \xi_2, 0)$ is exactly the Radon transform of the function

$$\phi(x_1, x_2) = \dfrac{f(x)}{x_3} = \dfrac{f(x)}{\sqrt{1 - x_1^2 - x_2^2}} .$$

So (1.9) is just the Radon inversion formula for ϕ. If

$$f(x_1, x_2, x_3) = -f(x_1, x_2, -x_3)$$

then $\widehat{f}(\xi_1, \xi_2, \xi_3, 0) = 0$ and we can reconstruct $f(x)$ knowing only $\widehat{f}'_3(\xi_1, \xi_2, \xi_3, 0)$.

Example 2. Let now $\gamma = \{\xi_0 = 0\}$. We already mentioned that this case corresponds to the Minkowski-Funk transform (integration on great circles). Similar to the first example we have:

$$f(x) = \int_\gamma \varkappa \widehat{f}$$

(1.10)
$$\varkappa f\Big|_\gamma = \frac{1}{16\pi^2} \frac{1}{\langle x, \xi \rangle^2} [\widehat{f}(0, \xi_1, \xi_2, \xi_3) + \langle x, \xi \rangle \widehat{f}'_0(0, \xi_1, \xi_2, \xi_3) \omega(\xi_1, \xi_2, \xi_3)]$$

and so to reconstruct generic functions we need not only $\widehat{f}(0, \xi_1, \xi_2, \xi_3)$ but also $\widehat{f}'_0(0, \xi_1, \xi_2, \xi_3)$. A regularized version of this formula does the trick:

$$\xi_1 = \cos\phi, \quad \xi_2 = \sin\phi, \quad \xi_3 = -p, \quad \xi_0 = 0,$$

(1.11)
$$\widehat{f}(\phi, p) \triangleq \widehat{f}(\cos\phi, \sin\phi, -p, 0), \quad \widehat{f}'_0(\phi, p) \triangleq \widehat{f}'_0(\cos\phi, \sin\phi, p, 0)$$

$$f(x) = \frac{1}{16\pi^2} \int_0^\pi d\phi \int_{-\infty}^\infty dp \frac{\widehat{f}'_p(p, \phi) + x_3 \widehat{f}'_0(p, \phi)}{x_3^2(p - x_1 \cos\phi - x_2 \sin\phi)}.$$

If f is an even function:

$$f(x) = f(-x)$$

then $\widehat{f}'_0(0, \xi_1, \xi_2, \xi_3) \equiv 0$ and we need only $\widehat{f}(\phi, p)$. This corresponds to the Minkowski-Funk transform of an even function. In the general case we can use this formula to reconstruct the even part of f: $1/2(f(x) + f(-x))$. The formula has the structure of the Radon inversion formula and the reason for this is that if in (1.2) we take the variables

$$y_1 = \frac{x_1}{x_3}, \quad y_2 = \frac{x_2}{x_3}, \quad \phi(y_1, y_2) = x_3^2 f(x) = (1 - x_1^2 - x_2^2) f(x),$$

then for $\xi_0 = 0$, (1.2) becomes the Radon transform of the function ϕ. If $f(x)$ is an odd function then $\widehat{f}(\phi, p) \equiv 0$ and we can reconstruct f through $\widehat{f}'_0(\phi, p)$.

Example 3. Both examples above involve a family of all planes going through a point outside S^2 (in example 1 this point is at infinity). Next we consider the family of planes going through a point $x \in S^2$. Let x be $(0,0,1)$ and then (1.1) has the form

(1.12)
$$\xi_0 + \xi_3 = 0$$

and

(1.13) $\varkappa f\Big|_\gamma = \frac{1}{16\pi^2} \frac{(x_3 - 1)\widehat{f}(\xi_0, \xi_1, \xi_2 - \xi_0) + (\widehat{f}'_3 - \widehat{f}'_0)(\xi_0, \xi_1, \xi_2 - \xi_0)\langle x, \xi \rangle}{\langle x, \xi \rangle^2} \omega(\xi_0, \xi_1, \xi_2).$

We can compute $\widehat{f}'_3 - \widehat{f}'_0\big|_\gamma$ knowing $\widehat{f}\big|_\gamma$ so that we need to differentiate $\widehat{f}$ only along the submanifold (1.12). Some can reconstruct $f(x)$ knowing only the restriction of $\widehat{f}$ on γ. If $\widehat{f}(\eta_1, \eta_2, p) \triangleq \widehat{f}(-p, \eta_1, \eta_2, p)$ then

(1.14) $\varkappa f\Big|_\gamma = \frac{1}{16\pi^2} \frac{\widehat{f}(\eta, p)(x_3 - 1) + f'_p(\eta, p)(\eta_1 x_1 + \eta_2 x_2 + p(x_3 - 1))}{(\eta_1 x_1 + \eta_2 x_2 + p(x_3 - 1))^2} \omega(p, \eta_1, \eta_2)$

and we again obtain a formula similar to the Radon inversion formula.

The explanation for this coincidence is the following: Stereographic projection transforms the sections γ into lines on $\mathbb{R}^2$. The corresponding coordinates

$$y_1 = \frac{x_1}{1-x_3}, \quad y_2 = \frac{x_2}{1-x_3}$$

makes the transform (1.2) coincide with Radon transform of the function

$$\phi(y) = \frac{1}{2}f(x)(1+x_3)$$

and $\int_\gamma \varkappa \widehat{f}$ gives the reconstruction of ϕ through its Radon transform.

Example 4. We give another example where $\varkappa \widehat{f}|_\gamma$ can be computed through $\widehat{f}|_\gamma$ alone and as a result we can reconstruct f through $\widehat{f}|_\gamma$ alone. Let γ be the cone

(1.15) $$\xi_0^2 - \xi_1^2 - \xi_2^2 = 0.$$

The planes $\langle \xi, x \rangle = 0$, $\xi \in \gamma$ can be characterized by the condition that

$$\{\langle \xi, x \rangle = 0\} \cap \{x_3 = 0\}$$

is tangent to S^2. If $\xi_0 = 1$, $\xi_1 = \cos\phi$, $\xi_2 = \sin\phi$, $\xi_3 = p$ and

$$\widehat{f}(\phi, p) \triangleq \widehat{f}(1, \cos\phi, \sin\phi, -p),$$

then

$$\varkappa \widehat{f}\Big|_\gamma = \frac{1}{16\pi^2 \langle x_0 \xi \rangle^2} \left[(\widehat{f}(\xi)(\xi_1 + x_1) + \langle x, \xi \rangle(\widehat{f}'_0 \xi_1 + \widehat{f}'_1)) d\xi_2 \wedge d\xi_3 \right.$$
$$\left. - (\widehat{f}(\xi)(\xi_2 + x_2) + \langle x, \xi \rangle(\widehat{f}'\xi_2 + \widehat{f}'_2)) d\xi_1 \wedge d\xi \right].$$

The differential operator $\xi_j \frac{\partial}{\partial \xi_0} + \frac{\partial}{\partial \xi_j}$ is tangential to (1.15), so we can compute $\varkappa \widehat{f}|_\gamma$ through $\widehat{f}|_\gamma$ alone.

Under stereographic projection, sections in γ transform into circles tangent to a fixed circle. So we can interpret them as horocycles on the hyperbolic plane. We thus obtain the inversion formula for the horocyclic Radon transform on the hyperbolic plane.

We have considered only a few of many possible inversion formulas for the spherical Radon transform for different 2-cycles all based on the universal differential form $\varkappa \widehat{f}$.

In the following section, we review the application of Example 1 to a problem in NMR crystallography studied in [R-S-D-M], and indicate its numerical solution, first given there.

2. Spherical tomography and NMR chemistry

In the application, $f(\mathbf{x})$, $\mathbf{x} \in S$, represents (in one typical instance) the number of deuterium nuclei in chemical environments in a sample (crystal or polymer) where the local field gradient at each nucleus (induced by its neighboring atoms) has a fixed magnitude, is axially symmetric, and is oriented by the direction of a deuterium-carbon bond which makes an angle θ with some fixed direction $\boldsymbol{\alpha}$. From a nuclear magnetic resonance (NMR) measurement (using a homogeneous field only), we can then estimate the number of atoms for which $\cos^2 \theta$ has any specified value. As seen below, this gives the integrals $P_g(t, \boldsymbol{\alpha})$ where $g(\mathbf{x}) = f(\mathbf{x}) + f(-\mathbf{x})$ and $-\mathbf{x}$ is the antipode of $\mathbf{x}$. Since it is thus impossible to separate $f(\mathbf{x})$ from $f(-\mathbf{x})$ we can assume we are dealing with g rather than f, but we prefer to consider the general problem, where $f(\mathbf{x}) \neq f(-\mathbf{x})$.

The application to crystallography thus uses certain solid-state NMR data to study partially oriented, or otherwise anisotropically oriented materials such as drawn polymers and defective crystals. Because the NMR data reflects site-specific, or very short range features of the chemical or nuclear environment, we expect that this new technique will be generally complementary to the results given by X-ray scattering and X-ray crystallography for exploring the structure of materials.

To expand on the above, in one mathematical model (of one particular experiment) of the above type arising in NMR spectroscopy, we assume we can measure the following integrals of f, a (nonnegative) function on the unit sphere S, over circles — not just great circles — on S. In more detail, we assume the measured NMR signal (from the current induced in a coil by the resonating nuclei) is

$$(2.1) \qquad S_\alpha(\tau) = \frac{1}{4\pi} \int_S f(\mathbf{x}) \exp(i\tau(3(\mathbf{x} \cdot \boldsymbol{\alpha})^2 - 1)) d\mathbf{x}, \quad -\infty < \tau < \infty$$

where τ is a dimensionless time parameter and $\mathbf{x} = (x_1, x_2, x_3)$ runs over the unit sphere $S = \{|x| = 1\}$, and $d\mathbf{x}$ is the element of area on S. The $3(x \cdot \alpha)^2 - 1$ coefficient in the exponent is a property of the Bloch equation for NMR physics [M, D]. Several approximations are made in using (2.1) to model the experiment. For more details see [R-S-D-M].

Letting P_f denote the integral of f over latitudinal circles,

$$(2.2) \qquad P_f(t, \alpha) = \int f(\mathbf{x}) \chi((x \cdot \alpha) = t) ds, \quad -1 \leq t \leq 1$$

where ds is the element of arc-length on the circle $\mathbf{x} \cdot \boldsymbol{\alpha} = t$, $|x| = 1$ (and χ indicates that the integral is only over this circle). We see that (2.1) is just

$$(2.3) \qquad \begin{aligned} S_\alpha(\tau) &= \frac{1}{2} \int_0^\pi P_f(\cos\theta, \alpha) \exp(i\tau(3\cos^2\theta - 1)) \sin\theta d\theta \\ &= \frac{1}{2} \int_{-1}^1 P_f(t, \alpha) \exp(i\tau(3t^2 - 1)) dt \end{aligned}$$

where we have set $t = \cos\theta$, $0 \leq \theta \leq \pi$ to get the second integral. Since $S_\alpha(t)$ is known, we may multiply by $\exp(i\tau)$, change t to $\sqrt{|t|}$ and invert the Fourier transform to obtain

$$(2.4) \qquad P_f(t, \boldsymbol{\alpha}) + P_f(-t, \boldsymbol{\alpha}) = P_g(t, \boldsymbol{\alpha}) = P_g(-t, \boldsymbol{\alpha})$$

where

(2.5) $$g(\mathbf{x}) = f(\mathbf{x}) + f(-\mathbf{x}),$$

with $-\mathbf{x}$ the antipode of $\mathbf{x}$, because $3t^2 - 1$ confounds t and $-t$. From the point of view of the NMR problem we would like to reconstruct g (one cannot even hope to reconstruct f because of the confounding above), from a knowledge of $P_g(t, \boldsymbol{\alpha})$ for $n \approx 100$ values of $\boldsymbol{\alpha}$, and for each $\boldsymbol{\alpha}$ for $m \approx 100$ values of t.

Each choice of $\boldsymbol{\alpha}$ corresponds to a separate choice of the direction of the main magnetic field or, equivalently, of a rotation of the sample to a new direction in a fixed magnetic field (homogeneous). It is most convenient to place the sample to be imaged in a test tube and to simply rotate the test tube to n discrete, equally-spaced $\boldsymbol{\alpha}$'s; this however is not a representative sampling of "direction space" since all the $\boldsymbol{\alpha}$'s obtained in this way lie in the one fixed plane. Nevertheless this choice of $\boldsymbol{\alpha}$'s is also most convenient mathematically as we saw in Example 1 of §1, and this seems a rather pleasant surprise. Indeed, one might naively think that the n $\boldsymbol{\alpha}$'s ought best be distributed somehow uniformly over S in order to best reconstruct f from $P_f(t, \boldsymbol{\alpha})$ for the 100×100 values of $(t, \boldsymbol{\alpha})$. Note that if one knows the integrals of f over *all* small circles, then f can be reconstructed everywhere, but this is not usable in practice for two reasons: first the small circle integrals tend to be very noisy, and second there are only 200 small circles among the 100 directions available, which gives poor resolution.

We have seen in §1, Example 1, that choosing all α's in one fixed plane (or in two "adjacent" planes, is *mathematically* natural. Also in the discussion in the opening paragraphs of §1 we saw that the choice of all $\boldsymbol{\alpha} \in S$ is "too many" for the problem at hand because f depends on 2 parameters but there are three parameters in $(t, \boldsymbol{\alpha})$ since $\boldsymbol{\alpha}$ is two-dimensional. This gives some theoretical basis for the measurement scheme used in [R-S-D-M].

We next show an elementary but ad hoc way to actually invert the spherical Radon transform, i.e. to recover f from $P_f(t, \boldsymbol{\alpha})$ where $\boldsymbol{\alpha}$ lies in one fixed plane, say the equatorial plane. Actually, as indicated, in §1 we cannot reconstruct $f(\mathbf{x})$ for all $\mathbf{x} \in S$, but merely $f(\mathbf{x}) + f(\mathbf{x}^*)$ where $\mathbf{x}$ and $\mathbf{x}^*$ are reflections in the common plane of the $\boldsymbol{\alpha}$'s. Clearly, if we know only the integrals of f over circles perpendicular to one fixed plane then we can never separate $\mathbf{x}$ and $\mathbf{x}^*$ since any circle through $\mathbf{x}$ contains $\mathbf{x}^*$ and they contribute in the same way. A moment's thought, also indicated already in Example 1 in (1.8) and (1.9) shows that if $g(x_1, x_2) = f(x_1, x_2, x_3) + f(x_1, x_2, -x_3)$, is a function on the equatorial plane $(x_1, x_2, 0)$, where $x_3 = \sqrt{1 - x_1^2 - x_2^2}$, and where the plane of the $\boldsymbol{\alpha}$'s is the equatorial plane, then the ordinary line integrals of $g(x_1, x_2)\sqrt{1 - x_1^2 - x_2^2}$ in this plane are exactly (up to a constant) the circle integrals we have called $P_f(t, \boldsymbol{\alpha})$. Thus the problem of reconstructing $f(\mathbf{x}) + f(\mathbf{x}^*)$ with $\mathbf{x} = (x_1, x_2, x_3)$, $\mathbf{x}^* = (x_1, x_2, -x_3)$ reduces to ordinary Radon inversion of a function in the plane from its line integrals [S-K, S-L, H, N]. Once $g(x_1,x_2)\sqrt{1-x_1^2-x_2^2}$ is reconstructed, we may divide by the known (Jacobian) $\sqrt{1-x_1^2-x_2^2}$ to obtain $g(x_1,x_2) = f(\mathbf{x}) + f(\mathbf{x}^*)$. For details, see [R-S-D-M].

Figure 1 is an example of the reconstruction of g using the method of Example 1 of §1 where f consists of 4 spherical caps each of constant density. The streaking is due mostly to noise in the data. For more details of the experiment underlying Figure 1, see [R-S-D-M].

What if we want to reconstruct $f(\mathbf{x})$, not merely $f(\mathbf{x})+f(\mathbf{x}^*)$? One needs then two "nearby" planes of $\boldsymbol{\alpha}$'s. In this way we obtain $f(\mathbf{x}) + f(\mathbf{x}^*)$ for the two nearby planes and it is then a simple matter to reconstruct $f(\mathbf{x})$ itself. This is because (again it is clear from the discussion below (1.7)) we know $f(\theta) + f(-\theta)$ in each circle perpendicular to both of the $\boldsymbol{\alpha}$-planes, and also $f(\theta + \epsilon) + f(-\theta + \epsilon)$, obtained by a small rotation of the first plane, and this "Cauchy data" allows us to find $f(\theta)$ in each such plane, i.e. to find f itself. In practice, this seems to suffer some small artifacts, of [R-S-D-M] and so it may turn out that the determination of $f(\mathbf{x})+f(\mathbf{x}^*)$ will be deemed adequate in practice to deduce $f(\mathbf{x})$ from side chemical knowledge — especially since tilting the test tube containing the sample may also present experimental difficulties. This remains to be seen.

Before two of us came into contact with the third (Simon Gindikin), we had a different way to reconstruct $f(\mathbf{x})$ from $f(\mathbf{x})+f(\mathbf{x}^*)$ involving 3-planes of $\boldsymbol{\alpha}$'s all mutually orthogonal. This method is described in [R-S-D-M], but it is not as simple, and is also artifacted in practice, as is the method of nearby planes discussed above. It is also less convenient experimentally.

3. Conclusion about the interplay between pure and applied mathematics

At the present time we see no way to utilize the many other consequences of the general theory of spherical integral geometry such as Example 2 of §1. But it is nice to see abstract theory and practical applications meld so neatly. In fact, in retrospect, it is true that the authors of [R-S-D-M] understood the phenomenon of the two nearby planes only after the International Meeting on Tomography and Integral Geometry of AMS-SIAM in Mount Holyoke, MA in the summer of 1993. This was aimed at bringing together practical and theoretical tomographers. It was clearly a successful meeting!

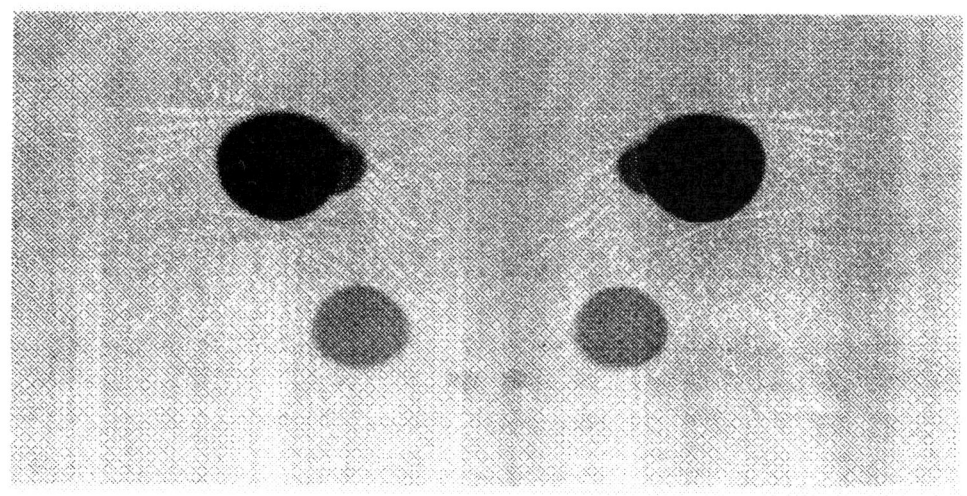

References

[D] Douglass, D. C., Schneemeyer, L. F., Spengler, S. E., Phys. Rev. B, **36**, 1831–1842, 1987.

[G-G-S] Gelfand, I., Graev, M., Shapiro, Z., Integral geometry on k-dimensional planes, Funct. Anal. Appl. **1** (1967), 14–27.

[G-S] Gelfand, I. M. and Shilov, G. E., Generalized Functions, vol. 1, Academic, New York, 1964.

[G] Gindikin, S., Spherical integral geometry, in preparation.

[H] Herman, G. T., Image Reconstruction from Projections, Academic Press, 1980.

[J] John, F., Plane Wares and Spherical Means Applied to Partial Differential Equations, Interscience, New York, 1955.

[M] Mansfield, P., Morris, P. G., NMR Imaging in Biomedicine: Supplement 2, Advances in Magnetic Resonance, Academic Press, New York, 1982.

[N] Natterer, F., The Mathematics of Computerized Tomography, Wiley, 1986.

[R-S-D-M] Reeds, J. A., Shepp, L. A., Douglas, D. C., Mirau, P. A., A spherical tomography for solid-state NMR, manuscript.

[S-K]   Shepp, L. A., Kruskal, J. B., Computerized tomography: the new medical X-ray technology, Amer. Math Monthly **85** (1978) 420–439.

[S-L]   Shepp, L. A., Logan, B. F., The Fourier reconstruction of a head section, IEEE Trans. Nucl. Sci. **NS-21** (1974), 21–43

Department of Mathematics
Rutgers University
New Brunswick, NJ 08903

AT&T Bell Laboratories
Murray Hill, NJ 07974

That Kappa Operator:

Gelfand-Graev-Shapiro inversion and Radon transforms on isotropic planes

E.L. GRINBERG *

ABSTRACT. We review the procedure first outlined by I.M. Gelfand, M.I. Graev, and Z.ßa. Shapiro for inverting Radon transforms using the ubiquitous kappa operator. We then apply this procedure to the Radon transform on isotropic 2-planes in $\mathbb{R}^4$ to obtain an inversion formula similar in spirit to those obtained by Gelfand and his collaborators.

§1. Introduction

The kappa operator enjoyed repeated mention at the 1993 AMS-SIAM Summer Seminar on the mathematics of tomography, impedance imaging and integral geometry. The air of mystery that surrounded its appearance indicates that there is room for review and revival of this multifarious object. The construction of the operator, its significance and method of application is well documented in the works of I.M. Gelfand and his collaborators. We will take this opportunity to review its basic realization in a fairly simple concrete case. Along the way, we hope to motivate some of its key features. We will conclude by giving an inversion formula in the spirit of the original applications of κ. We emphasize that the aim of this paper is exposition through the working-out of an example.

Let $f(x)$ be a continuous function on $\mathbb{R}^n$ (a "point function") that is small at infinity. Generally, we will assume that f is rapidly decreasing, but other decay conditions are certainly workable. The k-dimensional Radon transform, or k-plane transform maps f to the "plane function"

1991 *Mathematics Subject Classification.* Primary 44A12 ; Secondary 43A75, 58C75.
Key words and phrases. Integral Geometry, Lagrangian Grassmannian, Admissibility.
*Supported by a grant from the National Science Foundation
This paper was written while the author was visiting the Institute for Advanced Study. He wishes to thank the I.A.S. for its hospitality.
This paper is in final form and no version of it will be published elsewhere

© 1994 American Mathematical Society
0075-8485/94 $1.00 + $.25 per page

$$Rf(L) \equiv \int_L f.$$

Here L is an affine k-dimensional plane in $\mathbb{R}^n$. The collection of all such L's forms the affine Grassmann manifold $AG(k,n)$. This is distinguished from what is sometimes called the projective Grassmannian, or simply the Grassmann manifold $G(k,n)$ which denotes the set of all k-dimensional vector subspaces of $\mathbb{R}^n$. The structure of these spaces will be discussed in detail below.

The definition of Rf begs the question: what measure is used in the integration? There are various answers to this question and they lead to a variety of interesting studies. The most classical approach is to use Euclidean measure on each k-plane H. Allowing a fairly general measure leads to some interesting investigations. See the work of Quinto [**Q**], Boman [**B**], and Boman-Quinto [**BQ**] in which the effect of the properties of the measure strongly influence the properties of the transform R. In a somewhat different emphasis, one can "absorb" a measure into the data function f and then R becomes an operator on sections of line bundles. Gelfand has used this approach in the projective category. The original construction of the kappa operator involves a Radon transform that uses measures that are but slight modifications of Euclidean measure. For an overview of this style of integral geometry see [**Gi**].

Let A be an $(n-k) \times k$ matrix and let c denote a vector in $\mathbb{R}^k$. A generic k-plane L in $\mathbb{R}^n$ is a graph over the standard $\mathbb{R}^k \subset \mathbb{R}^n$ and so can be parameterized as
$$L = \{(x, Ax+c) | x \in \mathbb{R}^k\}.$$
This leads to what L. Ehrenpreis [**E**] calls the parameterized Radon transform:
$$Rf(A,c) = \int_{x \in \mathbb{R}^k} f(x, Ax+c) dx.$$

This is almost the same as the Euclidean Radon transform, except that the parameterization excludes a (thin) set of planes and introduces a Jacobian factor. The parameterized Radon transform has very useful applications to partial differential equations, as first shown by F. John [**J**]. Once this integral transform is defined some canonical questions are raised: Is R injective? What is its range? Is there an inversion formula? Is R overdetermined? If so, what are minimal Cauchy data for R? The synthesis of the kappa operator makes use of answers to some of these questions and sheds light on others.

The paper [**GGS**] gives the first construction of the kappa operator. While the construction has been much expanded and generalized we find great appeal and motivation in the basic ideas contained in this early work. The setting in [**GGS**] is *complex*. That is, the ambient space is $\mathbb{C}^n$, which we can view as $\mathbb{R}^{2n}$ endowed with a complex structure, and the integration is over complex k-planes L, which we can regard as special real $2k$-planes in $\mathbb{R}^{2n}$. The choice of a complex setting is justified by its relevance to the representation theory of semi-simple Lie groups, a topic deeply explored by the Gelfand school. Additional justification emerges in the inversion formula developed in [**GGS**]: it involves the algebraic topology of the complex Grassmannian, as exposed by S.S. Chern [**Ch**]. The complex Grassmannian is topologically simpler than its real counterpart and this is reflected in the Radon inversion problem. The link with algebraic topology is no coincidence and is sure to resurface again and again.

§2. The Radon transform on isotropic planes

We will develop the kappa operator in a context that is different from that of [**GGS**] so as to obtain a new result. But this will also show the flexibility and generality of the original approach. Rather than integrate over complex k-planes in $\mathbb{C}^n$ we will single out a different class of even-dimensional Euclidean spaces. The ambient space will be $\mathbb{R}^{2n}$ and points in it will be coordinatized by (x, y), where x and y are vectors in $\mathbb{R}^n$. In contrast with the complex structure in [**GGS**] we endow our copy of $\mathbb{R}^{2n}$ with the following quadratic form:

$$Q((x,y),(x',y')) = x \cdot y' - x' \cdot y.$$

The dot-product on the right above is the Euclidean inner product on $\mathbb{R}^n$. The skew symmetric form Q is non-degenerate and is the standard *symplectic form* on $\mathbb{R}^{2n}$. Let L be a vector subspace of $\mathbb{R}^{2n}$. The restriction $Q|_L$ need not be non-degenerate. In fact, it can vanish identically. In this case, we say that L is *isotropic*. The maximal isotropic planes are called *Lagrangian* planes and are necessarily n-dimensional. Our standard such L will be $\mathbb{R}^n \equiv \mathbb{R}^n \times 0 \subset \mathbb{R}^{2n}$. We can endow our ambient space $\mathbb{R}^{2n}$ with a complex structure by declaring $\mathbb{R}^n \times 0 \subset \mathbb{R}^{2n}$ to be the *real* coordinates and $0 \times \mathbb{R}^n \subset \mathbb{R}^{2n}$ to be the *purely imaginary* ones. Thus we have $\mathbb{R}^{2n} \approx \mathbb{C}^n$ and

$$\sqrt{-1} \cdot (\mathbb{R}^n \times 0) = 0 \times \mathbb{R}^n.$$

Now $\mathbb{C}^n$ has a standard Hermitian inner product $<\cdot,\cdot>$. The group of complex-linear transformations preserving $<\cdot,\cdot>$ is the unitary group and is denoted by $U(n)$. Decomposing $<\cdot,\cdot>$ into real and imaginary parts one sees that $U(n)$ preserves the Euclidean inner product on the underlying $\mathbb{R}^{2n}$ (this comes from the real part of $<\cdot,\cdot>$) and also the skew-symmetric form $Q(\cdot,\cdot)$ (this comes from the imaginary part of $<\cdot,\cdot>$). Thus $U(n) \subset O(2n)$ is precisely the subgroup preserving $Q(\cdot,\cdot)$. Linear algebra now shows that any Lagrangian plane L can be presented as $A\mathbb{R}^n$, where A is a unitary matrix viewed as a linear transformation in $\mathbb{R}^{2n}$. The unitary matrices A that preserve the subspace $\mathbb{R}^n \subset \mathbb{R}^{2n}$ are precisely the real orthogonal ones: $O(n) \subset U(n)$. So the collection of Lagrangian vector subspaces of $\mathbb{R}^{2n}$, the so-called *Lagrangian Grassmannian*, can be presented as the homogeneous space $U(n)/O(n)$. See [**Hö**] for the construction of the Lagrangian Grassmannian and its significance in the theory of oscillatory integrals. We will denote $U(n)/O(n)$ by $\Lambda(n)$. Another linear-algebraic check shows that the plane $\{(x, Ax) | x \in \mathbb{R}^n\}$ is Lagrangian precisely when the $n \times n$ matrix A is symmetric.

We will focus on the affine Lagrangian Radon transform. If f is a rapidly decreasing function on $\mathbb{R}^{2n}$ then, for a symmetric $n \times n$ matrix A and a vector $c \in \mathbb{R}^n$ we define

$$Rf(A,c) = \int_{x \in \mathbb{R}^n} f(x, Ax + c) \, dx.$$

Here dx is the standard Lebesgue measure on $\mathbb{R}^n$. Using Fourier transforms we showed in [**G1**] that this R is injective. As written, Rf is a function only on a dense open set of affine Lagrangian planes. However, aside from the Jacobian factor $\sqrt{|I + A^2|}$ the function Rf is just the integral of f over a Lagrangian plane with respect to the canonical Euclidean measure. Thus Rf extends smoothly to a function on the full collection of affine Lagrangian planes. The function $g(A,c) = Rf(A,c)$ has some special properties. Indeed, differentiating under the integral sign we have

$$\frac{\partial^3 g}{\partial c_k \partial c_l \partial a_{kl}} - \frac{\partial^3 g}{\partial c_k^2 \partial a_{ll}} - \frac{\partial^3 g}{\partial c_l^2 \partial a_{kk}} = 0. \tag{1}$$

Here $1 \leq k, l \leq n$ and, to interpret this equation correctly for A symmetric one must note that (for $k \neq l$) the operator $\frac{\partial}{\partial a_{kl}}$ is really an abuse of notation for $\frac{\partial}{\partial a_{kl}} + \frac{\partial}{\partial a_{lk}}$. These identities were first observed in [**DG**]; we are indebted to R.S. Strichartz for this reference. In [**G1**] we showed that these differential equations, along with some moment conditions, characterize the range of R. A note added in proof in [**G1**] indicates that the moment conditions are implied by these differential equations. In hindsight, this can be seen by several distinct arguments. L. Ehrenpreis gives a particularly simple approach to the elimination of moment conditions from range characterizations [**E**]. In similar contexts F. Gonzalez has shown that the ideal of range-characterizing differential operators has a (higher order) single generator that admits additional invariance properties. A corresponding result is likely to hold in this context as well.

We will not need the range characterization here, but only the fact that the above differential equations are satisfied. The group theoretic interpretation of these equations is given in [**G2**]. It is clear from [**GGS**] that the range characterization is the key to a good inversion formula for R and, perhaps, to *all* aspects of R. This is illustrated for a combinatorial analog of the Radon transform in [**G3**].

The first step towards an inversion formula is to reinterpret the differential equations satisfied by the range using differential forms. The idea of converting partial differential equations into systems of differential forms, or *differential systems*, is not new. E. Cartan and E. Kaehler developed an effective theory for such systems with numerous applications to differential geometry; see [**BGC**].

However, the Cartan-Kaehler theory is local, while the kappa operator below is global.

To simplify the arguments we will now restrict the ambient dimension to 4. Thus we will consider the Radon transform on (affine) Lagrangian 2-planes in $\mathbb{R}^4$. We will parameterize such planes by $L = \{(x, Ax + c) | x \in \mathbb{R}^2\}$. The Lagrangian Grassmannian $\Lambda(2) = U(2)/O(2)$ is locally parameterized by symmetric 2×2 matrices A and differential 1-forms on $\Lambda(2)$ are locally spanned by the basis $\{da_{11}, da_{22}, da_{12}\}$. Now let $g(A, c)$ be a function of parameterized affine Lagrangian planes. The moment has arrived–we are about to define the kappa operator! Let

$$\kappa_c g(A) = g_{c_1 c_2} da_{11} \wedge da_{22} + g_{c_1 c_1} da_{11} \wedge da_{12} + g_{c_2 c_2} da_{12} \wedge da_{22}.$$

The subscripts of g denote partial differentiation in the c-variables. In principle, κ is a differential form defined only on a dense open set of the full collection of Lagrangian planes $\Lambda(2)$. However, one can write the local formula for κ in another coordinate patch and verify that the form is in fact globally defined. (Actually, the reader who calculates the effect of the coordinate change on κ will find consistency only up to sign. We can take care of this by passing to a covering space; see the topological discussion below.)

We view κ_c as a differential form on $\Lambda(2)$ parameterized by c. An inspection now shows that if g is of the form Rf then the form $\kappa_c(g)$ is closed. In fact, this uses only the differential equations (1) we recorded above. Thus the κ-operator has the following mapping properties:

$$\{\text{functions of planes in } \mathbb{R}^4\} \xrightarrow{\kappa} \{\text{differential 2-forms on } \Lambda(2)\}$$

$$\{\text{image of Radon transform}\} \xrightarrow{\kappa} \{\text{closed 2-forms}\}$$

Once we have a closed differential form it is natural to integrate it over some cycle. In the next section we will single out a 2-dimensional cycle that gives the "right" pairing for κ_c and leads to a Radon inversion formula analogous to [**GGS**]'s. In closing this section we point out that the Gelfand approach produces a "universal" kappa operator. Our operator can be obtained from the universal one by restriction. Here we have chosen to construct κ_c directly from the range-characterizing differential equations.

§3. The algebraic topology of the Lagrangian Grassmannian

In the fundamental paper [**GGS**] the κ-operator gives a differential form on the Grassmann manifold of complex k-dimensional vector subspaces of $\mathbb{C}^n$, or complex Grassmannian $G_{\mathbb{C}}(k, n)$ for short. The homology of this space is generated by Schubert varieties and is described by S.S. Chern in the classic monograph

[**Ch**]. It is shown in [**GGS**] that the integrals of the complex κ vanish over all but one of the Schubert cells of the appropriate dimension. The special cell reduces the complex k-plane Radon transform to the hyperplane transform and an earlier (Fourier transform based) inversion formula can be used to integrate κ over this cell and thereby invert the complex Radon transform.

The complex Grassmannian has perhaps as nice a cellular decomposition as can be hoped for: there are cells only in even dimensions, and these are enumerated using classic algebraic geometry. While the topology of the Lagrangian Grassmannian is not as simple, it is nonetheless quite manageable. The space $\Lambda(n) = U(n)/O(n)$ is double covered by the "oriented" Lagrangian Grassmannian $\tilde{\Lambda}(n) \equiv U(n)/SO(n)$. This is the set of pairs $(A, \mathcal{O})$, where A is a Lagrangian subspace of $\mathbb{R}^{2n}$ and $\mathcal{O}$ is a choice of orientation on A. In our formulation of the Radon transform we have interpreted $Rf(A, c)$ as a function on $\Lambda(2) + \mathbb{R}^2$ (translates of Lagrangian planes). But we can just as easily view Rf as a function of translated *oriented* Lagrangian planes: change of orientation simply changes the sign of the integral defining R. Thus R becomes a multi-valued function of Lagrangian planes, or, an odd function (with respect to orientation) of oriented Lagrangian planes. It is certainly more convenient to work with $\tilde{\Lambda}(2)$ for the reasons that will become apparent below. In fact, if we were to insist on working globally on $\Lambda(2)$ and not $\tilde{\Lambda}(2)$ then we would have to abandon the differential forms approach altogether.)

The homology of the space $\tilde{\Lambda}(n)$ depends strongly on the parity of n: when n is odd $\tilde{\Lambda}(n)$ has the homology of a product of odd-dimensional spheres; when n is even, $\tilde{\Lambda}(n)$ has the homology of a product of odd-dimensional spheres and the even-dimensional sphere S^n. For a systematic treatment of the homology theory of symmetric spaces, including various forms of Grassmannians, see [**MT**], especially chapter 3, section 6. The results were originally obtained by A. Borel, R. Bott, H. Samelson, and J.P. Serre.

It is clear *a-priori* that we can only expect a local (differential) inversion formula for the Lagrangian Radon transform on $\mathbb{R}^{2n}$ for n even (the conclusion follows from, say, pseudodifferential operator considerations, or direct Fourier transform computations). This is one aspect of *Huygens' principle* and is confirmed by the algebraic topology in the appearance of the even homology sphere S^n when n is even. It turns out that this is the key homology class over which we need to integrate our form κ_c. Since we are dealing with a concrete low-dimensional example, we can present the homology class directly, without appeal to the general theory.

As we remarked above, $\Lambda(2) = U(2)/O(2)$ is double covered by $U(2)/SO(2)$. This last space, while not simply connected, has a connected isotropy group: the circle group $SO(2)$. There is a simple map from $U(2)$ to $SU(2) \times S^1$:

$$A = \begin{pmatrix} a_{11} a_{12} \\ a_{21} a_{22} \end{pmatrix} \longrightarrow \left(\begin{pmatrix} \det^{-1}(A) & 0 \\ 0 & 1 \end{pmatrix} \begin{pmatrix} a_{11} a_{12} \\ a_{21} a_{22} \end{pmatrix}, \det(A) \right),$$

where $\det(A)$ is the complex determinant of the 2×2 matrix A. This map is a diffeomorphism and induces a diffeomorphism between $U(2)/SO(2)$ and $(SU(2)/(SO(2)) \times S^1$. Now $SU(2)/SO(2)$ is diffeomorphic to the 2-sphere by standard identifications. In fact, if we view the group-manifold $SU(2)$ as the sphere S^3 then the natural map $SU(2) \longrightarrow SU(2)/SO(2)$ is the classical *Hopf fibration* :

$$S^1 \longrightarrow S^3$$
$$\downarrow$$
$$S^2$$

Hence $U(2)/SO(2)$ is diffeomorphic to the sphere product $S^2 \times S^1$. The Künneth theorem now implies that the second singular homology group of $\tilde{\Lambda}(2)$ has a single generator. Clearly, the generator comes from the inclusion $SU(2) \subset U(2)$; we will think of this as a unit determinant condition. The parameterization $\{(x, Ax) | x \in \mathbb{R}^2\}$ of Lagrangian planes is essentially a linearization of $\Lambda(2)$. So the unit determinant condition above translates to a zero trace condition for this parameterization. In what follows we should always use the oriented $\tilde{\Lambda}(2)$ and not $\Lambda(2)$. However, for local considerations the two are equivalent and so we will allow an occasional abuse of notation. It is worth noting that the issue of orientation never comes up in [**GGS**] since there the setting is entirely complex and hence canonically orientable.

§4. An inversion formula

With the topological motivation above in mind, we now consider the integral of the differential form κ_c over the cycle

$$\gamma = \{2 \times 2 \text{ matrices } A \,|\, tr(A) = 0\}.$$

On this cycle, we have $a_{11} = -a_{22}$ so $\kappa_c(g)$ is just $(-2)(g_{c_1 c_1} + g_{c_2 c_2})\, da_{11} \wedge da_{12}$. We will compute $\int_\gamma \kappa_c(g)$ when g is the Radon transform of a Gaussian function in $\mathbb{R}^4$. This will lead to an inversion formula.

Let $f(x_1, x_2, x_3, x_4) = e^{-(x_1^2 + x_2^2 + x_3^2 + x_4^2)}$ and put $g(A, c) = Rf(A, c)$. Using the notation $a^2 \equiv a_{11}^2 + a_{12}^2$ we have

$$g_{c_1 c_1} + g_{c_2 c_2} = -2 \int_{\mathbb{R}^2} (4[(a_{11} x_1 + a_{12} x_2)^2 + (a_{12} x_1 - a_{11} x_2)^2] - 4) \times$$

$$\times e^{-(x_1^2 + x_2^2 + (a_{11}^2 + a_{12}^2) x_1^2 + (a_{11}^2 + a_{12}^2) x_2^2)}\, dx_1 \wedge dx_2.$$

$$= -8 \int_{\mathbb{R}^2} \left(\frac{a^2(x_1^2 + x_2^2)}{1 + a^2} - 1 \right) \frac{e^{-x_1^2 + x_2^2}}{1 + a^2}\, dx_1 \wedge dx_2$$

We now use the Liouville integrals

$$\begin{cases} \int\limits_{-\infty}^{\infty} e^{-x^2}\,dx\ \sqrt{\pi} \\ \int\limits_{-\infty}^{\infty} x^2 e^{-x^2}\,dx\ \sqrt{\pi}/2 \end{cases}$$

to obtain

$$g_{c_1 c_1} + g_{c_2 c_2}(A, 0) = -8\left[\frac{a^2}{1+a^2}\left(\frac{\sqrt{\pi}}{2}\sqrt{\pi} - \frac{\sqrt{\pi}}{2}\sqrt{\pi}\right) - \pi\right](1+a^2)^{-1}$$
$$= \frac{8\pi}{(1+a^2)^2}.$$

Next, we integrate $\kappa_c(g)$ over our contour. This contour is parameterized by matrices of the form $\begin{pmatrix} a_{11} & a_{12} \\ a_{12} & -a_{11} \end{pmatrix}$ so we will integrate over the scalars a_{11} and a_{12}:

$$phantom = \int_{\mathbb{R}^2} (g_{c_1 c_1} + g_{c_2 c_2})(A, 0)\,da_{11} \wedge da_{12}$$

$$\int_{\mathbb{R}^2} \frac{8\pi}{(1+a_{11}^2+a_{12}^2)^2}\,da_{11} \wedge da_{12}$$

$$8\pi^2.$$

The calculation works out more simply than one might expect at the outset. This gives a heuristic confirmation that we have chosen the correct contour. There is no analog to this calculation in [**GGS**]. There the general inversion problem is reduced to a complex hyperplane inversion formula which was proved via Fourier transforms in an earlier paper. Here there is no "earlier" case to invoke. Rather, we suspect that this case can serve as a base for a higher-dimensional result. We now give an "abstract nonsense" argument proving that the following identity is valid not only for Gaussians and our "zero-trace" contour, but for all rapidly decreasing functions and homology 2-cycles:

$$\int_\nu \kappa_c(Rf) = 8\pi^2 \deg(\nu)\,f(0),$$

where $\deg(\nu)$ denotes the homology class of ν in $H_2(\tilde{\Lambda}(2), \mathbb{R})$ expressed as a multiple of our distinguished class above. Indeed, if f is a rapidly decreasing function on $\mathbb{R}^4$, the operation

$$f \longrightarrow \int_\nu \kappa_c(Rf)$$

is a clearly a Schwartz distribution of order at most two. This distribution is also invariant under translation and unitary rotations (so it has no first order differentiation terms). For a positive real scalar λ let $f^\lambda(x)$ denote the dilated function $f(\lambda x)$. Then a change of variables shows that $R(f^\lambda) = \lambda^{-2}(Rf)^\lambda(A,c) \equiv \lambda^{-2} Rf(A, \lambda c)$. The kappa operator is a partial differential operator which enjoys the property $\kappa_c(g^\lambda)(A, 0) = \lambda^2 \kappa_c(g)(A, 0)$. This shows that the Schwartz distribution above is positively homogeneous of degree zero. Our Gaussian calculation, along with a standard check involving homogeneous distributions, now implies that the distribution is simply $8\pi^2 \delta_0$. Of course, we can use translations to recover values of a function at any point in $\mathbb{R}^4$ from their integrals over Lagrangian planes. As with Cauchy's formula in several complex variables, the advantage of having an inversion formula involving integration of a closed differential form is that we can vary the cycle (contour) of integration within a homology class to obtain new (but equivalent) formulas.

§5. Admissibility

In this concluding section we discuss a question which follows naturally from the existence of inversion formulas as above. We have shown that a rapidly decreasing function on $\mathbb{R}^4$ is determined by its integrals over affine Lagrangian planes. Now the family of such planes is 5-dimensional: the orientation of a plane is a member of the 3-manifold $\tilde{\Lambda}(2)$ and the planes with a given orientation form a 2-dimensional coset space. Thus the Lagrangian Radon inversion problem is overdetermined. The *admissibility problem*, championed by Gelfand and his collaborators, asks for minimal families of planes (4-dimensional in our case) so that the Radon inversion problem, restricted to such planes, is still soluble by a local inversion formula. Much of the literature on this problem can be found in, or emanates from [**Gel**]. For an elementary analog of the admissibility problem on finite sets see [**G3**]. The admissibility theory in $\mathbb{C}^n$ enabled the Gelfand school to derive the Plancherel formula for complex semi-simple Lie groups; see [**GS**], appendix to chapter 6.

One of the earliest admissibility results [**K**] states that a rapidly decreasing function f on $\mathbb{C}^3$ is determined by its integrals over complex lines meeting a fixed (but arbitrary) complex algebraic curve. The beautiful article [**K**] gives an inversion formula for such *line complexes* (that is, families of lines that are minimal dimensional for Radon invertability). Although the analysis is based entirely on elementary Fourier transform computations the formula obtained involves a formidable-looking integral kernel. In hindsight this is nothing but a parameterized integral of an explicit coordinatization of the complex variant of the kappa operator. It seems likely that [**K**] provided the motivation for [**GGS**]. In turn, a special case of the main result in [**K**] was obtained earlier by Gelfand and used to give a Plancherel formula for the group $SL(2, \mathbb{C})$.

In our setting we cannot avail ourselves of the algebraic geometry of complex curves, but the symplectic geometry is nonetheless workable. We begin with a real curve $\Gamma \subset \mathbb{R}^4$ which we view as a proper smooth image of the real line. Fixing a base point $w \in \mathbb{R}^4$ we consider the real lines ℓ through the point w which meet the line Γ. Assume that w is a generic point (e.g., $w \notin \Gamma$). For each line ℓ and each angle θ we can canonically associate a Lagrangian plane L containing ℓ. For this, we can use the quaterionic structure on $\mathbb{R}^4$. A similar approach is available for $\tilde{\Lambda}(n)$ when n is even. Let $\mathbf{1}, \mathbf{i}, \mathbf{j}, \mathbf{k}$ denote the standard quaternion units. Earlier we defined a complex structure on $\mathbb{R}^4$ so this implicitly gives a realization for $\mathbf{i}$. Multiplication by our $\mathbf{i}$ sends the x_i axis to the x_{i+2} axis, where the subscripts are to be interpreted mod 4. To be consistent we realize $\mathbf{j}$ by the linear transformation which sends the x_i to the x_{i+3} axis and $\mathbf{k}$ as the map sending x_i to x_{i+1}. It is easy to check that for every angle θ the plane

$$\text{span}(\ell, (\cos(\theta)\mathbf{j} + \sin(\theta)\mathbf{k})\ell)$$

is a Lagrangian plane. This gives a map

$$\Gamma \times S^1 \longrightarrow \tilde{\Lambda}(2) + w.$$

It is not difficult to see that the image consists of *all* Lagrangian planes through w that meet Γ (we can handle oriented planes in this way as well). Let us call the resulting cycle $\gamma(\Gamma)$ and view it as an element of $H_2(\tilde{\Lambda}(2), \mathbb{Z})$. If we think of Γ as an image of the circle into $\mathbb{R}^4$ with one point at infinity then the cycle $\gamma(\Gamma)$ is the image of a torus into a 2-sphere hence has a chance of being homologically essential.

THEOREM. *Let Γ be a proper real curve in $\mathbb{R}^4$ and let f be a rapidly decreasing function on $\mathbb{R}^4$. Then for generic $w \in \mathbb{R}^4$ we have*

$$\int_{\gamma(\Gamma)} \kappa_c(Rf) = 8\pi^2 \, deg(\gamma(\Gamma), w) \, f(w),$$

where $deg(\cdot, w)$ counts the multiplicity of a cycle relative to the fundamental cycle in $H_2(\tilde{\Lambda}(2) + w, \mathbb{Z})$. Also, there exist curves $\Gamma \subset \mathbb{R}^4$ for which $deg(\gamma(\Gamma), w) \neq 0$ for almost all w.

PROOF. We have already proved nearly every part of the theorem. To exhibit a particular Γ for which the invariant $deg(\gamma(\Gamma), w)$ is generically non-zero, let Γ be a real affine line. We wish to show that the 2-cycle $\gamma(\Gamma)$ is homologous to our fundamental cycle. One way to do this is to parameterize $\gamma(\Gamma)$ explicitly. Instead, we will use the underlying symmetries. By our earlier topological considerations it will suffice to show that the cycle is an $SU(2)$ orbit of Lagrangian planes (we ignore points at infinity here). Given any two real lines ℓ_1 and ℓ_2 through w and Γ there is a rotation about w in $SU(2)$ that moves ℓ_1 to ℓ_2 (because $SU(2)$ acts transitively on the sphere S^3). This unitary rotation carries Lagrangian planes through ℓ_1 to Lagrangian planes through ℓ_2. Now take two Lagrangian planes L_1 and L_2 through w and the real line ℓ. Then the real 2-planes L_1 and L_2 span an affine real 3-plane P through w and there is a real transformation in $SO(P) \approx SO(3)$ in the 3-plane P moving L_1 to L_2 while keeping ℓ fixed. The usual double covering map $SU(2) \to SO(3)$ shows that we can achieve this by a matrix in $SU(2)$ acting on all of $\mathbb{R}^4$ and preserving our Lagrangian configurations. This completes the proof. $\square$

The topological invariant $\deg(\gamma(\Gamma), w)$ leads to the *Crofton symbol* which has played a fundamental role in the Gelfand school's analysis of admissibility problems in the real category [**GGR**]. Our analysis raises a number of questions (certainly more than it answers): Are there other algebraic curves Γ that lead to admissibility? (probably so, although the $\deg(\cdot, w)$ invariant will generally have jumps in w), Can this be carried out in higher dimensions? (certainly, if appropriate invariant constructions are substituted for the concrete computations presented here), Can this be carried out for geometries other than complex or symplectic? (very likely so, especially for geometries related to Lie groups and symmetric spaces). We emphasize that Gelfand and his collaborators have given answers to such questions in great generality in the literature. Thus one way to settle the questions raised here is to interpret the general theory in some special situations. In any event, we have given confirmation in a particular case of the general principle that whenever a sufficiently nice local inversion formula exists, it can be obtained via the "universal" κ-operator construction.

References

[**B**]. J. Boman, *Holmgren's Uniqueness Theorem and Support Theorems for Real Analytic Radon Transforms*, Contemp. Math. **140** (1992), 23-30.

[**BGC**]. R.L. Bryant, P.A. Griffiths, S.S. Chern, *Exterior Differential Systems*, M.S.R.I. Publ. # 8, Springer Verlag, 1991.

[**BQ**]. J. Boman and E.T. Quinto, *Support Theorems for Real Analytic Radon Transforms*, Duke Math. J. **55** (1987), 943-948.

[**Ch**]. S.S. Chern, *Complex Manifolds without Potential Theory*, Van Nostrand, Princeton, NJ, 1967.

[**DG**]. A. Debiard and B. Gaveau, *Formule d'inversion en geometrie integrale Lagrangienne*, C.R. Acad. Sc. Paris **296 Serie I** (1983), 423-425.

[**E**]. L. Ehrenpreis, *The Radon Transform*, (Book to appear).

[**G1**]. E.L. Grinberg, *Euclidean Radon Transforms: Ranges and Restrictions*, Integral Geometry, Contemp. Math. **63** (1987), 109-133.

[**G2**]. E.L. Grinberg, *On Images of Radon Transforms*, Duke J. Math. **52 no. 4** (1985), 939-972.

[**G3**]. E.L. Grinberg, *The Admissibility Theorem for the Hyperplane Transform over a Finite Field*, J. Combinatorial Th., Series A **53 no. 2** (1990), 316-320.

[**Gel**]. I.M. Gelfand, *Collected Works*, vol. III, Springer-Verlag, New Bork, 1987.

[**GGR**]. I.M. Gelfand, M.I. Graev, and R. Rosu, *The Problem of Integral Geometry and Intertwining Operators for a Pair of Real Grassmannian Manifolds*, J. Oper. Th. **12 (2)** (1984), 359-383.

[**GGS**]. I.M. Gelfand, M.I. Graev, and Z.ßa. Shapiro, *Integral Geometry on k-Dimensional Planes*, Funct. Anal. Appl. **1** (1967), 14-27.

[**Gi**]. S.G. Gindikin, *Integral Geometry as Geometry and as Analysis*, Integral Geometry, Contemp. Math. **63** (1987), 75-107.

[**GS**]. V. Guillemin and S. Sternberg, *Geometric Asymptotics*, Amer. Math. Soc., 1978.

[**Hö**]. L. Hörmander, *Fourier Integral Operators I*, Acta Math. (1970).

[**J**]. F. John, *The Ultrahyperbolic Differential Equation with Four Variables*, Duke J. Math. **4** (1938), 300-322.

[**K**]. A.A. Kirillov, *On a Problem of I.M. Gelfand*, Dokl. Akad. Nauk SSSR **137 no. 2** (1961), 276-277.

[**MT**]. M. Mimura and H. Toda, *Topology of Lie Groups, I and II*, Amer. Math. Soc. Transl. Vol. 91, 1991.

[**Q**]. E.T. Quinto, *The dependence of The Generalized Radon Transform on defining measures*, Trans. Amer. Math. Soc. **257 no. 2** (1980), 331-346.

DEPARTMENT OF MATHEMATICS, TEMPLE UNIVERSITY, PHILADELPHIA, PA 19122, USA
E-mail address: grinberg@.math.temple.edu

On uniqueness in the inverse conductivity problem with one boundary measurement

VICTOR ISAKOV

ABSTRACT. We give two uniqueness results for discontinuity surface of the conductivity coefficient with given one set of complete boundary data. We obtain a global result for interior sources and a local one for exterior sources.

In this note we describe two recent results on uniqueness of recovery of the coefficient

$$(1) \qquad a = 1 + k\chi(D)$$

of the conductivity equation

$$(2) \qquad div(a\nabla u) = f \quad \text{in } \Omega$$

1991 Mathematics Subject Classification. Primary 35R30

Supported by the NSF Grant DMS-9101421

This paper is a final form and no version of it will be submitted for publication somewhere else.

satisfying the condition

(3) $$\lim u(x) = 0 \text{ as } |x| \to +\infty$$

Here $\chi(D)$ is the characteristic function of a domain $D \subset \Omega$, k is a constant, $k > -1, k \neq 0$. In the first result we assume that $\Omega = \mathbf{R}^3$. Let B be a bounded domain with the C^1-boundary. When $f \in L_2(\Omega)$ and $\text{supp} f \subset B$, there is an unique solution $u \in H_{(1)}(B)$ to the equation (2) which is a harmonic function outside B and satisfies the condition (3) at infinity. The equation (2) is understood in the integral sense:

$$-\int_B a \nabla u \cdot \nabla \phi + \int_{\partial B} \partial u/\partial \nu \, \phi = 0$$

for any function $\phi \in C^1(\bar{B})$. By ν we denote the unit outward normal to the boundary of a domain. Referring to the book [8] we claim that when $\partial D \in C^{2+\lambda}$ ($0 < \lambda < 1$) and $f \in C^\lambda$ the function u^e defined as u on $\Omega \backslash D$ is contained in $C^{2+\lambda}(\Omega \backslash D)$ and the function u^i defined as u on D is contained in $C^{2+\lambda}(\bar{D})$. Then the equation (2) is equivalent to the harmonic equations for u^e, u^i and to the refraction conditions on ∂D:

(2$_d$)
$$\Delta u^e = f \quad \text{in } \Omega \backslash \bar{D}, \quad (1+k)\Delta u^i = f \quad \text{in } D$$

$$u^e = u^i, \quad \partial u^e / \partial \nu = (1+k) \partial u^i / \partial \nu \quad \text{on } \partial D$$

Let Γ be a surface in $\Omega \backslash \bar{B}$. Assume that we are given also

(4) $$u = g_0, \quad \partial u / \partial \nu = g_1 \quad \text{on } \Gamma$$

THE INVERSE CONDUCTIVITY PROBLEM.

Find a domain D entering the problem (2),(3) from the additional Cauchy data (4)

THEOREM 1. *Assume that $f \geq 0, f \in L^1(\Omega)$, is not identically zero and is zero outside D. Assume that*

(5) $$0 < k$$

Then a convex domain $D \in C^{2+\lambda}$ is uniquely determined by the data (4).

The proof is based on the following auxiliary result

LEMMA 1. *If two domains D_1 and D_2 produce the same data* (4) *then*

$$\int_{\partial D_1} v \partial u^i_1/\partial \nu = \int_{\partial D_2} v \partial u^i_2/\partial \nu$$

for all functions $v \in C^1(\bar{\Omega})$ harmonic in Ω.

PROOF. We have $div(a_1 \nabla u_1) = div(a_2 \nabla u_2)$ on Ω. According to the definition of a weak solution to the equation (1) we have

(5) $$\int_{\partial B} \partial u_1/\partial \nu \, v - \int_B a_1 \nabla u_1 \cdot \nabla v = \int_{\partial B} \partial u_2/\partial \nu \, v - \int_B a_2 \nabla u_2 \cdot \nabla v$$

for any function $v \in C^1(\bar{B})$. Here B is a ball containing D_1, D_2. The functions u_1 and u_2 are harmonic on $\Omega \backslash (\bar{D}_1 \cup \bar{D}_2)$ and according to (4) they have the same Cauchy data on Γ, by the uniqueness in the Cauchy problem for elliptic equations we conclude that $u_1 = u_2$ on $\Omega \backslash (D_1 \cup D_2)$. The condition (1) and the identity (5) now imply that

$$(6) \quad -\int_B \nabla u_1 \cdot \nabla v - k\int_{D_1} \nabla u_1 \cdot \nabla v = -\int_B \nabla u_2 \cdot \nabla v - k\int_{D_2} \nabla u_2 \cdot \nabla v$$

Using that the function v is harmonic in Ω and integrating by parts we conclude that

$$-\int_B \nabla u_1 \cdot \nabla v = -\int_{\partial B} u_1 \partial v/\partial \nu + \int_B u_1 \Delta v = -\int_{\partial B} u_1 \partial v/\partial \nu =$$

$$-\int_{\partial B} u_2 \partial v/\partial \nu = -\int_B \nabla u_2 \cdot \nabla v$$

because $u_1 = u_2$ on ∂B. Therefore (6) gives

$$\int_{D_1} \nabla u^i_1 \cdot \nabla v = \int_{D_2} \nabla u^i_2 \cdot \nabla v$$

Using that u^i_j are harmonic in D_j and intergrating by parts again we complete the proof.

LEMMA 2. Under the conditions of Theorem 1 we have $\partial u^i/\partial \nu > 0$ on ∂D.

PROOF. Let h be a solution to the problem $\Delta w = f/(1+k)$ in Ω, $w(x) \to 0$ as $|x| \to +\infty$. This solution is the volume potential

$$h(x) = -(1+k)^{-1} \int f(y) \, G(x,y) \, dy$$

where $G(x,y) = 1/(4\pi|x-y|)$ is the classical fundamental solution to the Laplace operator $-\Delta$. Since D is convex it is easy to observe that $\partial G/\partial \nu_x \leq 0$ when $x \in \partial D$ and $y \in D$, so $\partial h/\partial \nu > 0$ on ∂D.

Consider $w = u - h$. According to the refraction conditions (2_d)

this function is a solution to the problem

$$\Delta w^e = 0 \text{ in } \Omega\backslash D, \quad \Delta w^i = 0 \text{ in } D, \quad w(\infty)=0$$

(7)

$$w^e = w^i, \quad \partial w^e/\partial \nu - (1+k)\partial w^i/\partial \nu = k\partial h/\partial \nu \text{ on } \partial D$$

Moreover if w solves this problem then $u = h + w$ solves the original problem (2),(3). A solution to the problem (7) is a potential of the simple layer

$$w(x) = U_1(x;\sigma) = \int_{\partial D} \sigma(y)\, G(x,y)\, d\Gamma(y)$$

By the well-known jump relations

$$\partial w^e/\partial \nu = -\sigma/2 + \partial U_1/\partial \nu, \quad \partial w^i/\partial \nu = \sigma/2 + \partial U_1/\partial \nu$$

on ∂D (see, e.g. [6], section 1.6) where the term with U_1 means the potential with respect to the kernel $\partial G(x,y)/\partial \nu_x$, $x \in \partial D$, we conclude from the refraction conditions (7) that the density σ satisfies the following integral equation

(8) $\quad -\sigma/2 - (1+k)\sigma/2 - k\,\partial U_1/\partial \nu_x = k\,\partial h/\partial \nu \quad$ on ∂D

or

(9) $\quad (I - K)\sigma = -k/(1 + k/2)\, \partial h/\partial \nu$

where I is the identity operator and

$$K\sigma(x) = -k/(1+k/2) \int_{\partial D} \sigma(y)\, \partial G(x,y)/\partial \nu_x\, d\gamma(y), \quad x \in \partial D$$

The right side of the equation (9) is non-positive on ∂D according to the assumption (5) and the above property of the function h. Since $\partial G/\partial \nu \leq 0$ the operator K maps non-positive functions into non-positive functions. From the classical methods of potential theory it follows that K is a contraction in $C(\partial D)$, so the solution σ to the equation (8) is the sum of the Neumann series $h_1 + K h_1 + K^2 h_1 + \ldots$ where h_1 is the right side in (8). We have $h_1 < 0$, so $\sigma < 0$.

To conclude the proof we write

$$\partial u^e/\partial \nu = \partial h/\partial \nu + \partial w/\partial \nu = \partial h/\partial \nu - \sigma/2 + \partial U_1/\partial \nu$$

then express $\partial U_1/\partial \nu$ from (8) and obtain that $\partial u^e/\partial \nu = -(1/k+1)\sigma > 0$.

The proof is complete.

PROOF OF THEOREM 1. Let D_1, D_2 be two different solutions to the inverse problem and u_1, u_2 are corresponding solutions to the Dirichlet problems (2),(3). Denote exterior and interior parts of their boundaries $\partial D_2 \backslash \bar{D}_1, \partial D_1 \cap D_2, \partial D_1 \backslash \bar{D}_2, \partial D_2 \cap D_1$ by $\Gamma_{2e}, \Gamma_{2i}, \Gamma_{1e}, \Gamma_{1i}$. By using harmonic approximation and stability in the Dirichlet problem we can find a sequence of v_m such that $0 \leq v_m \leq 1$ on $D_1 \cup D_2$, $v_m \to 1$ in $L_1(\Gamma_{2e})$, and $v_m \to 0$ in $L_1(\Gamma_{1e})$. Moreover $v_m < 1 - \epsilon(F)$ on any compact set $F \subset D_1 \cup D_2$ where ϵ is a positive number which does not depend on m. For a complete proof we refer to Lemma 1.7.4 in the book [6].

By using Lemmas 2 and 1 we obtain

$$0 \geq \lim \left(\int_{\Gamma_{1e}} v_m \partial u^i_1/\partial \nu - \int_{\Gamma_{1i}} v_m \partial u^i_2/\partial \nu \right) =$$

$$\lim \left(\int_{\Gamma_{2e}} v_m \partial u^i_2/\partial \nu - \int_{\Gamma_{2i}} v_m \partial u^i_1/\partial \nu \right) >$$

(use the choice of v_m and Lemma 2 again)

$$\int_{\Gamma_{2e}} \partial u^i{}_2/\partial\nu - \int_{\Gamma_{2i}} \partial u^i{}_1/\partial\nu =$$

$$(1+k)^{-1}(\int_{\Gamma_{2e}} \partial u^e{}_1/\partial\nu - \int_{\Gamma_{2i}} \partial u^e{}_1/\partial\nu) = 0$$

Observe that here ν is the normal outward to D_1 on Γ_{2i} and to D_2 on Γ_{1i}. We have used also the refraction boundary conditions (2_d) and the equality $u_1^e = u_2^e$ outside $D_1 \cup D_2$. The last integral is zero by the Green's formula because the function $u^e{}_1$ is harmonic in $D_2 \backslash \bar{D}_1$. We obtained a contradiction which shows that $D_1 = D_2$.

The orthogonality relations can be also helpful when obtaining an information on size of D.

We think that the assumption $\partial D \in C^{2+\lambda}$ can be removed due to the recent results of Escauriaza, Fabes, and Verchota [3] on regularity of solutions to the transmission problem fir Lipschitz ∂D. For simplicity we formulated and proved Theorem 1 in the threedimensional case, but it is true in the plane case as well. Probably, Theorem 1 can be obtained for some convex domans $\Omega \neq \mathbf{R}^n$.

Such global results are still not available when $f=0$ in D (no interior sources). We know global uniqueness results in this case for convex polyhedrons D or for so-called contact domains D (Friedman and Isakov [4]).

Even local uniqueness is not easy to obtain. A progress has been achieved only in the plane case.

Let Ω be a bounded domain in $\mathbf{R}^2$ with the C^2-smooth boundary. Consider the Dirichlet problem for the equation (2) with the boundary condition

(10) $\qquad\qquad u = g_0 \in C^2 \quad \text{on } \partial\Omega.$

Let Γ be a part of $\partial\Omega$. As an additional data in the inverse problem we now prescribe

(11) $$\partial u/\partial\nu = g_1 \text{ on } \Gamma$$

Let D_0 be a simply connected subdomain of Ω. Let $z(t)$ be the normalized conformal mapping of this domain onto the unit disk B. Let $\{\sigma\}$ be a family Σ of analytic functions on B such that $z(t)+\sigma(t)$ is the normalized conformal mapping of some simply connected domain D_σ onto B, $|\sigma|_{2+\lambda} \leq M$. We will assume that Σ is closed with respect to this norm.

THEOREM 2. *Assume that the Dirichlet data g_0 has a unique local maximum and a unique local minimum on $\partial\Omega$. For a family Σ there is a number ϵ_Σ such that if D_σ is a solution of the inverse conductivity problem (1),(2),(10),(11) and $|\sigma|_0(B)<\epsilon_\Sigma$ then $\sigma=0$.*

A proof of this result is given in the paper [1]. It is based on the idea from [2] (where it was obtained for analytic ∂D_0) and on the reduction to a boundary value problem for analytic functions given in [9]. In [1] the index of ∇u^e on ∂D_0 plays a very important role. Alessandrini made a substantial contribution by showing that zeros of ∇u^e are isolated in $\Omega\backslash D_0$, so that the index is well defined. Then our conditions on the boundary data guarantee that this index is zero. The inverse problem is completely equivalent to the following non-linear boundary value problem for analytic functions σ, ϕ in the unit disk

$$\phi(t) = \Im\, U^e(z(t)+\sigma(t)) + U^e(z(t)+\sigma(t)) \quad \text{when } |t|=1$$

where U^e is an analytic function in $\Omega \backslash \overline{D}_0$ with the real part u^e. The linearization around $\sigma = 0$ is a non-standard boundary value problem for analytic functions which can be reduced to two Riemann-Hilbert problems. It is equivalent to the oblique derivative problem for harmonic functions h in D_0 with the boundary condition $\nabla u^e \cdot \nabla h = g_1$ on ∂D_0.

By using arguments in [1] one can modify the proof in [9] and obtain local uniqueness when $\Omega = \mathbf{R}^2$.

A local result similar to Theorem 2 is unknown in the three-dimensional case. A partial explanation is that then the linearized problem is equivalent to the oblique derivative problem which is always non-elliptic in $\mathbf{R}^3$.

Global uniqueness of D in case of many boundary measurements (g_1 is given for any g_0) follows from the results of the papers of Kohn and Vogelius [7] (analytic ∂D) and Isakov (Lipschitz ∂D).

REFERENCES

1. Alessandrini, G., Isakov, V., Powell, J., Local Uniqueness in the Inverse Conductivity Problem with One Measurement, preprint, 1993.
2. Bellout, H., Friedman, A,. Isakov, V., Stability for an Inverse Problem in Potential Theory, Trans. of AMS, **332** (1992), 271-296.
3. Escauriaza, L., Fabes, E., Verchota, G., On a regularity theorem for weak solutions to transmission problems with internal Lipschitz boundaries, Proc. AMS, **115** (1992), 1069-1076.

4. Friedman, A., Isakov, V., On the Uniqueness in the Inverse Conductivity Problem with One Measurement, Indiana Univ. Math. J., **38** (1989), 563-579.

5. Isakov,V., On uniqueness of recovery of a discontinuous conductivity coefficient,Comm.Pure Appl. Math., **41**(1988), 865-877.

6. Isakov, V., *Inverse Source Problems*, Mathematical Surveys and Monographs,Vol.34, AMS, Providence, RI, 1990.

7. Kohn, R., Vogelius, M., Determining Conductivity by Boundary Measurements, II, Interior Results, Comm. Pure Appl. Math., **38** (1985), 643-667.

8. Ladyzenskaja, O.A., Uralceva, N.N., *Linear and quasi-linear elliptic equations*, Academic Press, London, 1968.

9. Powell, J., On a Small Perturbation in the Two-Dimensional Inverse Conductivity Problem, J.Math.Anal.Appl., **175** (1993), 292-304.

Department of Mathematics and Statistics,
Wichita State University
Wichita, KS 67260-0033

E-mail address: ISAKOV@TWSUVM.BITNET

A Method for Finding Discontinuities of Functions from the Tomographic Data

A. I. KATSEVICH AND A. G. RAMM

ABSTRACT. A new method is described for finding discontinuities of a function from its tomographic data. It is based on finding a subset $\hat{S}$ of the tomographic data which is in a one-to-one correspondence with the discontinuity surfaces S of the density function $f(x)$, and the mapping L which sends $\hat{S}$ onto S. A numerical scheme based on this approach and results of numerical experiment are presented.

1. Introduction

One of the major problems in tomography is to recover the discontinuity surfaces of the density of the object from the tomographic data. This is done currently by inverting the full tomographic data using FBP algorithm or local tomography algorithm ([1], [2], [4]). The discontinuity surfaces are then recovered visually from the reconstructed image of the object. Some related problems are discussed in [5]. In [6], another method to recover singularities of a function is proposed. It is based on an analysis of wavefront sets.

Our idea is different and new. We want to find a subset $\hat{S}$ of the tomographic data which is in a one-to-one correspondence with the discontinuity surfaces S of the density function $f(x)$, and the mapping L which sends $\hat{S}$ onto S. If this is done, then the recovery of the discontinuity surfaces S of $f(x)$ is possible by applying the mapping L to $\hat{S}$. There are two steps in the suggested method:

1) to find $\hat{S}$ from the tomographic data, and
2) to invert $\hat{S}$ for S.

1991 *Mathematics Subject Classification.* Primary 44A15; Secondary 62-07.

The authors thank ONR and NSF for partial support.

This paper is in final form and no version of it will be submitted for publication elsewhere

The subset $\hat{S}$ of the tomographic data which is in a one-to-one correspondence with the discontinuity surfaces of $f(x)$ is found in [8] and [9], and the mapping which maps $\hat{S}$ onto S is the Legendre transform or the generalized Legendre transform defined in [7], [9], and [11]. In [8] – [11], the asymptotics of the Radon transform and X-ray transform are given when the point (α, p) approaches $\hat{S}$, the singular locus of the Radon transform (or X-ray transform). In [3], a method is given for finding discontinuity surfaces of a function from the knowledge of the noisy values of this function on a grid. In this paper, for simplicity we will discuss the case of the Radon transform in $\mathbb{R}^2$, that is the tomographic data on the plane.

In section 2, the results concerning the relation between S and $\hat{S}$ are reviewed. In section 3, the algorithm for finding the discontinuity surface S from the tomographic data is described. In section 4, numerical experiments are described.

2. Relation between S and $\hat{S}$

Let $f(x) \in C^\infty(\mathbb{R}^n)$. Consider the function $\psi(x) := f(x)\chi_D(x)$, where $\chi_D(x) = \begin{cases} 1, & x \in D \\ 0, & x \notin D \end{cases}$, $D \subset \mathbb{R}^n$ is a bounded region whose boundary S is a union of smooth hypersurfaces S_j, $j \in \mathcal{J}$, $\mathcal{J}$ is a finite set of indices. Assume that $f(x) \neq 0$ on S. The case when $\psi(x)$ has several discontinuity surfaces can be reduced to the case when $\psi(x)$ has one discontinuity surface S, and for simplicity we assume that S is a connected piecewise-smooth surface. Define the dual surface $\hat{S}$ as the set of points (α, p), $p \in \mathbb{R}^1$, $\alpha \in \mathbb{R}^n$, of the projective space $\mathbb{RP}_n$, such that the plane $\alpha \cdot x = p$ is tangent to S at some point $\bar{x} \in S$ (see [9] for more details). Let $x_n = g(x')$, $x' := (x_1, \ldots, x_{n-1})$ be the equation of S in local coordinates in a neighborhood of a point $\bar{x} \in S$. Define the Legendre transform of g, $Lg := h$, as follows. Let $\beta \in \mathbb{R}^{n-1}$ and consider the system $\nabla_{x'} g = \beta$ (*). If the Hessian of $g(x')$ does not vanish at $x' = \bar{x}'$, then (*) defines $x' = x'(\beta)$. Define $h(\beta) := x'(\beta) \cdot \beta - g(x'(\beta)) := Lg$ and call it the Legendre transform of g. It is proved in [8] and [9] that $\hat{S}$ has the local equation $q = h(\beta)$, where $h(\beta) = Lg$ and $q := -p/\alpha_n$, $\beta := -\alpha'/\alpha_n$, $\alpha_n \neq 0$. The Legendre transform is involutive, so $Lh = g$. Thus, if $\hat{S}$ is known and its equation in local coordinates is $q = h(\beta)$, then the local equation of S is $x_n = g(x')$, where $g = Lh$. Thus, the algorithm of finding S consists of two steps: 1) One finds $\hat{S}$, the singular locus of the Radon transform $\hat{f}(\alpha, p) := \int_{\ell_{\alpha p}} f(x) ds$ of the function $f(x)$; 2) Write the local equation of $\hat{S}$ as $q = h(\beta)$ and calculate $Lh := g(x')$. Then the local equation of S, the discontinuity surface of $f(x)$, is $x_n = g(x')$. In the above definition of the Radon transform, ds is the Lebesgue measure on the plane $\ell_{\alpha p}$, $\alpha \cdot x = p$ is the equation of this plane. Let $(\bar{\alpha}, \bar{p}) \in \hat{S}$. Then in a neighborhood of this point one has (see [10, p. 544])

(1)
$$\hat{\psi}(\bar{\alpha}, p) = \begin{cases} \psi(\bar{x})(p - \bar{p})_\pm^{(n+m-2)/2} r_1 + r_2, & \text{if } (n+m-1)I \text{ is even} \\ \psi(\bar{x})(p - \bar{p})^{\frac{n+m-2}{2}} (\ln|p - \bar{p}|) r_1 + r_2, & \text{if } (n+m-1)I \text{ is odd} \end{cases}$$

Here $r_i := r_i(\alpha, p)$, $i = 1, 2$, are some smooth functions, m is the codimension of the submanifold $S_m \subset S$ on which the point of contact $\overline{x} \in S$ is situated, I is the number of negative eigenvalues of the Hessian matrix of the function $(\overline{\alpha} \cdot x - \overline{p})/|\overline{\alpha}|$ on the submanifold S_m at the point $\overline{x}$. The formula for $r_1(\overline{\alpha}, \overline{p})$ is obtained in [9], note that $r_1(\overline{\alpha}, \overline{p}) \neq 0$. The sign " $-$ " in (1) corresponds to the case when I and $n + m$ are both even or both odd, the sign " $+$ " corresponds to all other cases, $p_+ := \max(p, 0)$. Consider for simplicity the case when $n = 2$ and S is a strictly convex smooth curve, so that $m = 1$ and $I = 0$. Then (1) yields:

$$\hat{\psi}(\overline{\alpha}, p) = \psi(\overline{x})(p - \overline{p})_+^{1/2} r_1 + r_2, \qquad p \to \overline{p},$$

and

(1')
$$\frac{\partial^\nu \hat{\psi}}{\partial p^\nu} \sim \psi(\overline{x}) \frac{\partial^\nu \left[(p - \overline{p})_+^{1/2}\right]}{\partial p^\nu} r_1(\overline{\alpha}, \overline{p}), \qquad p \to \overline{p}.$$

Therefore the local maximum of $\left|\frac{\partial^\nu \hat{\psi}}{\partial p^\nu}\right|$ in the p-variable for $\nu \geq 1$ is $\overline{p}$. Thus, $\hat{S}$ can be found by locating the local maxima of $\left|\frac{\partial^\nu \hat{\psi}}{\partial p^\nu}\right|$ in the p-variable.

3. Numerical scheme for finding S

In this section, we consider the two-dimensional tomographic data and develop methods for numerical finding of $\hat{S}$ and for inversion of $\hat{S}$ for S.

1. Suppose one is given the complete data $\hat{f}(\alpha_i, p_j)$, $1 \leq i \leq N_\alpha$, $1 \leq j \leq N_p$, where N_α and N_p are the number of angles and the number of projections per angle, respectively. Let $\nu, n_\alpha, n_p \geq 1$ be fixed.

Step 1.1. Fix i, $1 \leq i \leq N_\alpha$, and j, $1 \leq j \leq N_p$. For each α_k, $i \leq k \leq i + n_\alpha$, find p_k such that $|\hat{f}^{(\nu)}(\alpha_k, p_k)| = \max_{\ell, j \leq \ell \leq j + n_p} |\hat{f}^{(\nu)}(\alpha_k, p_\ell)|$.

Suppose that n_α is sufficiently small, so that $\hat{S}$ can be approximated by straight lines on the intervals $[\alpha_i, \alpha_{i+n_\alpha}]$. Suppose also that n_p is sufficiently small, so that for a fixed α, each of the intervals $[p_j, p_{j+n_p}]$ contains at most one point of $\hat{S}$. Let $(\tilde{\alpha}_i, \tilde{p}_j)$, where $\tilde{\alpha}_i := (\alpha_i + \cdots + \alpha_{i+n_\alpha})/n_\alpha$ and $\tilde{p}_j := (p_j + \cdots + p_{j+n_p})/n_p$, be the center of the current $n_\alpha \times n_p$ window. If $(\tilde{\alpha}_i, \tilde{p}_j) \in \hat{S}$, then the points (α_k, p_k), $k = i, \ldots, i + n_\alpha$, determined in Step 1.1 also belong to $\hat{S}$. Using the assumptions about smallness of n_α and n_p, we see that these points lie close to a straight line through $(\tilde{\alpha}_i, \tilde{p}_j)$, i.e. close to a line which locally approximates $\hat{S}$. Let $\theta^{(0)} := (\theta_\alpha^{(0)}, \theta_p^{(0)})$ be the unit vector in the (α, p)-space perpendicular to $\hat{S}$ at $(\tilde{\alpha}_i, \tilde{p}_j)$. Then it can be found by solving the following minimization problem

(2) $$\Phi_{i,j}(\theta) := \sum_{k=i}^{i+n_\alpha} (\theta_\alpha(\alpha_k - \tilde{\alpha}_i) + \theta_p(p_k - \tilde{p}_j))^2 \to \min, \qquad \theta_\alpha^2 + \theta_p^2 = 1.$$

The solution to (2) is given by

(3)
$$\theta_\alpha^{(0)} = \cos\phi, \quad \theta_p^{(0)} = \sin\phi, \quad \tan(2\phi) = 2\frac{\sum_{k=i}^{i+n_\alpha}(\alpha_k - \tilde{\alpha}_i)(p_k - \tilde{p}_j)}{\sum_{k=i}^{i+n_\alpha}(\alpha_k - \tilde{\alpha}_i)^2 - \sum_{k=i}^{i+n_\alpha}(p_k - \tilde{p}_j)^2},$$

and the minimal value $\Phi_{i,j}^{(\min)} := \Phi_{i,j}(\theta^{(0)})$ is obtained by substituting (3) into (2). Therefore if $(\tilde{\alpha}_i, \tilde{p}_j) \in \hat{S}$, then $\Phi_{i,j}^{(\min)} \approx 0$. In the opposite case, when $(\tilde{\alpha}_i, \tilde{p}_j) \notin \hat{S}$, the computed value $\Phi_{i,j}^{(\min)}$ will be large (see below). Using this fact, we obtain a decision rule to distinguish between the two cases. Let the threshold $A > 0$ be fixed.

Step 1.2. By substituting (3) into (2), compute $\Phi_{i,j}^{(\min)}$. If $\Phi_{i,j}^{(\min)} \leq A$, we assume that $(\tilde{\alpha}_i, \tilde{p}_j) \in \hat{S}$. If $\Phi_{i,j}^{(\min)} > A$, we assume that $(\tilde{\alpha}_i, \tilde{p}_j) \notin \hat{S}$.

Repeating Steps 1.1 and 1.2 for all pairs (i,j), $1 \leq i \leq N_\alpha$, $1 \leq j \leq N_p$, we obtain the singularity curve $\hat{S}$. To find the threshold A, let us use a standard approach to statistical hypotheses testing. Fix a window centered at a point $(\tilde{\alpha}_i, \tilde{p}_j)$. We say that the null hypothesis H_0 holds if $(\tilde{\alpha}_i, \tilde{p}_j) \notin \hat{S}$. The alternative H holds if $(\tilde{\alpha}_i, \tilde{p}_j) \in \hat{S}$. Fix ϵ, $0 < \epsilon < 1$, the probability of the first type error: rejecting H_0 when H_0 holds, and determine A from the equation $P\{\Phi_{i,j}^{(\min)} > A | H_0\} = \epsilon$. Since the noise is supposed to be independent from the signal (exact tomographic data), we may assume that, if H_0 holds, there is no correlation between positions (α_k, p_k) of local maxima of $|\hat{f}^{(\nu)}|$ within the window. Thus, a convenient way to compute A is by using the Monte-Carlo method: one models random distributions of local maxima (α_k, p_k), $k = i, \ldots, i+n_\alpha$, within the window and computes $\Phi_{i,j}^{(\min)}$ for each distribution. A value of the threshold A is chosen so that $\Phi_{i,j}^{(\min)} > A$ in $100\epsilon\%$ cases. Clearly, this procedure is shift invariant, i.e. it does not depend on indices i and j, so it can be done only once. Using the argument very close to the one presented in [**3**], one can prove the local consistency of the proposed algorithm. Recall that $\psi(\overline{x})r_1(\overline{\alpha}, \overline{p}) \neq 0$ in (1). Let us formulate the result:

THEOREM. *Let ϵ, the probability of the first type error, be fixed. Suppose one is given the noisy values of the Radon transform*

$$\hat{g}(\alpha_i, p_j) = \hat{f}(\alpha_i, p_j) + \xi_{ij}, \quad \alpha_{i+1} = \alpha_i + \Delta\alpha, \quad p_{j+1} = p_j + \Delta p,$$

where ξ_{ij} are independent and identically distributed random variables with finite first and second moments. Consider an arbitrary point $(\tilde{\alpha}_i, \tilde{p}_j) \in \hat{S}$ and suppose that $\Delta\alpha, \Delta p \to 0$, $n_\alpha, n_p \to \infty$, and $n_\alpha\Delta\alpha, n_p\Delta p \to 0$. Then, the probability of accepting H_0 at this point goes to zero as $n_\alpha, n_p \to \infty$.

Now we may assume that the singularity curve $\hat{S}$ has been found. Since calculation of derivatives enhances noise, some of the points from $\hat{S}$ will be missing, and some erroneously detected points will appear. Thus, one needs a stable algorithm for the inversion of $\hat{S}$ to obtain its dual curve S, the discontinuity curve of $f(x)$. In order to calculate S, we will compute a function $\Phi(x)$, $x \in \mathbb{R}^2$, such that its maxima correspond to the points of S. Fix an arbitrary point $x \in \mathbb{R}^2$ and consider a circle $B_\delta(x)$ with radius $\delta > 0$ centered at x. First, consider a model in which S is a circle with radius R centered at $(0,0)$. Taking into account discretization, suppose that all the points $(\tilde{\alpha}_i, \tilde{p}_j) \in \hat{S}$ have been found in Step 1.2. Define the function $\Phi(x)$ as the number of lines $\tilde{\alpha}_i \cdot \tilde{x} = \tilde{p}_j$, $\tilde{x} \in \mathbb{R}^2$, which pass through $B_\delta(x)$, that is

(4) $$\Phi(x) := \#\{(i,j) : |\tilde{\alpha}_i \cdot x - \tilde{p}_j| \leq \delta,\ (\tilde{\alpha}_i, \tilde{p}_j) \in \hat{S}\}.$$

Suppose that $\Delta \alpha N_p \Delta p \ll \delta \ll R$. The following properties of $\Phi(x)$ can be established: $\Phi(x) = 0$ if $|x| < R - \delta$,

(5) $$\Phi(x) = \frac{1}{\Delta \alpha} \frac{4\delta}{|x|} \left(1 + O(|x|^{-2})\right) \quad \text{as} \quad |x| \to \infty,$$

and $\Phi(x)$ attains its maximum

(6) $$\Phi(x) = \frac{4}{\Delta \alpha} \sqrt{\frac{\delta}{R}} \left(1 + O(\delta/R)\right)$$

when $|x| = R + \delta$, that is when $B_\delta(x)$ touches S. One sees that if δ is sufficiently small, the value of the function $\Phi(x)$ is determined only by a small part of the boundary S, namely, by the part of S which can be touched by straight lines passing through $B_\delta(x)$. Thus, in the case of a more general discontinuity curve S, formulas (5) and (6) are replaced by

(5′) $$\Phi(x) = \frac{1}{\Delta \alpha} \frac{4\delta}{\text{dist}(x, S(x))} \left(1 + O(\text{dist}^{-2}(x, S(x)))\right)$$

and

(6′) $$\Phi(x) = \frac{4}{\Delta \alpha} \sqrt{\frac{\delta}{R(x)}} \left(1 + O(\delta/R(x))\right),$$

where $\text{dist}(x, S(x))$ denotes the distance between x and the part of S which is touched by lines through $B_\delta(x)$, and $R(x)$ is the radius of the curvature of S at a point of contact between $B_\delta(x)$ and S. Note also that $\Phi(x)$ is additive, i.e. if S is multiconnected, $\Phi(x)$ is a sum of contributions from each simple-connected component. Now we describe an algorithm of the second step.

Step 2. Let $(\tilde{\alpha}_i, \tilde{p}_j)$ be the points detected at Step 1.2 as belonging to $\hat{S}$. Compute the function $\Phi(x)$ by the formula

$$\Phi(x) := \#\{(i,j) : |\tilde{\alpha}_i \cdot x - \tilde{p}_j| \leq \delta,\ (\tilde{\alpha}_i, \tilde{p}_j) \in \hat{S}\}.$$

Points at which $\Phi(x)$ is large correspond to discontinuity curve S.

Let us estimate the number of operations needed for the algorithm. Steps 1.1 and 1.2 require $O(N_\alpha N_p)$ operations, Step 2 requires $O(NN_\alpha)$ operations, where N is the number of points on the (x_1, x_2) - plane, where the function $\Phi(x)$ is evaluated. Thus the total operation count is $O(N_\alpha(N_p + N))$. Note that the

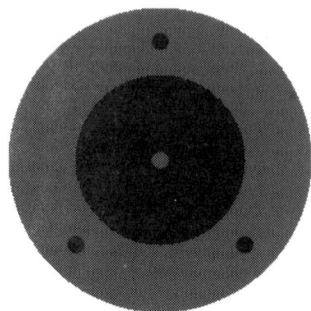

FIGURE 1. The phantom used for generating the Radon transform data.

filtered back-projection (FBP) algorithm requires $O(N_\alpha(N_p^2+N))$ operations or $O(N_\alpha(N_p \log N_p + N))$ if one uses FFT for the calculation of convolutions. Thus our algorithm is more economical than FBP.

4. Numerical experiments

On Fig. 1, one sees the phantom used for generating the Radon transform data. The densities are: exterior: 0, ellipse: 1.5, exterior annulus: 1, area between the annulus and the ellipse: 2, small circle inside the ellipse: 1, three small circles inside the annulus: 0.5. The Radon transform was computed for 250 angles (equispaced on $[0, \pi)$) and 301 projections per each angle. On Fig. 2, one sees an intensity plot of $|\partial^2 \hat{f}(\alpha, p)/\partial p^2|$ on the (α, p)-plane, and on Fig. 3 – an image of detected singularities by Steps 1.1 and 1.2. On Figs 2 and 3, the horizontal axis is the α - axis, and the vertical one is the p - axis. The second derivative was computed by the three-point scheme from the non-noisy data. The parameters of the algorithm were: $n_\alpha = 7$, $n_p = 7$, the probability of the first type error $\epsilon = 0.01$. On Fig. 4, an intensity plot of the function $\Phi(x)$ computed from the data on Fig. 3 is presented. The radius δ was chosen $\delta = \Delta p$. On Fig. 5, one sees an intensity plot of $\Phi(x)$ computed from the limited angle data. As the initial data we took detected singularities, which are represented on Fig. 3, and deleted angles from the range $[130°, 150°]$. On Figs 6 and 7, the further results for the limited-angle data inversion are presented. On Figs 8 and 9, the results for the exterior data problem are presented. The intervals of the missing data in p - variable are $[-0.3, 0.3]$ in Fig. 8, and $[-0.4, 0.4]$ in Fig. 9. The full data correspond to the interval $[-0.9, 0.9]$ in p - variable.

In the future, the authors plan to investigate the stability of the proposed algorithm with respect to noise and test it on real data.

REFERENCES

1. A. Faridani, L. E. Ritman, and K. T. Smith, *Local tomography*, SIAM J. Appl. Math **52** (1992), no. 2, 459-484.

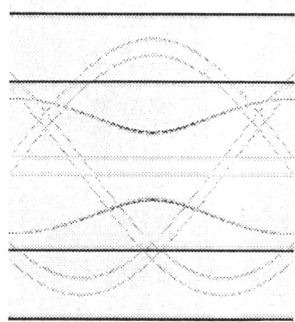

FIGURE 2. An intensity plot of $|\partial^2 \hat{f}(\alpha,p)/\partial p^2|$ on the (α,p)-plane.

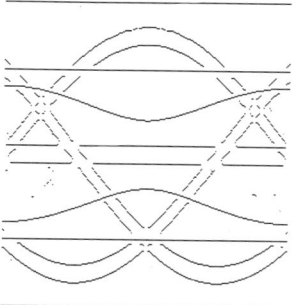

FIGURE 3. An image of detected singularities.

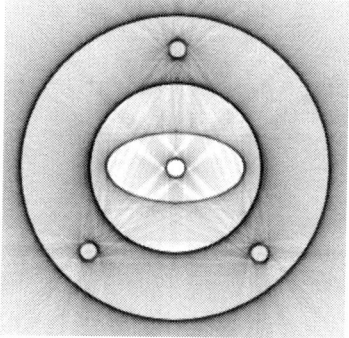

FIGURE 4. An intensity plot of $\Phi(x)$ computed from the data on Fig. 3.

2. A. I. Katsevich and A. G. Ramm, *FBP method for inversion of incomplete tomographic data*, Appl. Math. Lett. **5** (1992), no. 3, 77-80.
3. _____, *Multidimensional algorithm for finding discontinuities of functions from noisy data*, Math. Comp. Modeling **18** (1993), no. 1, 89-108.
4. F. Natterer, *The Mathematics of Computerized Tomography*, Teubner, Stuttgart, 1986.
5. V. Palamodov, *Nonlinear artifacts in tomography*, Soviet Physics Doklady **31** (1986), 888-

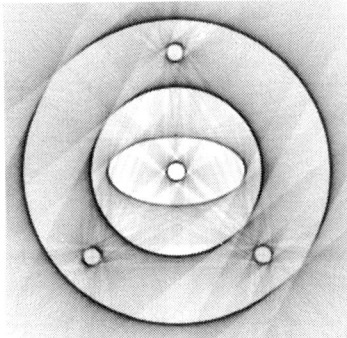

FIGURE 5. An intensity plot of $\Phi(x)$ computed from the limited angle data. The range of angles $[130°, 150°]$ is missing.

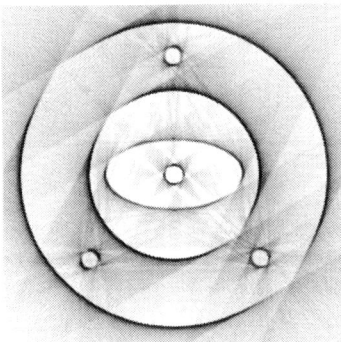

FIGURE 6. The same as on Fig. 5. The range of angles $[120°, 150°]$ is missing.

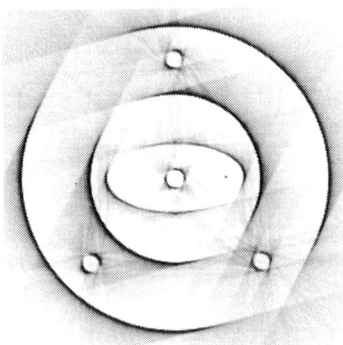

FIGURE 7. The same as on Fig. 5. The range of angles $[105°, 150°]$ is missing.

890.
6. E. T. Quinto, *Singularities of the x-ray transform and limited data tomography in* $\mathbb{R}^2$ *and*

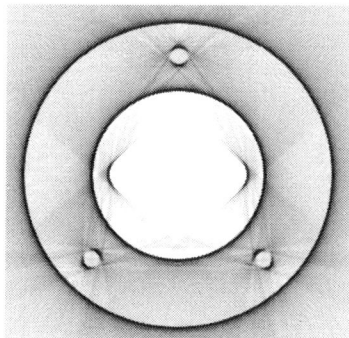

FIGURE 8. An intensity plot of $\Phi(x)$ for the exterior data problem with missing values of p in the interval $[-0.3, 0.3]$.

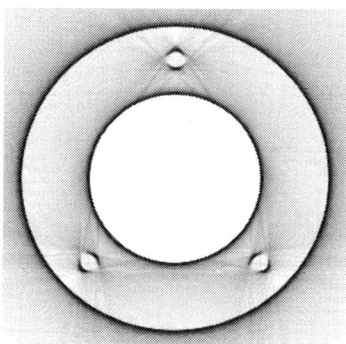

FIGURE 9. The same as in Fig. 8 with missing values of p in the interval $[-0.4, 0.4]$.

$\mathbb{R}^3$, SIAM J. Math. Anal. **24** (1993), 1215-1225.
7. A. G. Ramm, A. Steinberg, and A. I. Zaslavsky, *Stable calculation of the Legendre transform of noisy data*, J. Math. Anal. Appl **178** (1993), no. 2, 592-602.
8. A. G. Ramm and A. I. Zaslavsky, *Singularities of the Radon transform*, Bull. AMS **25** (1993), no. 1, 109-115.
9. _____, *Reconstructing singularities of a function given its Radon transform*, Math. Comput. Modeling **18** (1993), no. 1, 109-138.
10. _____, *Asymptotics of the Fourier transform of piecewise-smooth functions*, C.R. Acad. Sci., Paris **316** (1993), no. 1, 541-545.
11. _____, *X-ray transform, the Legendre transform and envelopes*, J. Math. Anal. Appl. (1993) (to appear).

DEPARTMENT OF MATHEMATICS, KANSAS STATE UNIVERSITY, MANHATTAN, KS 66506-2602, USA

E-mail address: KATSEV@KSUVM.KSU.EDU

DEPARTMENT OF MATHEMATICS, KANSAS STATE UNIVERSITY, MANHATTAN, KS 66506-2602, USA

E-mail address: RAMM@KSUVM.KSU.EDU

Probability Measure Estimation Using "Weak" Loss Functions in Positron Emission Tomography

ALVIN KURUC

April 21, 1994

ABSTRACT. Motivated by an idealized model of positron emission tomography, we consider the statistical problem of estimating an unknown probability measure, μ, given n independent observations distributed according to the probability measure $T\mu$, where T denotes the (scaled) Radon transform on measures. Instead of the usual loss functions based on metrics for probability measures which metrize convergence in total variation, we consider loss functions based on L^2 Sobolev norms which metrize weak convergence. We thereby obtain results on the rate of convergence of the minimax risk for this estimation problem as a function of n without smoothness assumptions on the probability measure μ. Moreover, we argue that metrics which metrize weak convergence are more relevant to the physical problem.

We describe one specific result. Let $L^2_\alpha(\mathbb{R}^2)$ denote the L^2 Sobolev space of functions on $\mathbb{R}^2$ of order α. Let $P(\bar{\Omega})$ denote the set of Borel probability measures on the unit disk $\bar{\Omega} \subset \mathbb{R}^2$. Define a metric on $P(\bar{\Omega})$ by

$$d_\alpha(\mu, \mu') = \sup\{|\int f d(\mu - \mu')| : f \in L^2_\alpha(\mathbb{R}^2) \text{ and } \|f\|_{L^2_\alpha(\mathbb{R}^2)} \leq 1\},$$

i.e., $d_\alpha(\mu, \mu') = \|\mu - \mu'\|_{L^2_{-\alpha}(\mathbb{R}^2)}$. Let $\hat{\mu}_n$ denote an estimator of μ based on n independent observations distributed according to $T\mu$. Then, for $\alpha > 3/2$,

$$\inf_{\hat{\mu}_n} \sup_{\mu \in P(\bar{\Omega})} E_{(T\mu)^n} d_\alpha(\mu, \hat{\mu}_n) = O(n^{-1/2}),$$

where $E_{(T\mu)^n}$ denotes expectation under the n-fold product of $T\mu$, i.e., the minimax risk is $O(n^{-1/2})$.

1991 *Mathematics Subject Classification.* Primary 62G07; Secondary 44A12, 92C55, 62G20, 62C20.

The author was supported by DoD National Defense Science and Engineering Graduate Fellowship Grant #DAAL03-91-G-0291.

This paper is in final form and no version of it will be submitted for publication elsewhere.

© 1994 American Mathematical Society
0075-8485/94 $1.00 + $.25 per page

1. Introduction

The motivating physical problem for this work is the medical imaging technique of positron emission tomography (PET). In PET, the goal is to characterize the spatial distribution of positron-emitting tracer molecules in a patient using external detectors. Shortly after a positron is emitted, it combines with an electron in an annihilation reaction. On the average, a positron travels only a very short distance between emission and annihilation, so the position of the annihilation reaction is approximately that of the positron's emission. The annihilation reaction results in the emission of a pair of annihilation photons traveling in (approximately) opposite directions along a line with uniformly-distributed random spatial orientation. These photons subsequently strike detectors at approximately the same time, forming what is known as a coincident pair. From a coincident pair, one can thus infer that a positron was emitted (approximately) on the line segment between the two detectors which detected the pair.

The positions of the positron emissions and the paths of the annihilation photons are naturally modeled as points and lines, respectively, in Euclidean 3-space. However, the most common detector configurations actually only detect coincident pairs whose paths are close to a fixed plane (and which therefore must originate from an annihilation reaction near that plane). In this case, it makes sense to think of the problem as being 2-dimensional. In what follows, we will, for simplicity, restrict ourselves to the 2-dimensional PET problem.

To construct a mathematical idealization of the PET problem, we will model the locations of positron emissions as independent random variables distributed according to a probability measure μ on the closed unit disk $\bar{\Omega} \subset \mathbb{R}^2$. Given that the jth positron emission occurs at $x_j \in \bar{\Omega}$, the line along which the resulting annihilation photons travel will be modeled as a random line l_j through x_j with uniformly-distributed random spatial orientation. It is assumed that these orientations are independent of the x_j and each other so that the l_j are independent random variables distributed according to a probability measure $\nu \stackrel{\text{def}}{=} T\mu$ on the set of lines in $\mathbb{R}^2$, where T is a (deterministic) function of μ. It is shown in sec. 4 that T is proportional to the Radon transform on measures. We are thus faced with the statistical inverse problem of trying to estimate the probability measure μ from n independent observations distributed according to the probability measure ν. We are interested in obtaining suitable notions of the inherent difficulty of this problem.

It should be emphasized that the model described here is a very idealized model of the PET problem. It ignores a number of physical effects which complicate PET in practice. Nevertheless, it appears to capture the essence of the problem of emission tomography.

DEFINITION 1.1. In order to put the various possible statistical approaches to the PET problem into a single theoretical framework, it is useful to introduce some standard notions of statistical decision theory. We follow [**Str85**]. A statistical experiment may be defined as an ordered triple $\mathcal{E} = (X, A, \{\mu_\theta : \theta \in \Theta\})$, where (X, A) is a measurable space, known as the sample space, and $\{\mu_\theta : \theta \in \Theta\}$ is a set of probability measures on (X, A) indexed by the set Θ, known as the parameter space. The set X is the set in which the observation is contained and μ_θ is the probability measure of the observations under the statistical model indexed by θ.

DEFINITION 1.2. Let $\mathcal{D}$ be a metric space, which we will refer to as the decision space. A function $\kappa : X \to \mathcal{D}$ is known as a (nonrandomized) decision function. A family of measurable functions $W_\theta : \mathcal{D} \to \mathbb{R}$, $\theta \in \Theta$ that are bounded below is called a loss function. For a decision function κ, $E_\theta W_\theta \kappa$ is called the risk of κ with respect to the loss function W_θ (E_θ denotes mathematical expectation with respect to the probability measure indexed by θ). The combination of a statistical experiment with a decision space and loss function is known as a statistical decision problem. Roughly speaking, the goal of a statistical decision problem is to find decision functions with small risk over a variety of $\theta \in \Theta$.

DEFINITION 1.3. We shall be exclusively interested in statistical decision problems in which W_θ depends on θ only through some function $\phi : \Theta \to \mathcal{D}$, i.e., we shall be interested in estimating $\phi(\theta)$. Such a statistical decision problem is called a statistical estimation problem. Most frequently, we shall take $\mathcal{D} = \Theta$ and ϕ equal to the identity function, i.e., we will be estimating θ. In statistical estimation problems, the decision function is called an estimator. In the problems considered here, the loss function is of the form $W_\theta = \ell \circ d(\cdot, \theta)$, where d is a metric on $\mathcal{D}$ and $\ell : [0, \infty) \to [0, \infty)$ is an increasing function (typically $\ell : x \mapsto x$ or $\ell : x \mapsto x^2$).

In the PET problem described above, the sample space (X, A) is the n-fold product of the set of lines through $\bar{\Omega}$. The parameter set Θ indexes a subset $\mathcal{P}$ of the set $P(\bar{\Omega})$ of probability measures on $\bar{\Omega}$. If the probability measure μ corresponds to θ, the probability measure of the observation is given by the n-fold product of $\nu = T\mu$. The major choices in selecting a statistical model for the PET problem are the choice of $\mathcal{P}$ (along with an appropriate parameterization) and the choice of a loss function.

The simplest models for PET are ones in which μ is assumed to belong to some predetermined finite-dimensional family of probability measures. Such models are termed parametric models. Most commonly, one "pixelizes" the image, that is, one divides the domain of interest $\bar{\Omega}$ into a finite number of squares on which the probability measure is assumed to be uniform (e.g., [**VSK85**, sec. 1.2]). Another possible approach, based on a singular value decomposition of the tomography process, is described in [**Bak91**]. The advantage of parametric models is that one can use the standard methods of parametric statistics to develop and evaluate estimators (e.g., maximum likelihood estimators and Cramér-Rao bounds). The main disadvantage of parametric models in PET is that, in practice, the actual μ is unlikely to conform to the assumed model, creating an error which falls outside the assumed statistical framework. Moreover, many natural questions about the PET problem, such as how potential spatial resolution increases with n, are difficult to formulate in a natural way using parametric models.

The limitations of parametric models may be transcended by allowing μ to lie in an infinite-dimensional family of probability measures. Such models are termed nonparametric models. Johnstone and Silverman [JS90] have recently described a statistical model where $\mathcal{P}$ was taken to be the subset of $P(\bar{\Omega})$ whose probability density functions with respect to (normalized) Lebesgue measure exist and lie in a certain ellipsoid in $L^2(\bar{\Omega})$, where $L^2(\bar{\Omega})$ denotes the space of square-integrable real-valued functions on $\bar{\Omega}$. The condition of lying in such an ellipsoid is essentially a smoothness and integrability constraint. If $\mu \in \mathcal{P}$, let f_μ denote the probability density associated with μ. Let $\hat{f}_n$ be an estimator of f_μ based on n independent observations distributed according to $T\mu$, with $\hat{f}(x)$ denoting the estimate of $f(x)$. The loss function, $W_\mu(\hat{\mu})$, was taken to be the squared L^2 distance between $\hat{f}_n$ and f_μ, resulting in a risk function given by $r(\mu, \hat{f}_n) \stackrel{\text{def}}{=} E_{(T\mu)^n} \|\hat{f}_n - f_\mu\|^2_{L^2(\bar{\Omega})}$, where $E_{(T\mu)^n}$ denotes expectation with respect to the n-fold product of $T\mu$. The overall difficulty of the problem was then assessed in terms of the minimax risk, $\inf_{\hat{\mu}_n} \sup_{\mu \in \mathcal{P}} r(\mu, \hat{\mu}_n)$. While Johnstone and Silverman were able to obtain quite precise characterizations of the functional form of the dependence of the minimax risk on n, the results were found to depend significantly on the specific smoothness and integrability constraints which were imposed. Moreover, the constraints used were, in all cases, quite restrictive from an applications point of view, e.g., they implied the density of interest always took values in the range $[0, 2]$.

In this paper, we will explore a different nonparametric approach to the PET problem. We will allow μ to be an *arbitrary* probability measure on $\bar{\Omega}$, i.e., we will take $\mathcal{P} = P(\bar{\Omega})$, and use loss functions that are based upon L^2 Sobolev metrics for probability measures of order < -1 (see sec. 5 for the definition). The significance of this change in loss function will be discussed in greater detail in the next section. Using this approach, we will see that it is possible to bound the minimax risk as a function of n without the use of smoothness assumptions. In fact, we shall see that, for L^2 Sobolev metrics of order $< -3/2$, the minimax risk is $O(n^{-1/2})$ (i.e., bounded above by $cn^{-1/2}$ for some constant c), as is typically the case in parametric models.

REMARK 1.4. Note added in proof: For the problem of estimating μ from n independent observations distributed according to μ itself, the minimax risk is $O(n^{-1/2})$ for loss functions based on Sobolev metrics of order < -1. Moreover, the minimax risk is *not* $O(n^{-1/2})$ for loss functions based on Sobolev metrics of order $\geq -3/2$ (resp. -1) for the problem of estimating μ from n independent observations distributed according to $T\mu$ (resp. μ). Proofs of these results are given in [**Kur94**].

2. Loss functions for estimation of probability measures

In this section, we will consider loss functions for the PET problem in the context of probability measure estimation problems in general. We start by recalling the definitions of some metrics and notions of convergence on spaces of probability measures.

DEFINITION 2.1. Let μ and μ' be probability measures on a measurable space (X, A). The distance in total variation between μ and μ' is defined by $d_v(\mu, \mu') \stackrel{\text{def}}{=} \sup_{A \in A} |\mu(A) - \mu'(A)|$. Convergence of a sequence of probability measures with respect to variational distance is called convergence in total variation or strong convergence.

DEFINITION 2.2. Let X be a topological space equipped with the Borel σ-algebra and $C_b(X)$ the set of bounded, continuous, real-valued functions on X. The sequence $\{\mu_n\}$ of probability measures on X is said to converge weakly to the probability measure μ if $\int f \, d\mu_n \to \int f \, d\mu$ for all $f \in C_b(X)$. If X is a compact subset of $\mathbb{R}^d$, then L^2 Sobolev metrics of order $< -d/2$ metrize weak convergence of probability measures on X, cf. [**Gin75**, thm. 2.2].

In most nonparametric probability measure estimation problems in the literature, the unknown probability measure is assumed to be representable as a probability density function and the loss function is based on the L^1 or L^2 distance between density functions. Convergence of density functions with respect to the L^1 metric is equivalent to strong convergence of the associated probability measures [**Str85**, lem. 2.4]. Under additional conditions, (e.g., density functions uniformly bounded above and below away from 0 and a finite common dominating measure, as in [**JS90**]) convergence of density functions with respect to the L^2 metric is also equivalent. Using these loss functions, it is, generally speaking, necessary to assume that the unknown probability density satisfies some smoothness condition in order to guarantee that the minimax risk for estimating the unknown probability measure converges to 0 as $n \to \infty$, cf. [**Dev87**, sec 5.3].

By using loss functions based on metrics, such as L^2 Sobolev norms, that metrize weak convergence, we are able to obtain upper bounds on the rate of convergence of the minimax risk without the need for smoothness assumptions. The obviation of smoothness assumptions fits in well with the spirit of nonparametric statistics and is thus an advantage of our approach. But what, if anything, do we lose by the change in loss functions? Clearly, loss functions based on metrics that metrize strong convergence are stricter than loss functions based on metrics that metrize weak convergence in the sense that convergence to 0 with respect to the former implies convergence with respect to the latter, but not vice versa. However, stricter does not necessarily imply more relevant in a physical application. Roughly speaking, the difference between the two classes of metrics is that metrics which topologize weak convergence consider measures which live on disjoint sets which are close together in the underlying space to be close together while metrics which topologize strong convergence consider them to be as far apart as can be. For example, consider measures on the real lines with respect to the usual Borel σ-algebra and let δ_x denote a point mass at x. Then the sequence of measures $\{\delta_{1/n}\}$ converges weakly to δ_0, but $d_v(\delta_{1/n}, \delta_0) = 1$ for all n. Which risk function is "better" in a particular application thus depends on whether or not "close counts" in that application. For general applications in PET and many other areas, it seems to the author that "close counts" and hence that loss functions for probability measures based on metrics inducing the weak topology are appropriate tools for studying these problems.

3. The Radon transform

In this section, we introduce the notions related to the Radon transform that are used in what follows. Our treatment parallels that of Hertle [**Her83**].

DEFINITION 3.1. Define the map $\omega : \mathbb{R} \to S^1$ by $\theta \mapsto (\cos\theta, \sin\theta)$. We shall use the map ω to define local coordinate systems on S^1, the local coordinate being denoted by θ. It will sometimes be convenient, by a slight abuse of language, to denote a function on S^1 by $f(\theta)$, where f is a function on $\mathbb{R}$ which is periodic with period 2π, e.g., $e^{-i2\pi\theta}$. Using this notation, the differential operator ∂_θ on S^1 is defined in the obvious way. The standard surface measure on S^1 induced by the differential 1-form $d\theta$ will be denoted by σ, so that $\int_{S^1} f\, d\sigma = \int_{-\pi}^{\pi} f[\omega(\theta)]\, d\theta$.

DEFINITION 3.2. Let $G_{1,2}$ denote the set of lines in $\mathbb{R}^2$. We define the standard double covering $\pi : S^1 \times \mathbb{R} \to G_{1,2}$ by taking $\pi(\omega, s) \in G_{1,2}$ to be the line in $\mathbb{R}^2$ through $s\omega$ which is perpendicular to ω. Note that $\pi(\omega, s) = \pi(-\omega, -s)$. We give $G_{1,2}$ the structure of a quotient manifold of $S^1 \times \mathbb{R}$ under π.

DEFINITION 3.3. For any function $g : S^1 \times \mathbb{R} \to \mathbb{R}$, define its drop $\check{g} : G_{1,2} \to \mathbb{R}$ by $\bar{g}(\pi(\omega, s)) \stackrel{\text{def}}{=} g(\omega, s) + g(-\omega, -s)$. For $g : G_{1,2} \to \mathbb{R}$ define the lift of g to $S^1 \times \mathbb{R}$ by $\tilde{g} \stackrel{\text{def}}{=} g \circ \pi : S^1 \times \mathbb{R} \to \mathbb{R}$.

DEFINITION 3.4. Let λ^d denote Lebesgue measure on $\mathbb{R}^d$. We will take λ^d to be the standard measure on $\mathbb{R}^d$ in the sense that $L^p(\mathbb{R}^d) \stackrel{\text{def}}{=} L^p(\mathbb{R}^d, \lambda^d)$. Similarly, we shall take the standard measures on $S^1 \times \mathbb{R}$ and $G_{1,2}$ to be $\sigma \times \lambda^1$ and the image measure $\frac{1}{2}(\sigma \times \lambda^1) \circ \pi^{-1}$, respectively.

DEFINITION 3.5. The Radon transform on $L^1(\mathbb{R}^2)$, which we shall denote by R, maps $f \in L^1(\mathbb{R}^2)$ to the function $Rf : G_{1,2} \to \mathbb{R}$ whose value at $\pi(\omega, s) \in G_{1,2}$ is equal to the integral of f with respect to Lebesgue measure on the line in $\mathbb{R}^2$ through the point $s\omega$ which is perpendicular to ω. The *standard* Radon transform on $L^1(\mathbb{R}^2)$, which we shall denote by $\widetilde{R}$, maps $f \in L^1(\mathbb{R}^2)$ to the lift of Rf to

$S^1 \times \mathbb{R}$. It can be shown that $\widetilde{R}f \in L^1(S^1 \times \mathbb{R})$ [**Her83**, p. 168]. It follows at once that $Rf \in L^1(G_{1,2})$.

REMARK 3.6. The standard Radon transform is most commonly used in the literature. However, in our statistical analysis of the PET problem, the observations are given as points in $G_{1,2}$. We will therefore need to go back and forth between the two definitions.

We next want to develop the adjoint of R.

PROPOSITION 3.7. *The map* $\widetilde{R}^* : L^\infty(S^1 \times \mathbb{R}) \to L^\infty(\mathbb{R}^2)$ *given by*

$$\widetilde{R}^* g(x) = \int_{S^1} g(\omega, x \cdot \omega) \, d\sigma(\omega)$$

for $g \in L^\infty(S^1 \times \mathbb{R})$ *is the adjoint of* $\widetilde{R} : L^1(\mathbb{R}^2) \to L^1(S^1 \times \mathbb{R})$ *in the sense that*

$$\int_{S^1 \times \mathbb{R}} \widetilde{R}f \, g \, d(\sigma \times \lambda^1) = \int_{\mathbb{R}^2} f \, \widetilde{R}^* g \, d\lambda^2$$

for all $f \in L^1(\mathbb{R}^2)$ *and* $g \in L^\infty(S^1 \times \mathbb{R})$. *The map* $R^* : L^\infty(G_{1,2}) \to L^\infty(\mathbb{R}^2)$ *given by*

$$R^* g(x) = \frac{1}{2} \widetilde{R}^* \tilde{g}(x)$$

for $g \in L^\infty(G_{1,2})$ *is the adjoint of* $R : L^1(\mathbb{R}^2) \to L^1(G_{1,2})$ *in the sense that*

$$\frac{1}{2} \int_{G_{1,2}} Rf \, g \, d\left[(\sigma \times \lambda^1) \circ \pi^{-1}\right] = \int_{\mathbb{R}^2} f \, R^* g \, d\lambda^2$$

for all $f \in L^1(\mathbb{R}^2)$ *and* $g \in L^\infty(G_{1,2})$.

PROOF. The result for $\widetilde{R}$ is given in [**Her83**, p. 169]. The result for R follows from this by the definitions. ∎

We will now develop the Radon transform on distributions and measures.

DEFINITION 3.8. Let X be $\mathbb{R}^d$, $G_{1,2}$, or $S^1 \times \mathbb{R}$. Define $C_0(X)$ to be the subset of $C(X)$ whose elements vanish at ∞ [**Fol84**, pp. 125-6]. Define $C_0^\infty(X)$ to be the subset of $C_0(X)$ whose derivatives of all orders are also in $C_0(X)$. The dual space to $C_0^\infty(X)$ is termed the space of integrable distributions and denoted by $D'_{L_1}(X)$ [**Itô85**, art. 125N]. If $g \in C_0^\infty(S^1 \times \mathbb{R})$, then $\check{g} \in C_0^\infty(G_{1,2})$. Thus if $v \in D'_{L_1}(G_{1,2})$, we can define its lift $\tilde{v} \in D'_{L_1}(S^1 \times \mathbb{R})$ by $\langle \tilde{v}, g \rangle \stackrel{\text{def}}{=} \langle v, \check{g} \rangle$, where the notation $\langle u, f \rangle$ indicates the operation of applying the distribution u to the test function f.

DEFINITION 3.9. For $u \in D'_{L_1}(\mathbb{R}^2)$, we define $Ru \in D'_{L_1}(G_{1,2})$ by $\langle Ru, g \rangle \stackrel{\text{def}}{=} \langle u, R^* g \rangle$ for any $g \in C_0(G_{1,2})$. We define $\widetilde{R}u \in D'_{L_1}(S^1 \times \mathbb{R})$ by $\widetilde{R}u \stackrel{\text{def}}{=} \widetilde{Ru}$. It is easily verified that $\langle \widetilde{R}u, g \rangle = \langle u, \widetilde{R}^* g \rangle$ for any $g \in C_0^\infty(S^1 \times \mathbb{R})$. By prop. 3.7, these definitions extend R and $\widetilde{R}$ from $L^1(\mathbb{R}^2)$ to $D'_{L_1}(\mathbb{R}^2)$. Moreover, since L^1 is dense in D'_{L_1}, these extensions are unique [**Her83**, rem. 1.5].

DEFINITION 3.10. Let $M(X)$ denote the space of (finite) signed measures on X. $M(X)$ is a Banach subspace of $D'_{L_1}(X)$ with respect to the total variation norm. That is, if μ is a signed measure on X, we can interpret μ as the integrable distribution $\langle \mu, f \rangle = \int_X f\,d\mu$, where $f \in C_0^\infty(X)$. Thus if $\mu \in M(\mathbb{R}^2)$, the Radon transform of μ is given by the integrable distribution $\langle R\mu, g \rangle = \int_{\mathbb{R}^2} R^* g\,d\mu$ for $g \in C_0^\infty(G_{1,2})$ and similarly for the standard Radon transform of μ. It is shown in [**Her83**, p. 171] that $\widetilde{R}\mu$ is actually a signed measure, i.e., that it can be extended to a continuous linear functional on $C_0(S^1 \times \mathbb{R})$. An analogous argument shows that $R\mu$ is also signed measure. If μ is a positive finite measure on $\mathbb{R}^2$, it is easy to see that $R\mu$ and $\widetilde{R}\mu$ are also positive finite measures.

REMARK 3.11. Def. 3.10 gives the Radon transform of a finite positive measure as a finite positive measure which is expressed in terms of its action on functions in $C_0^\infty(G_{1,2})$. The following proposition gives a more explicit expression for the Radon transform of a finite positive measure.

PROPOSITION 3.12. *Let μ be a finite positive measure on $\mathbb{R}^2$. Let E be a Borel set of $G_{1,2}$. Then $R\mu(E) = \int_{\mathbb{R}^2} R^* 1_E\,d\mu$, where 1_E denotes the indicator function of the set E.*

PROOF. For the sake of brevity, we will merely sketch the proof. The result is proved by first showing that it holds if E is open or if E is compact. This is done by approximating 1_E by monotone sequences of functions in $C_c(G_{1,2})$ and applying the Riesz representation theorem for positive measures [**Fol84**, thm. 7.2] and the dominated convergence theorem. The general result then follows by approximating an arbitrary Borel set from below by compact sets and above by open sets. This is possible since any finite Borel measure on a second-countable, locally-compact Hausdorff space is a regular Radon measure [**Fol84**, pp. 209, 210]. ∎

4. Probabilistic model for PET

In this section, we will show that the probability measure of the observations in our idealization of the PET problem is given by the (scaled) Radon transform of the probability measure of interest.

DEFINITION 4.1. The projective space $\mathbb{P}^1$ is the quotient space of S^1 obtained by identifying each point of S^1 with its antipodal point. We will denote the natural projection map by $p : S^1 \to \mathbb{P}^1$. We identify $\mathbb{P}^1$ with the set of lines through the origin in the obvious way.

DEFINITION 4.2. We will identify the set of lines in $\mathbb{R}^2$ through a point $x \in \mathbb{R}^2$ with the space $\mathbb{P}^1$ in the following way. If l is a line through x, we identify it with the unique line through the origin, i.e., the unique point $\bar{\omega} \in \mathbb{P}^1$, which is perpendicular to l. It is easy to see that this identification gives a bijective relation between the lines in $\mathbb{R}^2$ through x and $\mathbb{P}^1$.

DEFINITION 4.3. Given that a positron emission takes place at $x \in \mathbb{R}^2$, the line which its annihilation photons travel along is modeled as a line in $\mathbb{R}^2$ through x whose orientation is randomly distributed according to the image measure $\frac{1}{2\pi}\sigma \circ p^{-1}$ on $\mathbb{P}^1$ and is independent of x. The event of a positron emission occurring at $x \in \mathbb{R}^2$ and its annihilation photons having orientation $\bar{\omega} \in \mathbb{P}^1$ is thus described by the pair $(x, \bar{\omega}) \in \mathbb{R}^2 \times \mathbb{P}^1$. Thus the joint probability distribution of x and $\bar{\omega}$ is given by the product measure $\mu \times \left(\frac{1}{2\pi}\sigma \circ p^{-1}\right)$ on $\mathbb{R}^2 \times \mathbb{P}^1$.

DEFINITION 4.4. In the PET problem, one does not observe $(x, \bar{\omega})$, but rather only the point $\rho(x, \bar{\omega}) \in G_{1,2}$, where the function $\rho : \mathbb{R}^2 \times \mathbb{P}^1 \to G_{1,2}$ is given by $\rho : (x, p(\omega)) \mapsto \pi(\omega, x \cdot \omega)$. Thus, the probability measure of each observation in the PET problem is just the image measure, $\nu \stackrel{\text{def}}{=} \left[\mu \times \left(\frac{1}{2\pi}\sigma \circ p^{-1}\right)\right] \circ \rho^{-1}$ induced on $G_{1,2}$ by the map ρ. A calculation using prop. 3.12 shows that $\nu = \frac{1}{\pi}R\mu$. For convenience, we define $T\mu \stackrel{\text{def}}{=} \frac{1}{\pi}R\mu$.

5. Sobolev spaces

In this section, we will give the definitions of some of the Sobolev spaces which will be used in what follows.

DEFINITION 5.1. Let $\mathcal{S}(\mathbb{R}^d)$ denote the Schwartz space of smooth, rapidly decreasing functions on $\mathbb{R}^d$ [**Tre67**, p. 92, ex. IV] and $\mathcal{S}'(\mathbb{R}^d)$ its dual, the space of tempered distributions [**Tre67**, p. 271-2]. The Fourier transform of u, $\hat{u} : \mathbb{R}^d \to \mathbb{C}$, is defined by $\hat{u}(\xi) \stackrel{\text{def}}{=} \int_{\mathbb{R}^d} e^{-i2\pi x \cdot \xi} u(x)\, dx$ for $u \in \mathcal{S}(\mathbb{R}^d)$ [**Tre67**, p. 268, def. 25.1] and by duality for $u \in \mathcal{S}'(\mathbb{R}^d)$, i.e., $\langle \hat{u}, f \rangle \stackrel{\text{def}}{=} \langle u, \hat{f} \rangle$ for $f \in \mathcal{S}(\mathbb{R}^d)$ [**Tre67**, p. 275, def. 25.4]. For $\alpha \in \mathbb{R}$, the Sobolev space $L^2_\alpha(\mathbb{R}^d)$ is defined to be the subspace of $\mathcal{S}'(\mathbb{R}^d)$ whose elements u satisfy

$$\|u\|^2_{L^2_\alpha(\mathbb{R}^d)} \stackrel{\text{def}}{=} \int_{\mathbb{R}^d} (1 + 4\pi^2|\xi|^2)^\alpha |\hat{u}(\xi)|^2\, d\xi < \infty,$$

cf. [**Ste70**, subsec. V.3.1]. $L^2_\alpha(\mathbb{R}^d)$ is a Hilbert space with inner product

$$(u|v)_{L^2_\alpha(\mathbb{R}^d)} \stackrel{\text{def}}{=} \int_{\mathbb{R}^d} (1 + 4\pi^2|\xi|^2)^\alpha \hat{u}(\xi)\overline{\hat{v}(\xi)}\, d\xi$$

[**Tre67**, p. 330, prop. 31.7].

REMARK 5.2. The use of the circumflex to denote the Fourier transform conflicts with its use in denoting an estimate of an unknown quantity. Since both notations are quite standard, we shall just endure this ambiguity. It should be clear from context which meaning is intended.

DEFINITION 5.3. Let $\mathcal{E}'(S^1 \times \mathbb{R})$ denote the space of compactly supported distributions on $S^1 \times \mathbb{R}$, i.e., the space of continuous linear functionals on $C^\infty(S^1 \times \mathbb{R})$. Let $\mathcal{E}'(S^1 \times [-r/2, r/2])$ denote the subspace of $\mathcal{E}'(S^1 \times \mathbb{R})$ whose elements have support contained in $S^1 \times [-r/2, r/2]$.

DEFINITION 5.4. Let $C^\infty(S^1 \times r\mathbb{T}^1)$ denote the subspace of $C^\infty(S^1 \times \mathbb{R})$ whose elements are periodic with respect to the second variable with period r. $C^\infty(S^1 \times r\mathbb{T}^1)$ can be viewed as the set of smooth functions on the product space $S^1 \times r\mathbb{T}^1$, obtained by identifying points in $S^1 \times \mathbb{R}$ whose second coordinates differ by integer multiples of r. Let $\mathcal{E}'(S^1 \times r\mathbb{T}^1)$ denote the set of continuous linear functionals on $C^\infty(S^1 \times r\mathbb{T}^1)$. $\mathcal{E}'(S^1 \times r\mathbb{T}^1)$ can be viewed as the set of distributions on $S^1 \times r\mathbb{T}^1$. Since $C^\infty(S^1 \times r\mathbb{T}^1) \subset C^\infty(S^1 \times \mathbb{R})$, the elements of $\mathcal{E}'(S^1 \times \mathbb{R})$ can be considered as elements of $\mathcal{E}'(S^1 \times r\mathbb{T}^1)$ in a natural way. For $\kappa \in \mathbb{Z}^2$, we define the Fourier series coefficients of $v \in \mathcal{E}'(S^1 \times r\mathbb{T}^1)$ by

$$\hat{v}(\kappa) \stackrel{\text{def}}{=} \frac{1}{2\pi r} \langle v, e^{-i[\kappa_1 \theta + (2\pi/r)\kappa_2 s]} \rangle.$$

We define $L_\alpha^2(S^1 \times r\mathbb{T}^1)$ to be the subset of $\mathcal{E}'(S^1 \times r\mathbb{T}^1)$ such that

$$\|v\|_{L_\alpha^2(S^1 \times r\mathbb{T}^1)}^2 \stackrel{\text{def}}{=} 2\pi r \sum_{\kappa \in \mathbb{Z}^2} [1 + \kappa_1^2 + (2\pi/r)^2 \kappa_2^2]^\alpha |\hat{g}(\kappa)|^2$$

is finite.

DEFINITION 5.5. We shall define $G_{1,2}(r) \subset G_{1,2}$ to be $\pi(S^1 \times [-r,r])$. The Sobolev space $L_\alpha^2(G_{1,2}(r))$ is defined to be the subspace of $\mathcal{E}'(G_{1,2})$ whose elements v satisfy $\tilde{v} \in L_\alpha^2(S^1 \times 2r\mathbb{T}^1)$. The squared norm on $L_\alpha^2(G_{1,2}(r))$ is defined to be $1/2$ of the squared norm of the corresponding elements of $L_\alpha^2(S^1 \times 2r\mathbb{T}^1)$.

6. Estimation of probability measures in PET

The main theorem in this section shows that the minimax risk for estimating $\mu \in P(\bar{\Omega})$ with respect to the loss function generated by the Sobolev norm $\|\cdot\|_{L^2_{-\alpha}(\mathbb{R}^2)}$ for $\alpha > 3/2$ in the PET problem is $O(n^{-1/2})$. It is proved by constructing a sequence of estimators, $\{\hat{\mu}_n\}$, whose maximum risk over $P(\bar{\Omega})$ is $O(n^{-1/2})$.

DEFINITION 6.1. If $x_1, \ldots, x_n$ are independent samples of a random variable with observation space (X, A), we define the empirical probability measure generated by $x_1, \ldots, x_n$ to be the probability measure on (X, A) consisting of the sum of n point masses of measure $1/n$ located at $x_1, \ldots, x_n$.

THEOREM 6.2. Let $\alpha > 3/2$. There exists a sequence of estimators $\{\hat{\mu}_n\}$ of μ based on n independent observations distributed according to $T\mu$ such that $\sup_{\mu \in P(\bar{\Omega})} E_{(T\mu)^n} \|\hat{\mu}_n - \mu\|_{L^2_{-\alpha}(\mathbb{R}^2)} = O(n^{-1/2})$.

PROOF. We start by constructing the sequence of estimators. Fix n and let ν_n denote the empirical probability measure generated from n independent observations distributed according to ν. We first construct an auxiliary estimate, $\hat{\nu}_n$, of ν by choosing some $\hat{\nu}_n \in T[P(\bar{\Omega})]$ which satisfies

$$\|\hat{\nu}_n - \nu_n\|_{L^2_{-(\alpha-1/2)}(G_{1,2}(2))} \leq \inf_{\hat{\nu} \in T[P(\bar{\Omega})]} \|\hat{\nu} - \nu_n\|_{L^2_{-(\alpha-1/2)}(G_{1,2}(2))} + n^{-1/2}.$$

We then estimate μ by $\hat{\mu}_n = T^{-1}\hat{\nu}_n$. (The right-hand side of this equation makes sense since T is injective on $P(\bar{\Omega})$ and $\hat{\nu}_n \in T[P(\bar{\Omega})]$.)

We now show that $\hat{\mu}_n$ has the required behavior. By the triangle inequality, we have

$$\|\hat{\nu}_n - \nu\|_{L^2_{-(\alpha-1/2)}(G_{1,2}(2))}$$
$$\leq \|\hat{\nu}_n - \nu_n\|_{L^2_{-(\alpha-1/2)}(G_{1,2}(2))} + \|\nu_n - \nu\|_{L^2_{-(\alpha-1/2)}(G_{1,2}(2))}$$
$$\leq \inf_{\hat{\nu} \in T[P(\bar{\Omega})]} \|\hat{\nu} - \nu_n\|_{L^2_{-(\alpha-1/2)}(G_{1,2}(2))} + n^{-1/2} + \|\nu_n - \nu\|_{L^2_{-(\alpha-1/2)}(G_{1,2}(2))}$$
$$\leq 2\|\nu_n - \nu\|_{L^2_{-(\alpha-1/2)}(G_{1,2}(2))} + n^{-1/2}.$$

Since $\mu \in P(\bar{\Omega})$, the support of ν is contained in $G_{1,2}(1)$. It is shown below in prop. A.1 that this implies that $E_{\nu^n}\|\nu_n - \nu\|_{L^2_{-(\alpha-1/2)}(G_{1,2}(2))} \leq c_1(\alpha)n^{-1/2}$, where $c_1(\alpha)$ is a constant depending only on α. It follows that

$$E_{\nu^n}\|\hat{\nu}_n - \nu\|_{L^2_{-(\alpha-1/2)}(G_{1,2}(2))} \leq [2c_1(\alpha) + 1]n^{-1/2}.$$

To complete the proof, we use prop. B.13 below to obtain

$$\|\hat{\mu}_n - \mu\|_{L^2_{-\alpha}(\mathbb{R}^2)} \leq \pi c_2(\alpha)\|\hat{\nu}_n - \nu\|_{L^2_{-(\alpha-1/2)}(G_{1,2}(2))},$$

where $c_2(\alpha)$ is a constant depending only on α. It follows that

$$E_{(T\mu)^n}\|\hat{\mu}_n - \mu\|_{L^2_{-\alpha}(\mathbb{R}^2)} \leq \pi c_2(\alpha) E_{\nu^n}\|\hat{\nu}_n - \nu\|_{L^2_{-(\alpha-1/2)}(G_{1,2}(2))}$$
$$\leq \pi c_2(\alpha)[2c_1(\alpha) + 1]n^{-1/2}.$$

Since the right-hand side is independent of $\mu \in P(\bar{\Omega})$, the result follows. ∎

7. Estimation of linear functionals in PET

In this section, we will consider the estimation of linear functionals of the unknown probability measure μ of the form $\mu \mapsto \int_{\mathbb{R}^2} f \, d\mu$, for $f : \mathbb{R}^2 \to \mathbb{R}$. For convenience, we will write $\int_{\mathbb{R}^2} f \, d\mu$ as $\dot{f}(\mu)$.

Let $\alpha > 3/2$. If $\hat{\mu}_n$ is an estimator of μ satisfying the conditions given in thm. 6.2 and $\phi \in L^2_\alpha(\mathbb{R}^2)$, then the estimate $\dot{\phi}(\hat{\mu}_n)$ of $\dot{\phi}(\mu)$ satisfies

$$\sup_{\mu \in P(\bar{\Omega})} E_{(T\mu)^n}|\dot{\phi}_n - \phi(\mu)| \leq c(\alpha)\|\phi\|^2_{L^2_\alpha(\mathbb{R}^2)} n^{-1/2},$$

where $c(\alpha)$ is a constant. Examination of this equation gives some insight into the meaning of thm. 6.2. For example, if f is a nonnegative function, $\dot{f}(\mu)$ is a weighted (by the magnitude of f) average of the mass contained in the support of f. One can thus think of f as representing a generalized pixel. Now a natural quantity that one might want to compute in the PET problem is the mass contained in some measurable set $S \subset \bar{\Omega}$, i.e., the mass in some (ordinary) pixel. This quantity can be represented as the linear functional $\dot{1}_S$, where 1_S denotes the indicator function of S. However, note that the last display says nothing about estimating this functional, since $1_S \notin L^2_\alpha(\mathbb{R}^2)$ (unless $S = \emptyset$). (This follows from the Sobolev embedding theorem [**Fol84**, thm. 8.54], which shows that $L^2_\alpha(\mathbb{R}^2) \subset C_0(\mathbb{R}^2)$ when $\alpha > 1$.) To get an approximate answer to how much mass is contained in S, one could apply the last display to some function in $L^2_\alpha(\mathbb{R}^2)$ which is close in some sense to 1_S. For example, for some $\epsilon > 0$, we might choose f_ϵ such that $0 \leq f_\epsilon(x) \leq 1$, $f_\epsilon(x) = 1$ for $x \in S$, and $f_\epsilon(x) = 0$ for any x whose distance from S is $\geq \epsilon$. It is easy to see that as ϵ becomes smaller, $\|f_\epsilon\|_{L^2_\alpha(\mathbb{R}^2)}$, and hence the bound in the last display, must become larger.

The fact that our theory says nothing about how well one can estimate the mass in an ordinary pixel is disappointing. However, it reflect an intrinsic property of the estimation problem. In fact, the minimax risk for the estimation of the mass in some very benign-looking ordinary pixels is bounded away from 0 as $n \to \infty$. For example, let $\rho\bar{\Omega}$ denote the closed disk of radius ρ centered at the origin.

PROPOSITION 7.1. *For $0 < \rho < 1$, there exists $c > 0$, independent of n, such that*
$$\inf_{\hat{1}_{\rho\bar{\Omega}}} \sup_{\mu \in P(\bar{\Omega})} E_{(T\mu)^n}|\hat{1}_{\rho\bar{\Omega}} - 1_{\rho\bar{\Omega}}(\mu)| \geq c.$$

PROOF. If ν and ν' are probability measures on the measurable space X, let $H(\nu, \nu')$ denote the Hellinger distance between them. If ν and ν' are represented by the densities g and g', respectively, with respect to some common measure η, then $H(\nu, \nu')$ is given by $\|\sqrt{g} - \sqrt{g'}\|_{L^2(X,\eta)}$ [**Str85**, def. 2.7]. Define the modulus of continuity
$$\omega(\epsilon) \stackrel{\text{def}}{=} \sup\{|1_{\rho\bar{\Omega}}(\mu) - 1_{\rho\bar{\Omega}}(\mu')| : H(T\mu, T\mu') \leq \epsilon, \mu, \mu' \in P(\bar{\Omega})\}.$$

We will use the lower bound
$$\inf_{\hat{1}_{\rho\bar{\Omega}}} \sup_{\mu \in P(\bar{\Omega})} E_{(T\mu)^n}|\hat{1}_{\rho\bar{\Omega}} - 1_{\rho\bar{\Omega}}(\mu)| \geq c\,\omega(n^{-1/2})$$
for some $c > 0$ [**DL91**]. We claim that $\omega(\epsilon) = 1$ for $\epsilon > 0$, which will prove the result. To prove the claim, let $\epsilon > 0$ be given. Let μ_r denote the probability measure on $\mathbb{R}^2$ which is uniformly distributed on the circle of radius r centered at the origin with respect to the measure $d\theta$. A calculation shows that $\nu_r \stackrel{\text{def}}{=} T\mu_r$ is given by the probability density
$$d\nu_r(\theta, s) = \begin{cases} \frac{1}{\pi^2} \frac{1}{\sqrt{r^2 - s^2}} \, d\theta \, ds & \text{if } |s| \leq r \\ 0 \, d\theta \, ds & \text{if } |s| > r \end{cases}.$$

For $r > \rho$, another calculation shows that $d_v(\nu_r, \nu_\rho) = 2 - (4/\pi)\arcsin(\rho/r)$, which approaches 0 as $r \searrow \rho$. Now, $H^2(\nu', \nu) \leq d_v(\nu', \nu)$ for any probability measures ν and ν' [**Str85**, lem. 2.15]. It follows that $\lim_{r \searrow \rho} H(T\mu_r, T\mu_\rho) = 0$. On the other hand $|1_{\rho\bar{\Omega}}(\mu_r) - 1_{\rho\bar{\Omega}}(\mu_\rho)| = 1$ for any $r > \rho$. This proves the claim that $\omega(\epsilon) = 1$. ∎

REMARK 7.2. This result contrasts sharply with the situation for the problem of estimating $\mu(\rho\bar{\Omega})$ given n independent observations distributed according to μ itself. In fact, let μ_n denote the empirical measure constructed from n independent observations distributed according to μ and define the estimator $\hat{f}_n \stackrel{\text{def}}{=} \mathbf{i}_{\rho\bar{\Omega}}(\mu_n)$. Then it is not difficult to show that $\sup_{\mu \in P(\mu)} E_{\mu^n}|\hat{\mathbf{i}}_{\rho\bar{\Omega}n} - \mathbf{i}_{\rho\bar{\Omega}}(\mu)| = O(n^{-1/2})$. We thus see that prop. 7.1 reflects an inherent loss of spatial resolution when only observations distributed according to $T\mu$ are available.

Appendix A. Convergence of empirical measures in $L^2(G_{1,2}(2))$

PROPOSITION A.1. *Suppose ν is a probability measure on $G_{1,2}$ with support on $G_{1,2}(1)$ and ν_n is the empirical distribution generated by n independent observations distributed according to ν. Suppose $\alpha > 1$. Then*

$$E_{\nu^n}\|\nu_n - \nu\|_{L^2_{-\alpha}(G_{1,2}(2))} \leq c_1(\alpha) n^{-1/2},$$

where $c_1(\alpha)$ is a constant depending only on α.

PROOF. Let $\tilde{\nu}$ denote the lift of ν to a distribution on $S^1 \times \mathbb{R}$ as in definition 3.8. Clearly $\tilde{\nu}$ has support on $S^1 \times [-1,1]$, hence on $S^1 \times [-2,2]$.

It is well-known that the set of functions $\{\frac{1}{\sqrt{8\pi}} e^{-i(\kappa_1\theta + (\pi/2)\kappa_2 s)}\}_{\kappa \in \mathbb{Z}^2}$ is an orthonormal basis for $L^2_0(S^1 \times 4\mathbb{T}^1)$. Since the map $U_\alpha : f \mapsto F^{-1}((1 + \kappa_1^2 + (\pi/2)^2\kappa_2^2)^{\alpha/2} F(f))$, where F denotes the Fourier transform, is an isometric isomorphism of $L^2_0(S^1 \times 4\mathbb{T}^1)$ onto $L^2_{-\alpha}(S^1 \times 4\mathbb{T}^1)$, cf. [**Tre67**, p. 330, prop. 31.8], the set of distributions

$$\{U_\alpha(\frac{1}{\sqrt{8\pi}} e^{-i(\kappa_1\theta + (\pi/2)\kappa_2 s)})\}_{\kappa \in \mathbb{Z}^2}$$
$$= \{\frac{1}{\sqrt{8\pi}} (1 + \kappa_1^2 + (\pi/2)^2\kappa_2^2)^{\alpha/2} e^{-i(\kappa_1\theta + (\pi/2)\kappa_2 s)}\}_{\kappa \in \mathbb{Z}^2}$$

is an orthonormal basis for $L^2_{-\alpha}(S^1 \times 4\mathbb{T}^1)$. For any distribution $v \in L^2_{-\alpha}(S^1 \times 4\mathbb{T}^1)$, we have

$$\|v\|^2_{L^2_{-\alpha}(S^1 \times 4\mathbb{T}^1)} = 8\pi \sum_{\kappa \in \mathbb{Z}^2} (1 + \kappa_1^2 + (\pi/2)^2\kappa_2^2)^{-\alpha} |\hat{v}(\kappa)|^2.$$

Since

$$[(\nu_n - \nu)^\sim]^\wedge(\kappa) = \frac{1}{\sqrt{8\pi}} \int_{S^1 \times 4\mathbb{T}^1} e^{-i(\kappa_1\theta + (\pi/2)\kappa_2 s)} d(\nu_n - \nu)^\sim$$
$$= \frac{1}{\sqrt{2\pi}} \int_{G_{1,2}} \cos(\kappa_1\theta + (\pi/2)\kappa_2 s) d(\nu_n - \nu),$$

it follows that

$$\|(\nu_n - \nu)^\sim\|^2_{L^2_{-\alpha}(S^1 \times 4\mathbb{T}^1)}$$
$$= 4 \sum_{\kappa \in \mathbb{Z}^2} (1 + \kappa_1^2 + (\pi/2)^2\kappa_2^2)^{-\alpha} \left(\int_{G_{1,2}} \cos(\kappa_1\theta + (\pi/2)\kappa_2 s) d(\nu_n - \nu)\right)^2.$$

By Jensen's inequality, we have

$$(E_{\nu^n}\|(\nu_n - \nu)^{\tilde{}}\|_{L^2_{-\alpha}(S^1 \times 4\mathbb{T}^1)})^2$$
$$\leq E(\|(\nu_n - \nu)^{\tilde{}}\|^2_{L^2_{-\alpha}(S^1 \times 4\mathbb{T}^1)})$$
$$= 4\sum_{\kappa \in \mathbb{Z}^2}(1 + \kappa_1^2 + (\pi/2)^2\kappa_2^2)^{-\alpha} E\left(\int_{G_{1,2}}\cos(\kappa_1\theta+(\pi/2)\kappa_2 s)\,d(\nu_n - \nu)\right)^2.$$

Now if ν is a probability measure with support on $G_{1,2}(1)$ and g is a measurable function on $G_{1,2}$ such that $|g| \leq 1$, $\int g\,d\nu_1$ (ν_1 denotes the empirical measure generated by one observations distributed according to ν) is a random variable with mean $\int g\,d\nu$ and variance

$$\int_{G_{1,2}} g^2\,d\nu - \left(\int_{G_{1,2}} g\,d\nu\right)^2.$$

Since the observations generating the empirical measure ν_n are independent, it follows that $\int g\,d\nu_n - \int g\,d\nu$ is a zero-mean random variable with variance

$$\frac{1}{n}\left[\int_{G_{1,2}} g^2\,d\nu - \left(\int g\,d\nu\right)^2\right] \leq \frac{1}{n}\int_{G_{1,2}} g^2\,d\nu$$
$$\leq n^{-1}.$$

Applying this result, it follows that

$$E_{\nu^n}\|(\nu_n - \nu)^{\tilde{}}\|_{L^2_{-\alpha}(S^1 \times 4\mathbb{T}^1)} \leq 2\left[\sum_{\kappa \in \mathbb{Z}^2}(1 + \kappa_1^2 + (\pi/2)^2\kappa_2^2)^{-\alpha}\right]^{1/2} n^{-1/2}.$$

An argument similar to the usual integral test shows that the infinite sum on the right-hand side of this inequality is finite. We now use def. 5.5 to conclude that

$$E\|\nu_n - \nu\|_{L^2_{-\alpha}(G_{1,2}(2))} \leq \sqrt{2}\left[\sum_{\kappa \in \mathbb{Z}^2}(1 + \kappa_1^2 + (\pi/2)^2\kappa_2^2)^{-\alpha}\right]^{1/2} n^{-1/2},$$

which is the desired result. ∎

REMARK A.2. We cannot take $\alpha \leq 1$ in prop. A.1 since $\|\nu_n - \nu\|_{L^2_{-\alpha}(G_{1,2}(2))}$ will not, in general, even be finite.

Appendix B. Radon transforms and Sobolev spaces

In this appendix, we will establish prop. B.13, which gives a bicontinuity result for the Radon transform with respect to topologies induced by certain Sobolev norms. This result is used in the proof of thm. 6.2. The starting point is prop. B.7, due to Hertle, which gives an estimate for the Radon transform and its inverse in terms of a different Sobolev norm on $S^1 \times \mathbb{R}$.

DEFINITION B.1. The Schwartz space $\mathcal{S}(S^1 \times \mathbb{R})$ is defined to be the subspace of $C^\infty(S^1 \times \mathbb{R})$ consisting of functions g such that

$$|g|_m \stackrel{\text{def}}{=} \sup_{j+k \leq m} \sup_{(\omega,s) \in S^1 \times \mathbb{R}} (1+s^2)^m |\partial_\theta^j \partial_s^k g(\omega,s)|,$$

where $j,k \in \mathbb{N}$, is finite for all $m \in \mathbb{N}$. We equip $\mathcal{S}(S^1 \times \mathbb{R})$ with the topology induced by the seminorms $|\cdot|_m$. The space of tempered distributions on $S^1 \times \mathbb{R}$, $\mathcal{S}'(S^1 \times \mathbb{R})$, is defined to be the space of continuous linear functionals on $\mathcal{S}(S^1 \times \mathbb{R})$.

DEFINITION B.2. On $\mathcal{S}(S^1 \times \mathbb{R})$, we take the Fourier transform to be the usual Fourier transform with respect to the second variable only, i.e.,

$$\hat{g}(\omega,\eta) \stackrel{\text{def}}{=} \int_\mathbb{R} e^{i2\pi\eta s} g(\omega,s)\, ds.$$

The Fourier transform on $\mathcal{S}'(S^1 \times \mathbb{R})$ is defined by duality.

DEFINITION B.3. The Sobolev space $L^2_{(0,\alpha)}(S^1 \times \mathbb{R})$ is defined to be the subspace of $\mathcal{S}'(S^1 \times \mathbb{R})$ whose elements v satisfy

$$\|v\|^2_{L^2_{(0,\alpha)}} \stackrel{\text{def}}{=} \int_{S^1} \int_\mathbb{R} (1+4\pi^2\eta^2)^\alpha |\hat{v}(\omega,\eta)|^2 \, d\eta \, d\sigma(\omega) < \infty,$$

where $\hat{v}(\theta,\eta)$ is defined as in definition B.2. $L^2_{(0,\alpha)}(S^1 \times \mathbb{R})$ is a Hilbert space with inner product

$$(v|w)_{L^2_{(0,\alpha)}} \stackrel{\text{def}}{=} \int_{S^1} \int_\mathbb{R} (1+4\pi^2\eta^2)^\alpha \hat{v}(\omega,\eta) \overline{\hat{w}(\omega,\eta)} \, d\eta \, d\sigma(\omega).$$

DEFINITION B.4. The Sobolev space $L^2_{(0,\alpha)}(G_{1,2})$ is defined to be the subspace of tempered distributions $v \in \mathcal{S}'(G_{1,2})$ such that $\tilde{v} \in L^2_{(0,\alpha)}(S^1 \times \mathbb{R})$. The squared norm on $L^2_{(0,\alpha)}(G_{1,2})$ is defined to be $1/2$ the squared norm of the corresponding elements of $L^2_{(0,\alpha)}(S^1 \times \mathbb{R})$.

LEMMA B.5. *The norms* $\|\cdot\|_{L^2_\alpha(S^1 \times 2r\mathbb{T}^1)}$ *and* $\|\cdot\|_{L^2_{(0,\alpha)}(S^1 \times \mathbb{R})}$ *are equivalent on* $\tilde{R}[L^2_{\alpha-1/2}(r\bar{\Omega})]$ *for* $\alpha \geq 0,$.

PROOF. The proof is fairly straightforward, but somewhat lengthy. The details may be found in [**Kur94**]. ∎

DEFINITION B.6. We will use the notation $r\bar{\Omega} \subset \mathbb{R}^2$ to denote the closed disk of radius r centered at the origin. The subspace of $L^2_\alpha(\mathbb{R}^d)$ consisting of distributions with support on $r\bar{\Omega}$ will be denoted by $L^2_\alpha(r\bar{\Omega})$. Similarly, the subspace of $L^2_{(0,\alpha)}(S^1 \times \mathbb{R})$ (resp. $L^2_{(0,\alpha)}(G_{1,2})$) consisting of distributions with support on $S^1 \times [-r,r]$ (resp. $G_{1,2}(r)$) will be denoted by $L^2_{(0,\alpha)}(S^1 \times [-r,r])$ (resp. $L^2_{(0,\alpha)}(G_{1,2}(r))$).

PROPOSITION B.7. *The maps* $R: L^2_\alpha(r\bar{\Omega}) \to L^2_{(0,\alpha+1/2)}(G_{1,2}(r))$ *and* $\widetilde{R}: L^2_\alpha(\bar{\Omega}) \to L^2_{(0,\alpha+1/2)}(S^1 \times [-r,r])$ *are bicontinuous into for all real* α.

PROOF. The result for $\widetilde{R}$ is proved in [**Her83**, thm. 3.1] (note that $L^2_\alpha(S^1 \times [-r,r])$ in the notation used in [**Her83**] is equivalent to $L^2_{(0,\alpha)}(S^1 \times [-r,r])$ in our notation). From the definitions, the result carries over to R as well. ∎

The Sobolev norm $\|\cdot\|_{L^2_{(0,\alpha)}(G_{1,2})}$ on $G_{1,2}$ is a natural norm with which to describe continuity properties of the Radon transform. On the other hand, the Sobolev norm $\|\cdot\|_{L^2_\alpha(G_{1,2}(2))}$ is a natural norm for describing statistical convergence, as seen in prop. A.1. The goal of the following sequence of lemmas is to prove prop. B.13, which shows that we can replace the Sobolev norm $\|\cdot\|_{L^2_{(0,\alpha+1/2)}(G_{1,2})}$ on $G_{1,2}$ in prop. B.7 with $\|\cdot\|_{L^2_{\alpha+1/2}(G_{1,2}(2))}$.

LEMMA B.8. *The map* $\widetilde{R}: L^2_\alpha(r\bar{\Omega}) \to L^2_{\alpha+1/2}(S^1 \times 2r\mathbb{T}^1)$ *is continuous for all* $\alpha \in \mathbb{R}$ *and bicontinuous into for all* $\alpha \geq -1/2$.

PROOF. Bicontinuity for $\alpha \geq -1/2$ is proved by combining prop. B.7 with lemma B.5. Continuity for $\alpha < -1/2$ follows from the continuity of the natural injection $L^2_{(0,\alpha+1/2)}(S^1 \times [-r,r]) \hookrightarrow L^2_{\alpha+1/2}(S^1 \times 2r\mathbb{T})$. ∎

DEFINITION B.9. For real $\alpha < d$, we define the Riesz potential operator I^α by
$$(I^\alpha f)\hat{\,}(\xi) \stackrel{\text{def}}{=} (2\pi|\xi|)^{-\alpha}\hat{f}(\xi)$$
for functions f on $\mathbb{R}^d$ for which it makes sense (cf., [**Ste70**, sec. V.1]). For $f \in \mathcal{S}(\mathbb{R}^2)$, $(I^\alpha f)\hat{\,} \in L^1(\mathbb{R}^2)$, so, by the Riemann-Lebesgue lemma [**Fol84**, thm 8.22(f)], $I^\alpha f$ is well defined. For $f \in \mathcal{S}(\mathbb{R}^2)$ and $|\alpha| < d$, we have $I^\alpha I^{-\alpha} f = f$ [**Nat86**, p. 18], [**Hel80**, thm. I.8.6]. On $\mathcal{S}(S^1 \times \mathbb{R})$, we define I^α to act on the second, or "s" variable, i.e., the operator is applied fiberwise.

LEMMA B.10. *For* $f \in L^2_{\alpha+1}(\mathbb{R}^2)$, $\|I^{-1}f\|_{L^2_\alpha(\mathbb{R}^2)} \leq \|f\|_{L^2_{\alpha+1}(\mathbb{R}^2)}$.

PROOF. An easy calculation. ∎

LEMMA B.11. *The map* $\widetilde{R}^*\widetilde{R}$ *is equal to the map* $4\pi I^1$ *on* $\mathcal{S}(\mathbb{R}^2)$.

PROOF. For $f \in \mathcal{S}(\mathbb{R}^2)$, we have the Radon transform inversion formula
$$f = \frac{1}{4\pi} I^{-1} \widetilde{R}^* \widetilde{R} f$$
[**Nat86**, p. 18, thm. 2.1]. Applying the map I^1 to both sides of this equation gives the identity
$$I^1 f = \frac{1}{4\pi} \widetilde{R}^* \widetilde{R} f,$$
i.e., $\widetilde{R}^*\widetilde{R} = 4\pi I^1$ on $\mathcal{S}(\mathbb{R}^2)$. ∎

COROLLARY B.12. *For $f \in \mathcal{S}(\mathbb{R}^2)$, we have the identity*
$$f = \frac{1}{4\pi} \widetilde{R}^* \widetilde{R} I^{-1} f.$$

PROOF. Apply lem. B.11 to the identity $f = I^1 I^{-1} f$. ∎

PROPOSITION B.13. *The maps $R : L^2_\alpha(\bar{\Omega}) \to L^2_{\alpha+1/2}(G_{1,2}(2))$ and $\widetilde{R} : L^2_\alpha(\bar{\Omega}) \to L^2_{\alpha+1/2}(S^1 \times 4\mathbb{T})$ are continuous for all real α and bicontinuous into for all $\alpha < -1/2$. In particular, there exists a constant $c_2(\alpha)$ such that $\|u\|_{L^2_\alpha(\mathbb{R}^2)} \le c_2(\alpha) \|Ru\|_{L^2_{\alpha+1/2}(G_{1,2}(2))}$ for all $u \in L^2_\alpha(\bar{\Omega})$.*

PROOF. It suffices to establish the result for $\widetilde{R}$, since the result for R will then follow easily from the definitions. The result for $\widetilde{R}$ was established in lem. B.8, except for the continuity of the inverse map for $\alpha < -1/2$. To show that the inverse map is continuous for $\alpha < -1/2$, suppose $\alpha < -1/2$ and $u \in L^2_\alpha(\bar{\Omega})$. Since $L^2_\alpha(\mathbb{R}^2)$ and $L^2_{-\alpha}(\mathbb{R}^2)$ are dual to each other [**Tre67**, p. 331, prop. 31.10] and $\mathcal{S}(\mathbb{R}^2)$ is dense in $L^2_\alpha(\mathbb{R}^2)$ [**Tre67**, p. 330, prop. 31.9],

$$\|u\|_{L^2_\alpha(\mathbb{R}^2)} = \sup_{f \in \mathcal{S}(\mathbb{R}^2) : \|f\|_{L^2_{-\alpha}(\mathbb{R}^2)} \le 1} |\langle u, f \rangle|.$$

By cor. B.12, we can rewrite this as

$$\|u\|_{L^2_\alpha(\mathbb{R}^2)} = \frac{1}{4\pi} \sup_{f \in \mathcal{S}(\mathbb{R}^2) : \|f\|_{L^2_{-\alpha}(\mathbb{R}^2)} \le 1} \left| \langle u, \widetilde{R}^* \widetilde{R} I^{-1} f \rangle \right|$$

$$= \frac{1}{4\pi} \sup_{f \in \mathcal{S}(\mathbb{R}^2) : \|f\|_{L^2_{-\alpha}(\mathbb{R}^2)} \le 1} |\langle \widetilde{R} u, \widetilde{R} I^{-1} f \rangle|.$$

Applying lem. B.10, it follows that

$$\|u\|_{L^2_\alpha(\mathbb{R}^2)} \le \frac{1}{4\pi} \sup_{\phi \in L^2_{-(\alpha+1)}(\mathbb{R}^2) : \|\phi\|_{L^2_{-(\alpha+1)}(\mathbb{R}^2)} \le 1} |\langle \widetilde{R} u, \widetilde{R} \phi \rangle|.$$

We now want to employ the portion of lem. B.8 regarding the continuity of $\widetilde{R}$. To do so, we must first restrict the set over which the supremum is taken in the above inequality to functions whose support is contained in a fixed compact set. Let $\chi \in C_c^\infty(\mathbb{R}^2)$ such that $\chi = 1$ on $\bar{\Omega}$ and $\chi = 0$ on $\mathbb{R}^2 \setminus 2\Omega$. Then there exists a constant $d_1(-(\alpha+1))$ such that $\|\chi \phi\|_{L^2_{-(\alpha+1)}(\mathbb{R}^2)} \le d_1(-(\alpha+1)) \|\phi\|_{L^2_{-(\alpha+1)}(\mathbb{R}^2)}$ for all $\phi \in L^2_{-(\alpha+1)}(\mathbb{R}^2)$. Thus, for each $\phi \in L^2_{-(\alpha+1)}(\mathbb{R}^2)$ such that $\|\phi\|_{L^2_{-(\alpha+1)}(\mathbb{R}^2)} \le 1$, $\|\chi \phi\|_{L^2_{-(\alpha+1)}(\mathbb{R}^2)} \le d_1(-(\alpha+1))$ and $\phi = \chi \phi$ on $\bar{\Omega}$. It follows that

$$\|u\|_{L^2_\alpha(\mathbb{R}^2)} \le \frac{1}{4\pi} d_1(-(\alpha+1)) \sup_{\phi \in L^2_{-(\alpha+1)}(2\bar{\Omega}) : \|\phi\|_{L^2_{-(\alpha+1)}(\mathbb{R}^2)} \le 1} |\langle \widetilde{R} u, \widetilde{R} \phi \rangle|.$$

By lem. B.8, there exist a constant $d_2(\alpha)$ such that

$$\|\widetilde{R} f\|_{L^2_{-(\alpha+1/2)}(S^1 \times 4\mathbb{T})} \le d_2(\alpha) \|f\|_{L^2_{-(\alpha+1)}(\mathbb{R}^2)}$$

for all $\phi \in L^2_{-(\alpha+1)}(2\bar{\Omega})$. Thus

$$\|u\|_{L^2_\alpha(\mathbb{R}^2)} \leq \frac{d_1(-(\alpha+1))d_2(\alpha)}{4\pi} \sup_{\|g\|_{L^2_{-(\alpha+1/2)}(S^1\times 4\mathbb{T}^1)} \leq 1} |\langle \widetilde{R}u, g\rangle|$$

$$= \frac{d_1(-(\alpha+1))d_2(\alpha)}{4\pi} \|\widetilde{R}u\|_{L^2_{-(\alpha+1/2)}(S^1\times 4\mathbb{T}^1)}.$$

∎

References

[Bak91] J. R. Baker, *Spatially variant tomographic imaging: Estimation, identification, and optimization*, Ph.D. thesis, University of California at Berkeley, Berkeley, CA, 1991.

[Dev87] L. Devroye, *A course in density estimation*, Birkhäuser, Boston, 1987.

[DL91] D. L. Donoho and R. C. Liu, *Geometrizing rates of convergence, II*, Ann. Statist. **19** (1991), 633–667.

[Fol84] G. B. Folland, *Real analysis*, John Wiley & Sons, New York, 1984.

[Gin75] E. Giné, *Invariant tests for uniformity on compact Riemannian manifolds based on Sobolev norms*, Ann. Probab. **3** (1975), 1243–1266.

[Hel80] S. Helgason, *The Radon transform*, Birkhauser, Boston, 1980.

[Her83] A. Hertle, *Continuity of the Radon transform and its inverse on Euclidean space*, Math. Z. **184** (1983), 165–192.

[Itô85] K. Itô, *Encyclopedic dictionary of mathematics*, second ed., MIT Press, Cambridge, MA, 1985.

[JS90] I. M. Johnstone and B. W. Silverman, *Speed of estimation in positron emission tomography and related inverse problems*, Ann. Statist. **18** (1990), 251–280.

[Kur94] A. Kuruc, *Probability measure estimation in positron emission tomography using loss functions based on Sobolev norms*, Ph.D. thesis, Massachusetts Institute of Technology, Cambridge, MA, expected 1994.

[Nat86] F. Natterer, *The mathematics of computed tomography*, John Wiley & Sons, New York, 1986.

[Ste70] E. M. Stein, *Singular integrals and differentiability properties of integrals*, Princeton University Press, Princeton, NJ, 1970.

[Str85] H. Strasser, *Mathematical theory of statistics*, Walter de Gruyter, New York, 1985.

[Tre67] F. Treves, *Topological vector spaces, distributions, and kernels*, Academic Press, New York, 1967.

[VSK85] Y. Vardi, L. A. Shepp, and L. Kaufman, *A statistical model for positron emission tomography*, J. Amer. Stat. Assn. **80** (1985), 8–20.

Department of Mathematics, Massachusetts Institute of Technology, Cambridge, MA 02139

Current address: Center for Functional Imaging, Lawrence Berkeley Laboratory, Berkeley, CA 94720

E-mail address: kuruc@imasun.lbl.gov

On stability estimates in the exterior problem for the Radon Transform

SERGUEI LISSIANOI

ABSTRACT. We consider the problem of stability estimates for inversion of the Radon transform in the exterior of a disk. We show that there are no Hölder type stability estimates, even if we want to reconstruct a function in an annulus that is smaller than the one, where the Radon data is given.

1. Introduction

We consider the following problem. Let $F(x)$ be a compactly supported function in the plane $\mathbf{R}^2$, and $G=RF$ be its Radon transform. The following stability estimate is well known [6]:

$$\|F\|_{H_0^s} \leq C \|RF\|_{H_0^{s+1/2}}, \tag{1}$$

where H^α are the standard Sobolev spaces defined on natural domains. Let us assume now that the Radon data $G(s,\omega) = RF$ is given only for those lines $x \cdot \omega = s$ that do not intersect some fixed disk $D_Q = \{x \in \mathbf{R}^2 : |x| < Q\}$, i.e. for $|s| > Q$ (here $\omega \in S^1$, $x \in \mathbf{R}^2$ and $x \cdot \omega = x_1\omega_1 + x_2\omega_2$). It is known that (at least in the case of compactly supported functions) the values of $F(x)$ outside D_Q can be uniquely determined by the data (see [3], [6]). On the other hand, this exterior problem does not have nice stability property (1) any more [6]. In fact, it was shown in [2] and [6] that there is no estimate

$$\|F\|_{H_0^s(|x|>Q)} \leq C \|RF\|_{H_0^{s+t}(|s|>Q)} \tag{2}$$

1991 *Mathematics Subject Classification*. Primary 44A12, Secondary 35S30.

The work was partially supported by the Wesley Foundation Grant no.9012019 and NSF EPSCOR Grant.

This paper is in final form and no version of it will be submittedd for publication elsewhere

for a positive s, no matter how large t is. High instabilities are rather normal in many inverse problems. Sometimes, however, inverse problems admit a scale of estimates weaker than the Lipschitzian (2) ones (see [4]). For instance, sometimes there exist $C, s, m > 0$ and $0 < \gamma \leq 1$ such that for an operator A we have the following Hölder estimate:

$$\|F\|_{H^s} \leq C \|F\|_{H^m}^{1-\gamma} \|AF\|_{H^m}^{\gamma}. \tag{3}$$

Even weaker is the following logarithmic estimate:

$$\|F\|_{H^s} \leq d(\|F\|_{H^m}) (|\ln \|AF\|_{H^m}|)^{-\alpha} \tag{4}$$

for some $\alpha > 0$. Here $d(\cdot)$ is some bounded function.

It has been shown by P.Kuchment (unpublished) that there is no Hölder estimate (3) for the exterior Radon problem. In [5] V.Isakov and Ziqi Sun proved a result which implies the following logarithmic estimate for the exterior problem:

$$\|F\|_{L^2(|x|>Q)} \leq d\left(\|F\|_{C^1(\mathbf{R}^2)}\right) \left(|\ln \|RF\|_{H^1(|s|>Q)}|\right)^{-\alpha} \quad (0 < \alpha \leq 1).$$

Now the following question arises. *Assume that we need to recover only the values of $F(x)$ for $|x| > Q + \epsilon$ for some positive ϵ. Is it possible in this case to get at least a Hölder estimate of the following type:*

$$\|F\|_{L^2(|x|>Q+\epsilon)} \leq C \|F\|_{H^k(|x|>Q)}^{1-\gamma} \|RF\|_{H^k(|s|>Q)}^{\gamma} ?$$

We show that estimates of this kind do not exist.

2. The main result.

Theorem. *Let Q, P and ϵ be fixed, $0 < Q < P < \infty$, $\epsilon > 0, Q + \epsilon < P$. There exists a sequence of C^∞ functions F_l supported in the set $\{x \in \mathbf{R}^2 : Q \leq |x| \leq P\}$, for which no estimate of the form*

$$\|F_l\|_{L^2(|x|>Q+\epsilon)} \leq C \|F_l\|_{H^k(|x|>Q)}^{1-\gamma} \|RF_l\|_{H^k(|s|>Q)}^{\gamma}$$

can hold for any $C > 0$, $k \geq 0$, $0 < \gamma < 1$.

Proof. First of all, if the inequality is correct, then we can assume that k is an integer. Let $F_l(r, \varphi) = f(r) e^{il\varphi}, l = 2, 4, ..$, where $f(r) \in C^\infty(\mathbf{R}_+)$, $supp f \subset \{r \in \mathbf{R} : Q + \epsilon < r < P\}$, and $f(r) \geq 0$. We have: $\|F_l\|_{H^k(|x|>Q)} \leq M(k) l^k$ and $\|F_l\|_{L^2(|x|>Q+\epsilon)} = const \neq 0$. From the direct Cormack's formula (see, for instance [6]) we obtain:

$$G_l(\omega, s) := (RF_l)(\omega, s) = g_l(s) e^{il\varphi},$$

where $\omega = (\cos \varphi, \sin \varphi)$, and g_l is given by

$$g_l(s) = 2 \int_s^{+\infty} T_l\left(\frac{s}{r}\right) \left(1 - \frac{s^2}{r^2}\right)^{-1/2} f(r) dr$$

Here $T_l(t)$ is the Chebyshev polynomial of the first kind, i.e. $T_l(t) = \cos(l \arccos t)$ for $|t| \leq 1$. After some change of variables we obtain:

(5) $$g_l(s) = 2s \int_0^1 T_l(u) \frac{f\left(\frac{s}{u}\right)}{u^2 \sqrt{1-u^2}} du.$$

For any $k \in \mathbf{Z}+$ we consider the integral

(6) $$\int_0^1 T_l(u) \frac{f^{(k)}\left(\frac{s}{u}\right)}{u^{2+k} \sqrt{1-u^2}} du$$

as a function of s for $s \in [Q, P]$. The integral is proper at 0 and converges uniformly at 1, since: $\mathrm{supp} f^{(k)} \subset [Q, P]$, and $f^{(k)}(s/u) u^{-(2+k)} = 0$ when $u < Q/P$. Indeed, $u < Q/P$ implies $s/u > (sP)/Q \geq P$. Thus we have:

(7) $$\left| \frac{f^{(k)}\left(\frac{s}{u}\right)}{u^{2+k}} \right| \leq \left(\frac{P}{Q}\right)^{2+k} \max_{t \in \mathbf{R}+} \left| f^{(k)}(t) \right|$$

Therefore, we can differentiate (5) k times with respect to s and obtain:

$$g_l^{(k)}(s) = 2s \int_0^1 T_l(u) \frac{f^{(k)}\left(\frac{s}{u}\right)}{u^{2+k} \sqrt{1-u^2}} du + 2k \int_0^1 T_l(u) \frac{f^{(k-1)}\left(\frac{s}{u}\right)}{u^{1+k} \sqrt{1-u^2}} du.$$

The function f was originally defined on $[0, +\infty)$. We now extend it to $(-\infty, +\infty)$ as an even function. Then $f^{(k)}(s/u) (u^{2+k} \sqrt{1-u^2})^{-1}$ is also even and we can write

(8) $$g_l^{(k)}(s) = s \int_{-1}^1 T_l(u) \frac{f^{(k)}\left(\frac{s}{u}\right)}{u^{2+k} \sqrt{1-u^2}} du + k \int_{-1}^1 T_l(u) \frac{f^{(k-1)}\left(\frac{s}{u}\right)}{u^{1+k} \sqrt{1-u^2}} du.$$

Let us denote $f^{(k)}(s/u) u^{-(2+k)}$ by $b_{s,k}(u)$. Then (8) can be written as follows:

$$g_l^{(k)}(s) = s(T_l, b_{s,k}) + k(T_l, b_{s,k-1}).$$

Here the parenthesis denote the inner product in the space $L^2([-1,1], (1-u^2)^{-1/2})$. The Chebyshev polynomials T_l form (up to a constant factor) an orthonormal system in this space. Hence, $g_l^{(k)}(s)$ is the sum (up to the factors s and k) of the l-th coefficients of the Chebyshev expansion of the functions $b_{s,k}$

and $b_{s,k-1}$ on $[-1, 1]$. We now make use of the theorem 4.4.5 (i) from [1] (p.131), concluding that $\left|g_l^{(k)}(s)\right| \leq C(E_{l-1}(b_{s,k}) + E_{l-1}(b_{s,k-1}))$, where $E_n(h)$ denotes the error of the best uniform approximation of the function h by the polynomials of degree less than or equal to n. Now observe that for $s \in [Q, P]$ the functions $b_{s,k}$ belong to $C^\infty[-1, 1]$. Applying Jackson's Theorem IV ([1], p.145), we get for any $p \in \mathbf{Z}+$:

$$\left|g_l^{(k)}(s)\right| \leq C \frac{1}{l^p} \left(\left\|b_{s,k}^{(p)}\right\|_{C[-1;1]} + \left\|b_{s,k-1}^{(p)}\right\|_{C[-1;1]} \right). \tag{9}$$

The derivatives $b_{s,k}^{(p)}(u) = \frac{\partial^p}{\partial u^p} \left(f^{(k)}(s/u) u^{-(2+k)} \right)$ can be calculated by the Leibniz' rule as

$$\sum_{j=0}^{p} \binom{p}{j} \frac{\partial^j}{\partial u^j} \left(f^{(k)} \left(\frac{s}{u} \right) \right) \frac{d^{p-j}}{du^{p-j}} \left(\frac{1}{u^{k+2}} \right).$$

Applying the chain rule, we can represent this as a sum of expressions of the following type: $Cf^{(\alpha)}(s/u) s^\beta u^{-\delta}$, where the constants C, α, β and δ are bounded for fixed k and p. We recall now that $f(s/u) = 0$ for $u < Q/P$, so the norm of the whole sum representing $b_{s,k}^{(p)}$ is bounded for $s \in [Q, P]$ by a quantity which depends on k and p only. Combining this with (9), we get for any $p \in \mathbf{Z}+$:

$$\left|g_l^{(k)}(s)\right| \leq \frac{C_1(k,p)}{l^p} \tag{10}$$

Now we can estimate the Sobolev norms of the Radon transforms of the functions F_l:

$$\|G_l\|_{H^k(|s|>Q)} \leq C |l|^{2k} \|g_l(s)\|_{H^k([Q;P])}^2 = C |l|^{2k} \sum_{j=0}^{k} \int_Q^P \left(g_l^{(j)}(s) \right)^2 ds.$$

By the inequality (10) this is less than $C_2(k,p)/l^{2p-2k}$. Since p is arbitrary, we get:

$$\|G_l\|_{H^k(|s|>Q)} \leq C_3(k,p) |l|^{-p}. \tag{11}$$

Assume now that there exist C, k, γ such that for any l the following inequality is satisfied:

$$\|F_l\|_{L^2(|x|>Q+\epsilon)} \leq C \|F_l\|_{H^k(|x|>Q)}^{1-\gamma} \|RF_l\|_{H^k(|s|>Q)}^{\gamma}.$$

Then for any $p \in \mathbf{Z}+$ we have:

$$const = \|F_l\|_{L^2(|x|>Q+\epsilon)} \leq C \|F_l\|_{H^k(|x|>Q)}^{1-\gamma} \|RF_l\|_{H^k(|s|>Q)}^{\gamma} \leq C(k,p) l^{k(1-\gamma)-p\gamma}.$$

Choosing $p > (k(1-\gamma) + 1)\gamma^{-1}$, we get contradiction. The theorem is proved.

Acknowledgements

The author thanks Professor Peter Kuchment for his help and support.

References

1. Cheney, E. W., *Introduction to the approximation theory.* McGraw-Hill, New York, 1966.
2. Finch, D. V., *Cone beam reconstruction with sources on a curve.* SIAM J. Appl. Math. **43** 428-48.
3. Helgason, S., *Groups and Geometric Analysis.* Academic Press, New York, 1984.
4. Isakov, V., *Inverse source problems.* AMS, Providence, Rhode Island, 1990.
5. Isakov, V. and Ziqi Sun, *Stability estimates for hyperbolic inverse problems with local boundary data.* Inverse Problems **8** (1992) 193-206.
6. Natterer, F., *The mathematics of the computerized tomography.* Wiley, New York, 1986.

DEPARTMENT OF MATHEMATICS AND STATISTICS, WICHITA STATE UNIVERSITY, WICHITA, KS, 67260-0033

E-mail address: lissiano@twsuvm.bitnet

Data Correction and Restoration in Emission Tomography

SERGE J. LVIN

ABSTRACT. A method of correction of emission tomography data and of restoration of the unknown part of the data is obtained. The method forces the data to belong to the range of the exponential Radon transform.

1. Introduction

The problem of Single Photon Emission Computed Tomography (SPECT) in the case of a constant attenuation coefficient $\mu > 0$ and known boundary of the body can be reduced (see [1],[2]) to inverting the exponential Radon transform R_μ, that is, to solving the equation

$$(R_\mu F)(\phi, p) \equiv \int_{x \cdot \omega = p} F(x) \exp(\mu x \cdot \omega^\perp) d\sigma = G(\phi, p).$$

Here $F(x)$ is an unknown compactly supported function on the plane (tomogram), $G(\phi, p)$ is a known real valued function which is 2π-periodic in the angle variable ϕ and compactly supported in the variable p, $\omega = (\cos\phi, \sin\phi)$, $\omega^\perp = (-\sin\phi, \cos\phi)$, $d\sigma$ is the usual linear measure on the line $x \cdot \omega = p$, and μ is a nonzero constant. We suppose that F and G are infinitely smooth.

Let us denote by $g(\phi, \xi)$ the Fourier image with respect to the second variable of the function G:

$$g(\phi, \xi) = \frac{1}{\sqrt{2\pi}} \int G(\phi, p) \exp(-i\xi p) dp.$$

1991 *Mathematics Subject Classification.* Primary: 65R10, Secondary:44A12, 92C55.

The author thanks Prof. W. Bray and Prof. P. Kuchment for helpful discussions and Prof. Markovsky for his help with numerical examples.

This paper is in final form and no version of it will be submitted for publication elsewhere.

In this paper we will call the function g the emission tomography data. If G belongs to the range of the operator R_μ, then we will say that g is from the range of the operator $\widetilde{R_\mu}$.

Let us expand the function $g(\phi, \xi)$ into the complex Fourier series in the variable ϕ:

$$g(\phi, \xi) = \sum g_n(\xi) \exp(in\phi),$$

$$g_n(\xi) = \frac{1}{2\pi} \int g(\phi, \xi) \exp(-in\phi) d\phi.$$

The function g cannot be arbitrary. It was proved in [3] that the necessary and sufficient condition for g to belong to the range of the operator $\widetilde{R_\mu}$ is evenness of the functions $(\mu+\xi)^n g_n(\xi)$ in the variable ξ for all integers n, i.e. the fulfillment of the identity

(1) $$(\mu + \xi)^n g_n(\xi) = (\mu - \xi)^n g_n(-\xi), \ n \in \mathbf{Z}.$$

The data that we measure in emission tomography generally speaking does not satisfy condition (1) because the mathematical model cannot represent all real aspects of collection of the data (for instance, noise or measurement errors). Condition (1) enables us to correct the measured data, that is to decrease the discrepancy between the measured data and the ideal one. Using corrected data can bring us to a more precise tomogram F.

If we consider the emission tomography problem when the data is known only for $0 \leq \phi \leq \Delta$, where $\Delta < 2\pi$, then condition (1) gives us some additional information which helps to restore the unknown part of the data. This enables us to find the tomogram based on incomplete data.

In the case of transmission tomography, which corresponds to $\mu = 0$, methods of finding a tomogram based on incomplete data were discussed, for example, in [2], Chapter 6. Our approach is not appropriate in this case, since when $\mu = 0$ conditions (1) do not completely describe the range of the operator R_μ, but simply mean that $G(\phi + \pi, p) = G(\phi, -p)$. The last identity has been used before in transmission tomography for determining $G(\phi, p)$ for $\pi < \phi \leq 2\pi$ [2].

2. Data restoration

Let us suppose that the data $g^0(\phi, \xi)$ is measured only for $0 \leq \phi \leq \Delta$, where $\Delta < 2\pi$. Our problem is to restore the function $g^0(\phi, \xi)$ for all $0 \leq \phi \leq 2\pi$.

Let us introduce the following polynomials:

(2) $$a_n(\xi) = (\mu - \xi \, sgn \, n)^{|n|}, n \in \mathbf{Z},$$

where $a_0(\xi) = 1$. Then equality (1) can be rewritten in the form

(3) $$a_n(-\xi) g_n(\xi) = a_n(\xi) g_n(-\xi), n \in \mathbf{Z}.$$

We try to find $g(\phi, \xi)$ in the form of a finite Fourier series in the variable ϕ. It follows from (3) that coefficients of this series can be written in the form

$$g_n(\xi) = a_n(\xi) z_n(\xi)$$

where $z_n(\xi)$ are even functions in the variable ξ. So, we look for $g(\phi, \xi)$ of the form

(4) $$g(\phi, \xi) = \sum_{|n| \leq N} a_n(\xi) z_n(\xi) \exp(in\phi),$$

where $z_n(\xi)$ are even functions, which have to be found. It is also desirable that

(5) $$g(\phi, \xi) = g^0(\phi, \xi) \text{ for } 0 \leq \phi \leq \Delta, \xi \in \mathbf{R}.$$

However, generally speaking it is impossible to satisfy (5) even in the case $N = \infty$ unless $g^0(\phi, \xi)$ is the restriction onto the interval $0 \leq \phi \leq \Delta$ of a function from the range of the operator $\widetilde{R_\mu}$. That is why we change the condition (5) to the condition

(6) $$\|g(\phi, \xi) - g^0(\phi, \xi)\|_{L_2([0,\Delta] \times \mathbf{R})} \text{ is minimal.}$$

Let us denote by $z(\xi)$ the column vector

$$z(\xi) = col[z_n(\xi)]_{n=-N}^{N}.$$

Then (4) can be written as

$$g(\phi, \xi) = A(\phi, \xi) z(\xi),$$

where $A(\phi, \xi)$ is the row operator

(7) $$A(\phi, \xi) = row[a_n(\xi) \exp(in\phi)]_{n=-N}^{N}.$$

Using the evenness of $z(\xi)$, condition (6) can be written now in the form

(8) $$\|\widehat{A} z(\xi) - \widehat{g^0}\|_{L_2([0,\Delta] \times \mathbf{R})} \text{ is minimal,}$$

where

$$\widehat{A} = \begin{bmatrix} A(\phi, \xi) \\ A(\phi, -\xi) \end{bmatrix}, \widehat{g^0} = \begin{bmatrix} g^0(\phi, \xi) \\ g^0(\phi, -\xi) \end{bmatrix}.$$

We consider here $z(\xi)$ only for $\xi \geq 0$. After solving (8) we can extend $z(\xi)$ to all $\xi \in \mathbf{R}$ using evenness of this vector function.

Let us also mention that we would like the function $g(\phi, \xi)$ to be the Fourier image of a real valued function, that is, the coefficients $g_n(\xi)$ must satisfy the condition $\overline{g_n(\xi)} = g_{-n}(-\xi)$. The functions $z_n(\xi)$ have to satisfy the condition

(9) $$\overline{z_n(\xi)} = z_{-n}(\xi).$$

We will check this condition after solving (8).

It is known (see [4]) that instead of (8) it is sufficient to solve the equation

(10) $$\widehat{A}^+ \widehat{A} z = \widehat{A}^+ \widehat{g^0},$$

where $\widehat{A}^+$ is the dual operator to $\widehat{A}$. The operator $\widehat{A}^+$ can be found as

$$\widehat{A}^+ = [A^*(\xi), A^*(-\xi)],$$

where

$$A^*(\xi)g(\phi,\xi) = \int_0^\Delta \overline{A^\tau(\phi,\xi)} g(\phi,\xi) d\phi$$

(we use the notation A^τ for the transpose matrix to A). Then the right hand side in (10) is

(11) $$\widehat{A}^+ \widehat{g}^0 = \int_0^\Delta (\overline{A^\tau(\phi,\xi)} g^0(\phi,\xi) + \overline{A^\tau(\phi,-\xi)} g^0(\phi,-\xi)) d\phi.$$

Let us find now the left hand side of (10). The matrix operator $\widehat{A}^+ \widehat{A}$ can be represented as

(12) $$\widehat{A}^+ \widehat{A} = [b_{mn}(\xi) c_{mn}(\xi)]_{m,n=-N}^N,$$

where

(13) $$\begin{aligned} b_{mn}(\xi) &= a_m(\xi) a_n(\xi) + a_m(-\xi) a_n(-\xi), \\ c_{mm} &= \Delta, \\ c_{mn} &= i(n-m)^{-1}(1 - \exp(i(n-m)\Delta)) \text{ for } m \neq n. \end{aligned}$$

The matrix $\widehat{A}^+ \widehat{A}$ is self-adjoint and positive definite for all $\xi \geq 0$. Non obvious here is only that its kernel is trivial.

If some vector z is in the kernel of the operator $\widehat{A}^+ \widehat{A}$, then it is also in the kernel of the operator $\widehat{A}$, i.e.

$$A(\phi,\xi)z = 0 \text{ and } A(\phi,-\xi)z = 0 \text{ for } \phi \in [0,\Delta].$$

Analyticity of these expressions implies that they are equal to zero for all ϕ. Hence,

$$a_n(\xi) z_n = 0 \text{ and } a_n(-\xi) z_n = 0 \text{ for all } |n| \leq N.$$

When $\mu \geq 0$ this implies that $z_n = 0$, i.e. $z = 0$. Therefore, the kernel of the operator $\widehat{A}^+ \widehat{A}$ is trivial.

It is easy to see that if we consider the equation (10) for all $\xi \in \mathbf{R}$, then its right hand side is an even smooth function of ξ. The matrix functions $\widehat{A}^+ \widehat{A}$ and $(\widehat{A}^+ \widehat{A})^{-1}$ are also even and smooth. This proves that $z(\xi)$ is a smooth function at the origin, if we extend it to $\xi < 0$ as an even function.

Now, when expressions for the both sides of (10) are available, it is easy to check that if $g^0(\phi,\xi)$ is the Fourier image of a real valued function (i.e. $\overline{g^0(\phi,\xi)} = g^0(\phi,-\xi)$), then $\overline{z(\xi)}$ satisfies the same equation as the vector $[z_n(\xi)]_{n=-N}^N$. This proves that $z(\xi)$ satisfies the condition (9).

Let us denote by $C_{2\pi}^\infty S$ the subspace of 2π-periodic (in the variable ϕ) functions $g(\phi, \xi)$ in the space $C^\infty[0, 2\pi] \otimes S(\mathbf{R})$, where $S(\mathbf{R})$ is the Schwartz space. Then the following statement holds:

THEOREM 1. *Let $g^0(\phi, \xi)$ be a function in $C^\infty[0, \Delta] \otimes S(\mathbf{R})$. Then the N-th order trigonometrical polynomial $g(\phi, \xi)$ that satisfies (1) and (6) can be uniquely found by*

1) solving for all $\xi \geq 0$ the system (10) that has a positive definite matrix;
2) extending the solution $z(\xi)$ to all ξ as an even vector function;
3) substituting $z(\xi) = [z_n(\xi)]_{n=-N}^N$ into the formula (4).

This function $g(\phi, \xi)$ belongs to $C_{2\pi}^\infty S$ and it is the Fourier image of a real valued function, if the function $g^0(\phi, \xi)$ has the same property.

(We remind the reader that the expressions involved into (10) and (4) are given by formulas (11), (7), (12), (13), and (2).)

3. Data correction

We consider now the case when the measured data $g^0(\phi, \xi)$ is known for all values of the angle ϕ, but it does not belong to the range of the operator $\widetilde{R}_\mu$. We would like to correct g^0 in such a way that the corrected function belongs to that range, i.e. satisfies (1). This problem could be considered independently of the previous one. We prefer, however, to look at it as at the particular case of data restoration for $\Delta = 2\pi$.

Let us denote by $g_n^0(\xi)$ the Fourier coefficients of the function $g^0(\phi, \xi)$. Then the formula (11) can be written for $\Delta = 2\pi$ as

$$\widehat{A}^+ \widehat{g}^0 = [2\pi(a_n(\xi)g_n^0(\xi) + a_n(-\xi)g_n^0(-\xi))]_{n=-N}^N.$$

All the coefficients c_{mn} in (12) are zeros when $m \neq n$ and $\Delta = 2\pi$. Hence, the matrix $\widehat{A}^+ \widehat{A}$ is diagonal and we can easily find $z(\xi)$ from (10):

$$z(\xi) = [\beta_n(\xi)(a_n(\xi)g_n^0(\xi) + a_n(-\xi)g_n^0(-\xi))]_{n=-N}^N,$$

where

(14) $$\beta_n(\xi) = (a_n^2(\xi) + a_n^2(-\xi))^{-1}.$$

Using (4) we can find now the corrected data

(15) $$g(\phi, \xi) = \sum_{|n| \leq N} \beta_n(\xi)(a_n^2(\xi)g_n^0(\xi) + a_n(\xi)a_n(-\xi)g_n^0(-\xi)) \exp(in\phi).$$

We eliminated here all the coefficients $g_n^0(\xi)$ for $|n| > N$ and corrected each of the remaining coefficients by

$$g_n(\xi) - g_n^0(\xi) = \beta_n(\xi)(-a_n^2(-\xi)g_n^0(\xi) + a_n(\xi)a_n(-\xi)g_n^0(-\xi)).$$

If we do not eliminate the tail coefficients, we obtain the function

$$(16) \quad g^1 = g^0 - \sum_{|n| \leq N} \beta_n(\xi)(a_n^2(-\xi)g_n^0(\xi) - a_n(\xi)a_n(-\xi)g_n^0(-\xi)) \exp(in\phi).$$

The L_2-distance between g and g^0 is larger than between g^1 and g^0, but g is in the range of $\widetilde{R}_\mu$, while only the terms g_n^1 of g^1 for $|n| \leq N$ are in the range.

In the case $N = \infty$ there is no difference between g and g^1. There is no convergence problem when $N \to \infty$, since the absolute values of the coefficients $\beta_n(\xi)a_n^2(\xi)$, $\beta_n(\xi)a_n^2(-\xi)$, and $\beta_n(\xi)a_n(\xi)a_n(-\xi)$ in the series (15) and (16) are bounded by one.

THEOREM 2. *Let the function $g^0(\phi, \xi)$ belong to $C_{2\pi}^\infty S$. Then the function $g(\phi, \xi)$ given by (15) also belongs to $C_{2\pi}^\infty S$ and it is the L_2-nearest to $g^0(\phi, \xi)$ Nth order trigonometric polynomial whose Fourier coefficients satisfy (1).*

The function $g^1(\phi, \xi)$ given by (16) is the L_2-nearest to $g^0(\phi, \xi)$ function in $C_{2\pi}^\infty S$ whose Fourier coefficients satisfy (1) for all $|n| \leq N$.

Functions $g(\phi, \xi)$ and $g^1(\phi, \xi)$ are Fourier images (in the second variable) of real valued functions, if the function $g^0(\phi, \xi)$ has the same property.

The expressions involved in (15) and (16) above are given by the formulas (14) and (2).

4. Concluding remarks

1. Our procedure of data restoration is as a matter of fact the procedure of the orthogonal projection of the measured data onto the subspace of trigonometric polynomials of order N in the variable ϕ with coefficients satisfying the property (1). It is possible to avoid the most laborious part of this procedure, namely the inversion of the matrix $\widehat{A}^+(\xi)\widehat{A}(\xi)$ for all $\xi \geq 0$, if we divide the procedure into two steps. On the first step one finds the orthogonal projection $g^*(\phi, \xi)$ of the data $g^0(\phi, \xi)$ onto the subspace of general trigonometrical polynomials in the variable ϕ. On the second step one finds the orthogonal projection of $g^*(\phi, \xi)$ onto the subspace of trigonometric polynomials with the property (1). The second step is nothing but the procedure of data correction described in the section 3. On the first step we need to invert only a self-adjoint matrix which does not depend on the variable ξ. Alternatively, one can simply expand g into a series of functions $exp(in\phi)$ that have been orthogonalized first on the interval $[0, \Delta]$.

2. The procedure of data correction can be written as the sum of two convolutions:

$$g(\phi, \xi) = \int K_1(\phi - \psi, \xi) g^0(\psi, \xi) d\psi + \int K_2(\phi - \psi, \xi) g^0(\psi, -\xi) d\psi.$$

It can be also written as the sum of convolutions of the initial function $G^0(\phi,p)$ as follows:

$$G(\phi,p) = \int\int K_3(\phi-\psi,p-q)G^0(\psi,q)d\psi dq + \int\int K_4(\phi-\psi,p-q)G^0(\psi,-q)d\psi dq.$$

The kernels K_i can be found in advance.

References

[1] Markoe, A., *Fourier inversion of the attenuated X-ray transform*, SIAM J. Math. Anal. **15**(1984), 718-722.

[2] Natterer, F., *The Mathematics of Computerized Tomography*, Wiley, New York, 1986.

[3] Kuchment, P. and Lvin, S., *Paley-Wiener theorem for exponential Radon transform*, Acta Applicandae Mathematicae, **18**(1990), 251-260.

[4] Curtain, R. and Pritchard, A., *Functional Analysis in Modern Applied Mathematics*, Academic Press, New York, 1977.

Department of Mathematics, University of Maine, Orono, ME 04469
E-mail address: lvin@maine.maine.edu

On Problems of Integral Geometry in the non-Convex Domains

R. Mukhometov

ABSTRACT. This paper deals with the uniqueness and stability problem of integral geometry in bounded non-convex domains in R^2. At the end of the paper this problem is investigated in R^n, $n \geq 2$. We succeed in reducing this problem to a known problem which is considered in the convex domain.

1. Introduction

In [1–2] the following problem of integral geometry was considered. Suppose M is a bounded domain in R^n with a piecewise smooth boundary ∂M and a given Riemannian metric g. The domain M is convex relative to the geodesics with respect to the metric g, and the family K of all geodesics is regular in M. This means that the set of all geodesics that go out from a fixed point do not have caustics; any geodesic $k(y, y_1)$ goes out to its ends y, y_1 on the boundary of M; for each pair of points on M there is a unique geodesic that connects them. For any curve $k \in K$ we know the integral of the function $u = u(x)$, $x \in M \bigcup \partial M$. It is required to determine $u(x)$ from this information.

---

[0]1991 *Mathematical Subject Classification.* Primary 53C65. The author was supported by International Science Foundation. This paper is in final form and no version of this paper will appear elsewhere

A stability estimate is obtained for this problem. The same result is correct in $n = 2$ for a family K that consists of arbitrary curves (not geodesics) satisfying analogous regularity conditions. In [3] the same problem has been considered in the Finsler space.

In this paper, the same problem is considered but in the case of a non-convex domain, $M \subset R^2$.

2. The problem

For simplification let the domain M be as in Figure 1 and let the family K consist of all the linear segments with ends on ∂M and that entirely belong to M. The points b_1 and b_2 are the points of inflection. We separate the boundary ∂M into $\partial_1 M$ and $\partial_2 M$ where $\partial_1 M$ is the non-convex part of the boundary that is the closed arc $b_1 b_2$ and $\partial_2 M$ is the closure of the remaining part of ∂M. Otherwise the proofs will be made as if K are curves. Later we extend the result to this case. For $n = 2$, the curves of K do not have to be the geodesics of some metric. The family K must satisfy analogous regularity conditions excepting one condition. There are pairs of points on ∂M for which the curve connecting these points does not exist. Suppose that for every interior point $x \in M$ and every direction θ there is a curve in K that passes through x in the direction θ. Assume the same for the points $x \in \partial M$ and for the directions θ inside M.

Let M be a compact manifold with boundary ∂M. We denote by TM_x the tangent vectors $a \neq 0$ lying above the point $x \in M$ and by TM the join of these manifolds over all $x \in M$. As $M \subset R^2$, we introduce the global coordinate system (x^1, x^2) in M. This coordinate system defines coordinates (a^1, a^2) for every vector $a \in TM_x$. The collection of numbers (x^1, x^2, a^1, a^2) defines the coordinate system in TM.

Let $F = F(x, a)$ be the Finsler metric in M. This metric, F, is a smooth function on TM that satisfies the following conditions:

1) $F(x, ka) = |k| F(x, a)$, $k \in R$;

2) $F(x, a) > 0$, if $a \neq 0$;

3) The Hessian $\left(\frac{1}{2} \frac{\partial^2 F^2}{\partial a^i \partial a^j} \right)$ is positive definite.

A Finsler metric is said to be *smooth* as long as its derivatives up to order three exist. As a special case, F may be a Riemannian metric.

On TM a smooth function $Q(x,a)$ of (x,a) is given that satisfies the condition

$$Q(x, ta) = |t|Q(x, a), \quad t \in R, \quad t \neq 0.$$

We denote by $k(x,y)$ the arc of the curve of K connecting the points $x, y \in M$. Let $\tilde{x} = \tilde{x}(t)$ be a parameterization of this arc. For each arc $k(x,y)$ we define the function

$$w(x, y) = \int_{k(x,y)} u(\tilde{x}) Q(\tilde{x}, \tilde{a}) dt, \quad \tilde{a} = \frac{d}{dt}\tilde{x}(t),$$

where $u(x)$, $x \in \bar{M}$ is some function. Let $\rho(x, a) = Q(x,a)\big/F(x,a)$, we get

(2.1) $\quad w(x, y) = \int_{k(x,y)} u(\tilde{x}) \rho(\tilde{x}, \tilde{a}) ds, \quad ds = F(\tilde{x}, \tilde{a}) dt.$

The weight function ρ satisfies the condition

$$\rho(x, ta) = \rho(x, a), \quad t \in R, \quad t \neq 0.$$

We formulate the following problem of integral geometry. For any curve $k \in K$ we know the integral (2.1) of the function $u = u(x)$, $x \in \bar{M}$, over the whole curve k with given weight function $\rho = \rho(x, a)$, $(x, a) \in T\bar{M}$. It is required to determine $u = u(x)$, $x \in \bar{M}$.

As the domain M is non-convex with respect the family K then there are pairs $(x, y) \in \partial M \times \partial M$ for which the function $w(x, y)$ is not defined.

3. Preliminary information and the family of curves K

Many of the mentioned formulas for a Finsler metric in this section are given in [3, 5]. Some of the formulas will be given with proofs. We denote by

$$g_{ij} = \frac{1}{2} \frac{\partial^2 F^2}{\partial a^i \partial a^j}$$

and by the (g^{ij}) matrix inverse to (g_{ij}). The components g_{ij} form a covariant tensor of the second rank. For each $a \in TM$, we define the covector $b = (b_i)$, $b_i = g_{ij}(x, a)a^j$, and conversely $a^i = g^{ij} b_j$. As usual, we use summation notation and the summation from 1 to 2 is made for having the same indexes. Since $b_i = F\partial F/\partial a^i$, we have

$$(3.1) \qquad \frac{a^i}{F} = g^{ij}\frac{\partial F}{\partial a^j} \quad \text{and} \quad \frac{\partial F}{\partial a^i} = \frac{1}{F}g_{ij}a^j, \quad i = 1, 2.$$

We prove

$$(3.2) \qquad \frac{\partial}{\partial a^k}\left(g^{ij}\frac{\partial F}{\partial a^j}\right) = g^{ij}\frac{\partial^2 F}{\partial a^j \partial a^k}.$$

We have

$$\frac{\partial}{\partial a^k}\left(g^{ij}\frac{\partial F}{\partial a^j}\right) = g^{ij}\frac{\partial^2 F}{\partial a^j \partial a^k} + \frac{\partial g^{ij}}{\partial b^l}\frac{\partial F}{\partial a^j}\frac{\partial b^l}{\partial a^k}.$$

It is required to prove that the last term is equal to zero. Since

$$g^{ij}(x, b) = \frac{1}{2}\frac{\partial^2 H^2(x, b)}{\partial b_i \partial b_j},$$

where H is the Hamiltonian function for the Lagrangian $F(x, a)$, $H(x, b)$ is homogeneous of degree 1 in b. Hence, g^{ij} is homogeneous of degree zero. Since the tensor $\partial g^{ij}/\partial b^l$ is symmetric relative to all three indexes and $\partial F/\partial a^j = F^{-1}b_j$, we have

$$\frac{\partial g^{ij}}{\partial b_l}b_j = 0$$

and (3.2) follows. From the definition of the reciprocal matrix we have

$$(3.3) \qquad g_{11} = g^{22}\det(g_{ij}), \quad g_{22} = g^{11}\det(g_{ij}),$$
$$g_{12} = -g^{12}\det(g_{ij}).$$

Substituting these formulas in (3.1), we get

$$(3.4) \qquad \frac{\partial F}{\partial a^1} = \frac{\det(g_{ij})}{F}\left(g^{22}a^1 - g^{12}a^2\right),$$

$$\frac{\partial F}{\partial a^2} = \frac{\det(g_{ij})}{F}\left(g^{11}a^2 - g^{12}a^1\right).$$

The formula,

$$(3.5) \qquad \frac{\partial^2 F}{\partial a^i \partial a^j} = -\frac{1}{F}\frac{\partial F}{\partial a^i}\frac{\partial F}{\partial a^j} + \frac{1}{F}g_{ij}$$

that follows from the definition of g_{ij}, is necessary below.

Let SM be the manifold with boundary of all pairs (x, θ), $x \in M$, θ is a direction in TM_x. If the point x is fixed the set $\{(x, \theta)\}$ is denoted by SM_x.

Define the form

$$\eta = \frac{\partial F}{\partial a^1} dx^1 + \frac{\partial F}{\partial a^2} dx^2$$

on TM. This form does not depend on the choice of the coordinates. The function $F(x, a)$ is homogeneous by a therefore the form η is defined on SM and in this connection the vector $a = a(\theta)$ depends smoothly on θ. The form $\omega = -\eta \wedge d\eta$ on SM is a form of highest degree. It is easy to check that $\omega = -\eta \wedge d_a \eta$, since the form ω on SM contains terms that differ from zero only of the kind $dx^i \wedge dx^j \wedge da^k$, $i, j, k = 1, 2$.

Lemma 1. The form ω is positive on SM and

$$\omega = F^{-2} \det(g_{ij}) \, dx \wedge \left(a^1 da^2 - a^2 da^1 \right), \quad dx = dx^1 \wedge dx^2.$$

Proof. Using (3.1), (3.3) and (3.4) we obtain the required formula for ω:

$$\omega = -\frac{\partial F}{\partial a^i} dx^i \wedge \frac{\partial^2 F}{\partial a^k \partial a^j} da^k \wedge dx^j =$$

$$= \left(\frac{\partial F}{\partial a^1} \frac{\partial^2 F}{\partial a^2 \partial a^k} - \frac{\partial F}{\partial a^2} \frac{\partial^2 F}{\partial a^1 \partial a^k} \right) dx \wedge da^k =$$

$$= \frac{1}{F^2} \left(g_{11} g_{2k} a^1 + g_{12} g_{2k} a^2 - g_{21} g_{1k} a^1 - g_{22} g_{1k} a^2 \right) dx \wedge da^k =$$

$$= \frac{\det(g_{ij})}{F^2} dx \wedge \left(a^1 da^2 - a^2 da^1 \right).$$

From the last expression we see that the form ω is positive and the lemma follows.

Let $k(x, y)$ be the arc of some curve from K that goes out from the point $x \in M$ along the direction θ and intersects the boundary ∂M at the point y. The set of all $y \in \partial M$ that connect to some arc $k(x, y)$ with the fixed point x consists of subsets belonging to $\partial_1 M$ and ∂M_2. These subsets are denoted respectively by $D_1(x)$ and $D_2(x)$. We have $D_1(x) \bigcup D_2(x) = \partial M$ for the points x inside the domain $c_1 c_2 o$

and $D_1(x) \cup D_2(x) \neq \partial M$ for the points x inside ob_1b_2. Let S_iM_x be the set of directions θ from the point x corresponding to $y \in D_i(x)$, $i = 1, 2$. It is obvious that $S_1M_x \cup S_2M_x = SM_x$. Let $P_i = \{(x,y)|x \in M, y \in D_i(x)\}$ and $S_iM = \{(x,\theta)|x \in M, \theta \in S_iM_x\}$ ($i = 1, 2$). The mapping $\beta_i : (x,y) \in P_i \to (x,\theta) \in S_iM_x$ is a diffeomorphism. For the inverse mapping β_i^{-1} denote $y_i = y_i(x,a)$, $a = a(\theta)$, $a \in TM_x$, $a(\theta)$ depends smoothly on θ and $a = a(\theta)$ is a smooth convex hypersurface in TM_x. We shall write $y_i = y_i(x,\theta)$ instead of $y_i = y_i(x,a)$ also.

Consider the boundaries of the manifold with boundary P_1, P_2 and divide the boundary $\partial(P_1 \cup P_2)$ into B_{22}, B_{21}, B_{12}, B_0, B_{00}, $\tilde{B}_0$, $\tilde{B}_{00}$. The boundary B_{22} is that part of $\partial(P_1 \cup P_2)$ which belongs to $\partial_2 M \times \partial_2 M$. Analogously, $B_{21} \subset \partial_2 M \times \partial_1 M$ and $B_{12} \subset \partial_1 M \times \partial_2 M$. Note that the points of $\partial_1 M \times \partial_1 M$ are absent from $\partial(P_1 \cup P_2)$. In short, the set $B = B_{22} \cup B_{21} \cup B_{12} \subset \partial M \times \partial M$ consists of pairs of points on ∂M such that a curve in K connecting them exists. For every point $z \in \partial_1 M$ there exist three curves $k(z, y_1)$, $k(z, y_2)$ and $k(y_1, z, y_2)$ of K that touch $\partial_1 M$ in the point z. Here the curve passing through y_1, z, y_2 is denote by $k(y_1, z, y_2)$. Such a curve must exist in K. We denote by J_0 the set of all points of M that are covered by curves of the type $k(z, y_1)$ where $z \in \partial_1 M$ and y_1 belongs the arc $b_2 y_1 c_1$ (see Figure 1). Analogously let J_{00} denote the set of points in M that are covered by all curves of the type $k(z, y_2)$ where $z \in \partial_1 M$ and y_2 belongs the arc $c_2 y_2 b_1$. Note that the arc $b_1 b_2$ is the envelope for the curves of the type $k(z, y_1)$ and for the curves of the type $k(z, y_2)$. The sets

$$\tilde{B}_0 = \{(x,z)| z \in \partial_1 M, x \in k(z,y), y \in b_2 y_1 c_1\},$$
$$B_0 = \{(x,y)|x \in k(y,z,\tilde{y}) \& k(z,\tilde{y}), z \in \partial_1 M, \tilde{y} \in b_2 y_1 c_1\} \quad \text{and}$$
$$\tilde{B}_{00} = \{(x,z)|z \in \partial_1 M, x \in k(z,y) \, y \in c_2 y_2 b_1\},$$
$$B_{00} = \{(x,y)|x \in k(y,z,\tilde{y}) \& k(z,\tilde{y}) \, z \in \partial_1 M, \tilde{y} \in c_2 y_2 b_1\}$$

will be needed below. Note that
$\partial(P_1 \cup P_2) = B \cup (B_0 \cup \tilde{B}_0) \cup (B_{00} \cup \tilde{B}_{00})$.

On the curve ∂M we introduce the coordinate system $\{t\}$ with initial point on the arc $c_1 c_2$ where t is the length of the curve that is measured from the initial point counter-clockwise. Let the equation of the curve ∂M be $y = y(t)$. For the part $\partial_1 M$ of the curve ∂M we replace the variable y by z, so that the equation $\partial_1 M$ is $z = z(t)$.

We define the diffeomorphism Ψ mapping the pair $(x,y) \in B_0$ to the pair $(x,z) \in \tilde{B}_0$ as follows. For each $y \in c_2 y_2 b_1$, a point $z \in \partial_1 M$ exists such that the curve $k(y,z) \in K$ touches $\partial_1 M$ at the point z. Assume that the diffeomorphism $z = z_0(y)$ exists for these y and z. For every such curve $k(y,z)$ a curve $k(y,z,\tilde{y}) \in K$ exists that contains the curves $k(y,z)$ and $k(z,\tilde{y})$, $\tilde{y} \in b_2 y_1 c_1$. For fixed y and hence for $z = z_0(y)$ the mapping Ψ taking the pair (x,y) to the pair (x,z) can be evaluated for every $x \in k(z,\tilde{y})$. Thus the diffeomorphism Ψ is defined by the diffeomorphism $z = z_0(y)$ and $x \in k(z,\tilde{y})$ identically maps in x. The same holds for the diffeomorphisms Ψ_0 for the sets $B_{00}, \tilde{B}_{00}$ and $z = z_{00}(y)$.

B_0 and $\tilde{B}_0$ are bundle manifolds with different bases $\{y\}, \{z\} \subset \partial M$ but with the same fibers. In this connection the mapping Ψ is the mapping between the identical points of the fibers. We introduce the bundle map $(\tilde{t}, \tilde{\tau})$ on $\tilde{B}_0$ where $\tilde{t}$ is the other designation of the parameter t of the curve $\partial_1 M$ and $\tilde{\tau}$ is the arc length of the curve $k(z(\tilde{t}), \tilde{y})$, $\tilde{y} \in b_2 y_1 c_1$ from the point $z(\tilde{t})$ to the point $x \in k(z(\tilde{t}), \tilde{y})$. If M is the domain of the Euclidean space and K is the family of the linear segment then $x = z(\tilde{t}) + \tilde{\tau} z_{\tilde{t}}(\tilde{t})$, $y = z(\tilde{t})$. If F is the Finsler metric then $x = x(z(\tilde{t}), z_{\tilde{t}}(\tilde{t}), \tilde{\tau})$, $y = z(\tilde{t})$ or $x = x(\tilde{t}, \tilde{\tau})$, $y = z(\tilde{t})$ are the continuously differentiated functions. Analogously (t, τ) is the bundle map on B_0 where t is the parameter of the curve ∂M, τ is the arc length of the curve $k(y(t), z, \tilde{y})$, $\tilde{y} \in b_2 y_1 c_1$ from the point $y(t) \in \partial M$ to the point $x \in k(z, \tilde{y})$ and $z = z_0(y)$. If M is the domain of the Euclidean space and K is the family of the linear segment then $x = y(t) + \tau \xi(t)$, $y = y(t)$ where the vector $\xi(t)$ points so that $k(y(t), z, \tilde{y})$ touches $\partial_1 M$. If F is the Finsler metric then $x = x_0(t, \tau)$, $y = y(t)$ are continuously differentiated functions.

The mapping Ψ between the manifolds $B_0 \to \tilde{B}_0$ induces the mapping between the maps $\{(t, \tau)\} \to \{(\tilde{t}, \tilde{\tau})\}$ that has the view $\tilde{t} = \tilde{t}(t)$ $\tilde{\tau} = \tau - T(t)$ where $T(t)$ is the length of the curve $k(y(t), z)$, $z = z_0(y)$. We assume the Jacobian this mapping $J = \tilde{t}_t < 0$. Therefore the mapping Ψ does not preserve the orientations of B_0 and $\tilde{B}_0$.

4. The main result

THEOREM. For $u(x) \in C^1(\bar{M})$, $F(x,a) \in C^3(T\bar{M})$ and $\rho(x,a) \in C^1(T\bar{M})$,

(4.1) $$\int_M u^2(x) \int_S \left(F^{-2}\rho^2 - g^{ij}\frac{\partial \rho}{\partial a^i}\frac{\partial \rho}{\partial a^j} \right) \det(g_{ij}) d\theta dx < I,$$

$$I = -\int_B \frac{\partial w(y(t), y(l))}{\partial t}\frac{\partial w(y(t), y(l))}{\partial l} dt \wedge dl +$$
$$+ \int_{B_0} \rho u(x) \frac{\partial w(z_0(y(t)), y(t))}{\partial t} dt \wedge d\tau$$
$$- \int_{B_{00}} \rho u(x) \frac{\partial w(z_{00}(y(t)), y(t))}{\partial t} dt \wedge d\tau$$

where $x = x_0(t,\tau)$ on B_0 and on B_{00} $x = x_{00}(t,\tau)$ is the function that is analogous to $x = x_0(t,\tau)$; S is the unit sphere in TM_x, θ is the angular variable, $a = a(\theta)$, and the function w is the data of the problem.

Corollary 1. If in (4.1) the weight function $\rho(x,a)$ satisfies the condition

$$\int_S \left(F^{-2}\rho^2 - g^{ij}\frac{\partial \rho}{\partial a^i}\frac{\partial \rho}{\partial a^j} \right) \det(g_{ij}) d\theta \geq 0$$

and this integral may be equal to zero only on a subset of M of measure zero then the uniqueness of the solution of the problem follows.

Corollary 2. If F is the Riemannian metric and $\rho \equiv 1$ then

(4.2) $$2\pi \int_M u^2(x) dv \leq I,$$

where $dv = \sqrt{\det(g_{ij})} dx$ is the element of the Riemannian volume.

Let F be the Riemannian metric and the family K consists of the geodesics of this metric only. If $u \equiv 1$ then the function w, the data of our problem, is the length $\tau(y, y_1)$ of the geodesic that joins points $y, y_1 \in \partial M$. Using the method of the proof of the theorem above we obtain the next formula for the Riemannian volume of the non-convex domain M.

$$2\pi \int_M \sqrt{\det(g_{ij})}dx = -\int_B \frac{\partial \tau(y(t), y_1(l))}{\partial t} \frac{\partial \tau(y(t), y_1(l))}{\partial l} dt dl +$$

$$+ \int_{\partial_1 M} \tilde{T}(t) \frac{\partial (T_0 - T_{00})}{\partial t} dt,$$

where $T_0(t)$ is the length $\tau(z(t), y_0(z(t)))$, $T_{00}(t)$ is the length $\tau(y_{00}(z(t)), z(t))$, $\tilde{T}(t) = T_0(t) + T_{00}(t)$, $y = y_0(z)$ and $y = y_{00}(z)$ are the inverse mappings respectively for $z = z_0(y)$ and $z = z_{00}(y)$.

Remark 1. The stability estimate is not completely useful because the presence in (4.1) the integral of the product of the unknown function $u(x)$ and the derivative of the known function w. If $w(z_0(y(t)), y(t)) = 0$ and $w(z_{00}(y(t)), y(t)) = 0$, i.e., the integrals along the curves which are touched $\partial_1 M$ are equal zero, then the stability estimate is obtained. We may make the conclusion that the integrals along these curves must be count exacter.

5. The auxiliary statements

We do not introduce the index i for the function $w = w(x, y)$, $(x, y) \in P_i$, $i = 1, 2$, to simplify notation.

1-form $d_x w = (\partial w / \partial x^j) dx^j$ on P_i is preimage some form $w_j dx^j$ on $TS_i M$, $i = 1, 2$. Obviously

$$w_j(x, a(\theta)) = \left.\frac{\partial w(x, y)}{\partial x^j}\right|_{y = y(x, a(\theta))}, \quad j = 1, 2.$$

Lemma 2. We have the equality

$$\left(w_i w_j g^{ij} + 2Fug^{ij} w_i \frac{\partial \rho}{\partial a^j}\right)\omega = -d_x w \wedge d d_x w + d\left[w_i \frac{a^i}{F} d_x w \wedge \eta\right],$$

where $df = d_x f + d_a f$, $d_x f = (\partial f / \partial x^i) dx^i$, $d_a f = (\partial f / \partial a^i) da^i$ for every smooth function $f = f(x, a)$ on SM and $d_x w = w_i dx^i$.

Proof. Note that the forms $d_x w$, η and $w_i \frac{a^i}{F}$ (the derivative in the direction of $\frac{a}{F}$) do not depend on the coordinate system. Write the form $d_x w \wedge d\left(w_i \frac{a^i}{F}\right) \wedge \eta$ as follows

(5. 1) $$d_x w \wedge d\left(w_i \frac{a^i}{F}\right) \wedge \eta = A_1 + A_2,$$

$$A_1 = d_x w \wedge \frac{\partial w_i}{\partial a^j} \cdot \frac{a^i}{F} da^j \wedge \eta,$$

$$A_2 = d_x w \wedge w_i \frac{\partial}{\partial a^j}\left(\frac{a^i}{F}\right) da^j \wedge \eta.$$

On the other hand

(5. 2) $$d_x w \wedge d\left(w_i \frac{a^i}{F}\right) \wedge \eta = B_1 + B_2 + B_3,$$

$$B_1 = -d\left[\left(w_i \frac{a^i}{F}\right) d_x w \wedge \eta\right],$$

$$B_2 = \left(w_i \frac{a^i}{F}\right) d_a d_x w \wedge \eta,$$

$$B_3 = -\left(w_i \frac{a^i}{F}\right) d_x w \wedge d_a \eta.$$

The proof of the lemma is then reduced to the proof of the following equalities

(5. 3) $\qquad A_2 + B_3 = w_i w_j g^{ij} \omega$

(5. 4) $\qquad A_1 + B_2 = d_x w \wedge d d_x w$

(5. 5) $\quad -2 d_x w \wedge d\left(w_i \frac{a^i}{F}\right) \wedge \eta = 2 F u \left(g^{ij} w_i \frac{\partial \rho}{\partial a^j}\right) \omega.$

In fact, we obtain the lemma if we add (5.3)–(5.5) with the equality

$$B_1 = -d\left[\left(w_i \frac{a^i}{F}\right) d_x w \wedge \eta\right],$$

and note that the left-hand sides in (5.1), (5.2) and (5.5) add to give zero.

The proof of (5.5): letting $w_i \frac{a^i}{F} = -u\rho$ we have

$$-2 d_x w \wedge d_a\left(w_i \frac{a^i}{F}\right) \wedge \eta = 2u d_x w \wedge \frac{\partial \rho}{\partial a^i} da^i \wedge \frac{\partial F}{\partial a^j} dx^j.$$

Using $(\partial\rho/\partial a^i)\, a^i = 0$ and the formulas (3.4) for $(\partial F/\partial a^j)$ we get (5.5).

The proof of (5.3): Substituting a^i/F in A_2 and B_3 by the formulas (3.1) and using (3.2) we get

$$A_2 + B_3 = d_x w \wedge \left(w_i g^{il} \frac{\partial^2 F}{\partial a^l \partial a^j} \right) da^j \wedge \frac{\partial F}{\partial a^k} dx^k -$$

$$- \left(w_i g^{ik} \frac{\partial F}{\partial a^k} \right) d_x w \wedge \frac{\partial^2 F}{\partial a^i \partial a^j} da^j \wedge dx^i.$$

Using (3.1) and (3.5) for $\partial F/\partial a^i$ and $\partial^2 F/\partial a^i \partial a^j$ the equality

$$A_2 + B_3 = -\frac{1}{F^2} w_m dx^m \wedge \left(w_l a^l g_{ij} - w_j a^k g_{ik} \right) da^j \wedge dx^i$$

is obtained. Substituting here g_{ij} by g^{ij} in accord with (3.3), we get (5.3).

The proof of (5.4): Substituting $\partial F/\partial a^i$ by the forms (3.1) and using $F^2 = g_{ij} a^i a^j$ after the addition of similar terms, we have

$$A_1 + B_2 = (-1)^i \frac{\partial w_l}{\partial a^k} \frac{a^l}{F} w_i \sum_{m \neq i} g_{mj} dx \wedge da^k -$$

$$- \frac{(-1)^l}{F} \frac{\partial w_l}{\partial a^k} w_i \frac{a^i}{F} \sum_{m \neq l} g_{mj} a^j dx \wedge da^k =$$

$$= \left(w_2 \frac{\partial w_1}{\partial a^k} - w_1 \frac{\partial w_2}{\partial a^k} \right) dx \wedge da^k = d_x w \wedge d_a d_x w = d_x w \wedge dd_x w$$

Lemma 2 is proved.

Lemma 3*. We have the inequality

$$(5.\,6) \quad g^{ij} w_i w_j + F^2 u^2 g^{ij} \frac{\partial \rho}{\partial a^i} \frac{\partial \rho}{\partial a^j} + 2 F u g^{ij} w_j \frac{\partial \rho}{\partial a^i} - u^2 \rho^2 \geq 0$$

on SM.

Proof. Denoting by

$$\rho_i = \frac{\partial \rho}{\partial a^i}, \quad F_i = \frac{\partial F}{\partial a^i}, \quad \rho^i = g^{ij} \rho_j, \quad w^i = g^{ij} w_j$$

[0]V.A. Sharafutdinov orally informed the author of this lemma.

and using the formulas

$$F_i \frac{a^i}{F} = 1, \quad \frac{a^i}{F} = g^{ij} F_j$$

and also

$$w_i \frac{a^i}{F} = -u\rho, \quad \frac{a^i}{F} \rho_i = 0, \quad \rho^i F_i = 0,$$

we transform the left side in (5.6)

$$w_i w^i + (Fu\rho^i)(Fu\rho_i) + (u\rho F_i)\left(u\rho \frac{a^i}{F}\right) + 2\left(Fu\rho^i + u\rho \frac{a^i}{F}\right) w_i =$$

$$= \left(Fu\rho^i + u\rho \frac{a^i}{F} + w^i\right)(Fu\rho_i + u\rho F_i + w_i) =$$

$$= g^{ij}(Fu\rho_j + u\rho F_j + w_j)(Fu\rho_i + u\rho F_i + w_i) \geq 0$$

and the lemma follows.

6. The proof of the theorem

We deduct the inequality (5.6) multiplied on the positive form of the highest degree on SM from the equality in lemma 2 and get

$$(6.\,1) \quad u^2 \left(\rho^2 - F^2 g^{ij} \frac{\partial \rho}{\partial a^i} \frac{\partial \rho}{\partial a^j}\right) \omega \leq$$

$$\leq -d_x w \wedge dd_x w + d\left[w_i \frac{a^i}{F} d_x w \wedge \eta\right].$$

This inequality is integrated on the manifold with boundary SM.

$$(6.\,2) \quad \int_M u^2(x) \int_{SM_x} \left(F^{-2}\rho^2 - g^{ij} \frac{\partial \rho}{\partial a^i} \frac{\partial \rho}{\partial a^j}\right) \omega \leq I,$$

$$I = \int_{SM} -d_x w \wedge dd_x w + d\left[w_i \frac{a^i}{F} d_x w \wedge \eta\right].$$

We transform the right side of (6.2). With the help of the diffeomorphisms β_i we make the change of variables $(x, \theta) \mapsto (x, y)$ in the integrals to the right in (6.2), in this connection we suppress the indexes in P_i, β_i, and get

$$I = I_1 + I_2, \quad I_1 = \int_P -d_x w \wedge dd_x w, \quad I_2 = \int_P d\left[w_i \frac{a^i}{F} d_x w \wedge \beta^* \eta\right].$$

We prove that the form in the integral I_1 is exact integrand.

$$d_x w \wedge dd_x w = dw \wedge dd_x w = -d[dw \wedge d_x w] = d[d_x w \wedge d_y w].$$

Here the first equality holds since P has dimension 1 in y. So granting $w_i(a^i/F) = -\rho u$ we have

$$I = -\int_P d\varphi, \quad \varphi = \rho u d_x w \wedge \beta^* \eta + d_x w \wedge d_y w$$

and using Stokes formula we get

(6. 3) $$I = -\int_{\partial P} \varphi.$$

Recall that $\partial P = B \cup \left(B_0 \cup \tilde{B}_0\right) \cup \left(B_{00} \cup \tilde{B}_{00}\right)$. Our purpose is to express I by the data of the problem.

(6. 4) $$-\int_B \varphi = -\int_B d_x w \wedge d_y w =$$

$$= -\int_B \frac{\partial w(y(t), y(l))}{\partial t} \frac{\partial w(y(t), y(l))}{\partial l} dt \wedge dl$$

since B has dimension 1 for every x and y.

Consider the form φ on B_0 and $\tilde{B}_0$. We express the function $w = w(x, y)$ on B_0 by the function $w = w(x, z)$ on $\tilde{B}_0$ and the data of our problem with the help of the mapping $z = z_0(y)$ according to the formula

(6. 5) $$w(x, y) = w(x, z_0(y)) + w(z_0(y), y).$$

Here in the right side $w(z_0(y), y)$ is the known function from the data of the problem. The next equality is true.

(6. 6) $$\beta_2^* \eta|_{B_0} = \psi^* \beta_1^* \eta|_{\tilde{B}_0} = \frac{\partial F}{\partial a^1} dx^1 + \frac{\partial F}{\partial a^2} dx^2.$$

Note that

$$\beta_1^* \eta = -d_x \tau(x, z), \quad \beta_2^* \eta = -d_x \tau(x, y).$$

if the family K consists of the geodesics, where $\tau(x,z)$ is the length of the geodesic $k(x,z)$. Using (6.6) in the right side (6.3) we have the integral

$$-\int_{\tilde{B}_0} \varphi, \quad \varphi = \rho u d_x w(x,z) \wedge \left(\frac{\partial F}{\partial a^1}dx^1 + \frac{\partial F}{\partial a^2}dx^2\right) +$$
$$+ d_x w(x,z) \wedge d_z w(x,z).$$

On the other hand substituting $w(x,y)$ by the formula (6.5) in the form φ of the integral $-\int_{B_0}$ we have

(6.7) $$-\int_{B_0} \varphi = -\int_{B_0} \varphi_1 - \int_{B_0} \varphi_2,$$

$$\varphi_1 = \rho u d_x w(x, z_0(y)) \wedge \left(\frac{\partial F}{\partial a^1}dx^1 + \frac{\partial F}{\partial a^2}dx^2\right) +$$
$$+ d_x w(x, z_0(y)) \wedge d_y w(x, z_0(y)),$$

$$\varphi_2 = \rho u d_x w(z_0(y), y) \wedge \left(\frac{\partial F}{\partial a^1}dx^1 + \frac{\partial F}{\partial a^2}dx^2\right) +$$
$$+ d_x w(x, z_0(y)) \wedge d_y w(z_0(y), y) +$$
$$+ d_x w(z_0(y), y) \wedge d_y w(x, z_0(y)) +$$
$$+ d_x w(z_0(y), y) \wedge d_y w(z_0(y), y).$$

Lemma 4.

(6.8) $$\int_{\tilde{B}_0} \varphi - \int_{B_0} \varphi_1 = 0.$$

Proof. The form φ on $\tilde{B}_0$ is written as follows.

$$\varphi = \left[\rho u \left(\frac{\partial w}{\partial x^1}\frac{\partial F}{\partial a^2} - \frac{\partial w}{\partial x^2}\frac{\partial F}{\partial a^1}\right)\frac{D(x^1, x^2)}{D(\tilde{t}, \tilde{\tau})} - \right.$$
$$\left. - \left(\frac{\partial w}{\partial z^i}\frac{dz^i}{d\tilde{t}}\right)\left(\frac{\partial w}{\partial x^i}\frac{\partial x^i}{\partial \tilde{\tau}}\right)\right] d\tilde{t} \wedge d\tilde{\tau}.$$

Analogously, the form φ_1 on B_0 is written

$$\varphi_1 = \left[\rho u \left(\frac{\partial w(x, z_0(y))}{\partial x^1}\frac{\partial F}{\partial a^2} - \frac{\partial w}{\partial x^2}\frac{\partial F}{\partial a^1}\right)\frac{D(x^1, x^2)}{D(t, \tau)} - \right.$$

$$- \left(\frac{\partial w}{\partial z_0^j} \frac{dz_0^j}{dy^i} \frac{dy^i}{dt}\right) \left(\frac{\partial w}{\partial x^i} \frac{\partial x^i}{\partial \tau}\right)\bigg] dt \wedge d\tau.$$

In the form φ_1 we pass to the variables $(\tilde{t}, \tilde{\tau})$.

$$dt \wedge d\tau = \frac{D(t,\tau)}{D(\tilde{t},\tilde{\tau})} d\tilde{t} \wedge d\tilde{\tau} = t_{\tilde{t}} d\tilde{t} \wedge d\tilde{\tau}, \quad \frac{\partial x^i}{\partial \tau} = \frac{\partial x^i}{\partial \tilde{\tau}}.$$

Substituting these formulas in φ_1 this form and φ coincide, i.e.

(6. 9) $$\left(\psi^{-1}\right)^* \varphi_1 = \varphi$$

Since $t_{\tilde{t}} < 0$ the mapping Ψ does not preserve the orientation. From here and (6.9) the lemma follows.

Lemma 5.

(6. 10) $$-\int_{B_0} \varphi_2 = \int_{B_0} \rho u(x) \frac{\partial w\left(z_0(y(t)), y(t)\right)}{\partial t} dt \wedge d\tau$$

where $w(z(t), t)$ is the known function from the data of the problem.

Proof. Since $d_x w\left(z_0(y), y\right) = 0$ we have

$$\varphi_2 = d_x w\left(x, z_0(y)\right) \wedge d_y w\left(z_0(y), y\right).$$

It is obvious that

(6. 11) $$d_y w\left(z_0(y(t)), y(t)\right) = \frac{\partial w\left(z_0(y(t)), y(t)\right)}{\partial t} dt.$$

Therefore in the form $d_x w\left(x, z_0(y)\right)$ for us only the forms with $d\tau$ have meaning.

(6. 12) $$d_x w\left(x, z_0(y)\right) = \frac{\partial w}{\partial x^i} \frac{\partial x^i}{\partial \tau} d\tau + \ldots = \frac{\partial w}{\partial \tau} d\tau + \ldots =$$

$$= \rho u(x) d\tau + \ldots$$

From (6.11) and (6.12) the lemma follows.

For the form φ on the manifolds B_{00} and $\tilde{B}_{00}$ the statements that are analogs of Lemmas 4 and 5 are correct but in (6.10) the right side has a minus sign.

Using (6.4), (6.8) and (6.10) for obtaining the right side in (3.1) of the theorem and (6.2) for obtaining the left side in (3.1) we get the final estimate of the theorem.

In Sections 2 and 3 under the description of the family K we consider all curves k given by line segments. We describe the family K that consists of these following curves. The convex part $\partial_2 M$ and the family K must possess the following property. For every interior point $y \in \partial_2 M$ its neighborhood $U_y \subset \partial_2 M$ exists and the $k(y, y_1) \in K$ with the ends y and y_1 exists for every point $y_1 \in U_y$. The limit $k(y, y_1)$ is the point y as y_1 approaches y. Now, consider the concave part $\partial_1 M$. Every curve $k \in K$ may have no more one point on $\partial_1 M$. For every internal point $z \in \partial_1 M$ a unique curve $k(y_1, z, y_2) \in K$ exists with the ends $y_1, y_2 \in \partial_2 M$ such that $k(y_1, z, y_2)$ touches $\partial_1 M$ in a unique point z. In this connection the curves $k(y_1, z)$ and $k(z, y_2)$ belong to K also. The points y_1 or y_2 coincide with z if z is the end $\partial_1 M$. The ends b_1 and b_2 are analogs of the points of inflection for the curves of K. The curvature of the curve $\partial_1 M$ at the point b_1 must coincide with the curvature of the curve $k(c_1, b_1)$ at b_1, and analogously for the point b_2. This proves the theorem.

7. Remarks

1. In the proof of the theorem the function $t = t(\tilde{t})$ and its derivative $t_{\tilde{t}}$ that must be negative are used. We give an example of the part ∂M with a point of inflection. Let the equation ∂M be

$$y = \begin{cases} x^2, & x > 0 \\ -x^2, & x \leq 0. \end{cases}$$

It follows that the mapping $z = z_0(y)$ is

$$(x, x^2) \mapsto \left(-x(1+\sqrt{2}), -x^2(1+\sqrt{2})^2\right),$$

where x is the parameter of the curve ∂M, and

$$t_{\tilde{t}} = -(1+\sqrt{2}) \frac{\sqrt{1 + 4(1+\sqrt{2})^2 x^2}}{\sqrt{1 + 4x^2}} < 0,$$

$$\lim_{x \to 0} t_{\tilde{t}} = -(1+\sqrt{2}).$$

2. The theorem can be generalized in the case when there are several concave parts on ∂M.

3. Note that if M has dimension $n > 2$, difficulties appear which are not considered by the author.

8. Using the reflected rays to improve the estimate

In specific cases for the non-convex domains, the estimate is obtained as in case the convex domains [1–3] on n-dimensional manifolds. Let the domain M be the shell between two non-intersecting spheres, i.e.

$$\partial M = S_1^{n-1} \cup S_2^{n-1} \quad \text{and} \quad S_1^{n-1} \subset S_2^{n-1}.$$

In this connection the sphere S_1^{n-1} is non-convex relatively K, i.e. $\partial_1 M = S_1^{n-1}$. The family K consists of the geodesics of the Finsler metric F. For every geodesic $k(y, z) \in K$, $y \in S_2^{n-1}$, $z \in S_1^{n-1}$ a geodesic $k(y_1, z) \in K$, $y^1 \in S_2^{n-1}$, $z \in S_1^{n-1}$ exists which is considered as the reflected ray for $k(y, z)$. The pair of geodesics $k(y, z)$ and $k(y_1, z)$ are replaced the broken ray $k(y, z) \cup k(y_1, z)$. Thus all geodesics have their ends on S_2^{n-1}. For this problem in integral geometry, stability is obtained as in the case of convex domains (see [4]). The next case is analogous. We change the domain M on the Figure 1. Let $\partial_1 M$ and $\partial_2 M$ form in the points b_1 and b_2 the acute angle α, $0 \leq \alpha < \frac{\pi}{2}$. Then we also may utilize the broken rays that are reflected from $\partial_1 M$. This case also is considered in [4].

9. The other method obtaining of the estimate

There is another approach to the solution of the problem of integral geometry in the non-convex domain M relative to the family K of curves. Assume that the domain M may widen until the domain $M' \supset M$ and the curves of K continue toward the boundary $\partial M'$ so that the domain M' becomes convex relative to the new regular family K' of the curves. We may make this continuation when M is an arbitrary domain and K is the family of the linear segments as in Figure 1. To do this we need to continue linearly the segments k to $\partial M'$ where M' is the convex domain containing M. Now we obtain the integrals along the new curves $k' \in K'$. It is required to find the values of the function $u = u(x)$ and its derivatives on the boundary

∂M. In the beginning, we determine $u(x)$ on the convex part $\partial_2 M$. Let
$$w(y_1, y) = \int_{k(y_1,y)} u\rho\, ds, \quad y^1, y \in \partial_2 M,$$
be as in Figure 2. For simplification, the family K consists of the linear segments k of the Euclidean metric F and also $\rho|_{\partial M} \neq 0$. Since
$$u(y_1)\rho = \lim_{y \to y_1} \frac{w(y_1, y)}{\tau(y_1, y)},$$
where $\tau(y_1, y)$ is the length of $k(y_1, y)$, $u|_{\partial_2 M}$ is determined. Under fixed $y_1 = y_1(t_1)$ we have
$$\frac{\partial w(y_1, y(t))}{\partial t} = \frac{\sin \alpha}{\tau(y_1, y)} \cdot I(y_1, y) +$$
$$+ \cos \alpha(t_1, t) \cdot u(y)\rho, \quad I(y_1, y) = \int_{k(y_1,y)} \frac{\partial(u\rho)}{\partial h} \tau(y_1, \tilde{x}) ds,$$
where $\tilde{x}$ is the variable of integration on $k(y_1, y)$, h is the direction orthogonal to the ray $k(y_1, y)$ at the point $\tilde{x}$, $\alpha(t_1, t)$ is the angle between the tangent to $\partial_2 M$ at the point $\tilde{x}$ and the ray $k(y_1, y)$. From this equality the integral $I(y_1, y)$ is determined since $\partial w/\partial t$ is determined from the data of the problem and $u(y)|_{\partial_2 M}$ was determined earlier. According to the mean value theorem
$$I(y_1, y) = \frac{\partial(u\rho)}{\partial h}(x_0) \cdot \frac{\tau^2(y_1, y)}{2},$$
where x_0 is the internal point of $k(y_1, y)$, hence
$$\frac{\partial u\rho}{\partial n}(y_1) = 2 \lim_{y \to y_1} \frac{I(y_1, y)}{\tau^2(y_1, y)},$$
where n is the normal to $\partial_2 M$ at the point (y_1) and therefore $\partial u/\partial n|_{\partial_2 M}$ is determined. Similarly we may find every derivative of the function $u(x)$ along every direction on $\partial_2 M$. Now we find the function $u(x)$ and its derivatives on the non-convex part of $\partial_1 M$. Let $z(t)$ be an interior point of $\partial_1 M$ and $K \ni k(z, y_1)$ be the segment that is tangent to $\partial_1 M$ at the point z (see Figure 2). For the fixed y_1 we have

$$\frac{\partial w(z(t), y_1)}{\partial t} = \frac{1}{\tau(z, y_1)} \cdot \left(\lim_{\Delta t \to 0} \frac{\Delta l}{\Delta t} \right) \int_{k(z,y_1)} \frac{\partial (u\rho)}{\partial h} \tau(\tilde{x}, y_1) ds + u(z)\rho,$$

where Δl is the length of the arc $(x_0, z(t+\Delta t))$, h is the direction orthogonal to the ray $k(z, y_1)$ at the point $\tilde{x}$. Since $\Delta l \sim \Delta t^2$,

$$\lim_{\Delta t \to 0} \frac{\Delta l}{\Delta t} = 0$$

and $u(z)\rho$ remains to the right. So

$$u(z)|_{\partial_1 M} = \frac{1}{\rho} \cdot \frac{\partial w(z(t), y_1)}{\partial t}.$$

Similarly to $\partial_2 M$, the derivatives along every direction of the function $u(x)$ are obtained on $\partial_1 M$. We consider the function $u_0 = u_0(x) \in C^2(\bar{M})$ such that its values and the values of its derivatives of the first and second orders coincide with $u(x)$ on ∂M. The function

$$u_1(x) = \begin{cases} u(x) - u_0(x) & ; \quad x \in M \cup \partial M \\ 0 & ; \quad x \in M' \backslash M \end{cases}$$

belongs to $C^2(M')$. We extend the weight function ρ and its derivatives until the second order continuously on $T_0 M'$ and denote this by ρ_1. Obviously we may define

$$w = \int_{k'} u_1 \rho_1 ds$$

for every $k' \in K'$. For the resulting problem of integral geometry on the convex domain M' relatively the regular family K' of the curves the good stability estimate is obtained as in [1–3]. Certainly using this estimate the uniqueness theorem of the primary problem is obtained. Similarly the stability estimate is obtained for $n > 2$ but for the family K of the geodesics of the Finsler metric F.

The advantage in the proof of the theorem in §4 as compared with the one stated above is that one need not continue the curves in M' (or the family of the vector fields) and the estimate is obtained for the original function $u = u(x)$.

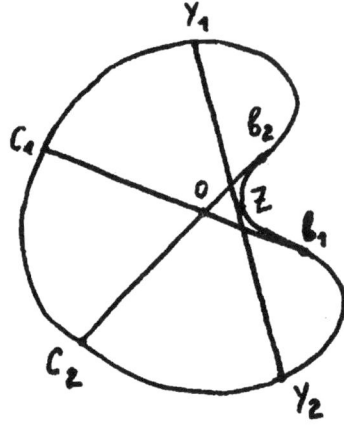

FIGURE 1 FIGURE 2

References

1. R.G. Mukhometov, *The problem of recovery of a two-dimensional Riemannian metric and integral geometry*, Soviet Math. Dokl., Vol. 18, **1** (1977), 27–31.

2. R.G. Mukhometov, *On integral geometry problem along the geodesics of the Riemannian metric*, In the transactions: Ill-Posed Mathematical Problems and Geophysics Problems, Computer Center, Academy of Science of SSSR, Novosibirsk 1979, pp. 96–110 (Russian).

3. I.N. Bernstein and M.L. Gerver, *A condition for distinguishing Metrics by travel times*, In the transactions: Methods and algorithms for interpretation of seismological data (Computational seismology, 13), Moscow 1980, pp. 50-73 (Russian).

4. R.G. Mukhometov, *On integral geometry problems in a domain with a reflecting part of the boundary*, Soviet Math. Dokl., Vol. 36, **2** (1988), 260–264.

5. H. Rund, *The differential geometry of Finsler spaces*, Springer-Verlag, Berlin, 1959, pp. 1–501.

Institute of Mathematics, Novosibirsk, 630090, Russia
E-mail address: mukhom@math.nsk.su

Recent developments in X-ray tomography

F. Natterer

Abstract: *We derive optimal sampling conditions for fan beam tomography and describe a novel fan beam reconstruction algorithm of the circular harmonic type. We give a unified derivation of the cone beam inversion formulas of Grangeat, B. Smith, Gelfand-Goncharov and Tuy based on a formula of Hamaker - K. Smith - Solmon - Wagner. We derive a Cormack type integral equation for cone beam tomography with sources on a circle.*

1 Introduction

Recently, many new types of tomography emerged: Polarization tomography [24], diffuse tomography [25], ultrasound tomography [6], impedance tomography [1], vector tomography [2]. All these new techniques require sophisticated new mathematics; in fact their final success depends crucially on the solution of difficult mathematical problems. On the other hand, ordinary X-ray CT still offers intruiging mathematical problems. In this paper we give some examples.

In section 2 we present some results on optimal sampling, mainly for fan beam geometry in the plane. However it is clear that every new scanning geometry, in particular in $3D$, raises similar questions. The method developed in section 2 seems well suited for dealing with such problems.

In section 3 we review some of the inversion formulas which have been

---

MR *Subject Classification.* Primary 92C55.

obtained by various authors in quite different ways. We show that these formulas can be obtained easily from an elementary identity for convolutions of the n-dimensional cone beam transform with distributions of degree $1-n$ which has been obtained as early as 1980 by Hamaker, K. Smith, Solmon and Wagner [11].

In section 4 we derive a Cormack type integral equation for cone beam tomography with sources on a circle. The integral equation is a Volterra equation of the Abel type. It reduces to Cormack's integral equation in the case of a flat object. The equation is obtained by a Mellin transform perpendicular to the circle and by a Fourier transform on the circle.

2 Resolution

Let f be a function supported in the ball $|x| < \rho$ of $I\!R^n$. Assume f to be essentially Ω-band-limited in the following sense: There is a positive number $\varepsilon \ll 1$ such that

$$\varepsilon_0(f, \Omega) = \int_{|\xi|>\Omega} |\hat{f}(\xi)| d\xi \le \varepsilon \int_{I\!R^n} |\hat{f}(\xi)| d\xi$$

where

$$\hat{f}(\xi) = (2\pi)^{-n/2} \int_{I\!R^n} e^{-ix\cdot\xi} f(x) dx$$

in the Fourier transform. A loose application of the Shannon sampling theorem (see e.g. Jerry [13]) shows that the smallest datail in f is of size $2\pi/\Omega$. In the spirit of this theorem the problem of resolution is how tomographic data of f have to be sampled in order to reconstruction f reliably.

In order to understand what we mean by reliable we give an example. Let R be the Radon transform, e.g.

$$(Rf)(\theta, s) = \int_{x\cdot\theta=s} f(x) dx, \quad \theta \in S^{n-1}, \quad s \in I\!R^1. \tag{2.1}$$

Assume $(Rf)(\theta_j, \cdot) = 0$ for p directions $\theta_1, \ldots, \theta_p$ which are sufficiently general. Then, for $0 < \vartheta < 1$,

$$\|f\|_{L_\infty(|x|<\rho)} \le \frac{(2\pi)^{-n/2}}{1 - \eta(\vartheta, \Omega)} \varepsilon_0(f, \vartheta\Omega) \tag{2.2}$$

provided that $p \geq \binom{\Omega + n - 1}{n - 1}$. Here, $\eta(\vartheta, \Omega)$ decays exponentially as $\Omega \to \infty$. More precisely, there are positive constants $C(\vartheta)$, $\lambda(\vartheta)$, $\Omega(\vartheta)$ such that

$$0 \leq \eta(\vartheta, \Omega) \leq C(\vartheta) e^{-\lambda(\vartheta)\Omega}$$

provided that $\Omega \geq \Omega(\vartheta)$, see Natterer [18], chapt. III. Since, for Ω large, $\binom{\Omega + n - 1}{n - 1}$ behaves like $\Omega^{n-1}/(n-1)!$, we may interpret (2.1) as follows: If the Radon transform of an essentially Ω-band-limited functions is know for $\Omega^{n-1}/(n-1)!$ sufficiently general directions, then f can be determined reliably, see Louis [16]. In order to avoid cumbersome notations we shall use these vague notions below. Just one more example: For the X-ray transform

$$Pf(\theta, x) = \int_{I\!R^1} f(x + t\theta) dt, \quad \theta \in S^{n-1}, \quad x \in \theta^\perp$$

Maaß [17] has shown that Ω directions $\theta \in S^{n-1}$ suffice to determine f reliably.

Let us now consider fan beam tomography in the plane. The source rotates around the reconstruction region $|x| < \rho$ on the circle $|x| = r$ where $r \geq \rho$. This gives rise to the fan beam transform

$$Df(\beta, \alpha) = \int_{L(\beta, \alpha)} f(x) dx$$

where $L(\beta, \alpha)$ is the straight line through the source $r \begin{pmatrix} \cos \beta \\ \sin \beta \end{pmatrix}$, making an angle α with the vector $r \begin{pmatrix} \cos \beta \\ \sin \beta \end{pmatrix}$.

Df is a periodic function of its arguments β, α. The sampling of periodic function in $I\!R^n$ has been studied in Natterer [19]. Let g be a function in $I\!R^n$ whose periods $p_1, \ldots, p_n$ are the columns of the non-singular matrix P. We sample g on the lattice $L_W = W Z\!\!\!Z^n$ generated by the non-singular matrix W. For this to make sense we must have $L_P \subseteq L_W$, i.e. $P = WM$ with an integer matrix M. The reciprocal lattice $L_W^\perp$ is generated by the matrix

$2\pi(W^{-1})^T$, and correspondingly for $L_P^\perp$. We have $L_P^\perp \supseteq L_W^\perp$. The Fourier transform of g is defined to be

$$\hat{g}(\xi) = |\det(P)|^{-1} \int_{P[0,1)^n} g(x) e^{-ix \cdot \xi} dx, \quad \xi \in L_P^\perp.$$

With all this notations we have the following variant of the Petersen - Middleton sampling theorem [22]:

Let K be a finite set in $L_P^\perp$ such that $K + \xi \cap K + \xi' = \phi$ for $\xi, \xi' \in L_W^\perp$ and $\xi \neq \xi'$.

(i) If g is a P-periodic function such that $\hat{g}$ vanishes outside K, then g is uniquely determined by its values on L_W/L_P.

(ii) If g_1, g_2 are P-periodic functions such that $\hat{g}_1$, $\hat{g}_2$ vanish outside K, then

$$\int_{P[0,1)^n} g_1(x) g_2(x) = |\det(W)| \sum_{y \in L_W/L_P} g_1(y) g_2(y).$$

We apply this result to the function $g = Df$ where $n = 2$ and $P = \begin{pmatrix} 2\pi & 0 \\ 0 & \pi \end{pmatrix}$. In [20] we have shown that $\hat{g}$ is small outside the set

$$K : |k - m| < \Omega r, \quad |k| r > |k - m|$$

where $\xi = \begin{pmatrix} k \\ m \end{pmatrix}$ and m even, see fig. 1.

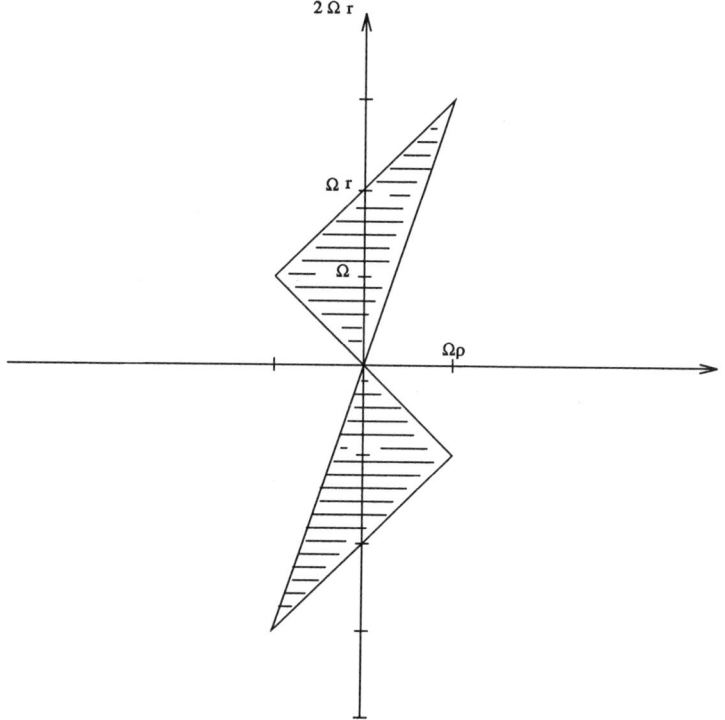

Fig. 1: The set K.

A matrix W satisfying the condition of the theorem is

$$2\pi (W^{-1})^T = 2\Omega r \begin{pmatrix} \frac{\rho}{r+\rho} & 0 \\ 0 & 1 \end{pmatrix}, \quad W = \frac{\pi}{\Omega r} \begin{pmatrix} \frac{\rho}{r+\rho} & 0 \\ 0 & 1 \end{pmatrix}. \quad (2.3)$$

This corresponds to the lattice

$$\beta = \beta_j = j\Delta\beta, \quad \Delta\beta = \frac{r+\rho}{\rho}\frac{\pi}{\Omega r},$$

$$\alpha = \alpha_\ell = \ell\Delta\alpha, \quad \Delta\alpha = \frac{\pi}{\Omega r}. \quad (2.4)$$

From the derivation it is clear that these conditions are best possible: Decreasing $\Delta\beta$, $\Delta\alpha$ below the values set by (2.4) causes the translates of K with respect to $L_W^\perp$ to overlap. The optimality of (2.4) has also been corroberated by numerous numerical examples in [19]. In fig. 2 we compare (2.4) with earlier results. The condition for $\Delta\alpha$ is precisely the Nyquist condition. So it does not come as a surprise that this condition is the same in all results. However the condition on $\Delta\beta$, hence the number $p = 2\pi/\Delta\beta$ of views, varies from author to author. (2.4) yields

$$p = \frac{2r}{r+\rho}\rho\Omega . \tag{2.5}$$

In [18], chapt. III we obtained

$$p = 2\rho\Omega . \tag{2.6}$$

Joseph and Schulz [14] obtained

$$p = \frac{2}{1-\rho/r}\rho\Omega , \tag{2.7}$$

while Rattey and Lindgren [23] found

$$p = \max\left(1, \frac{2}{1+3\rho/r}\right)\rho\Omega . \tag{2.8}$$

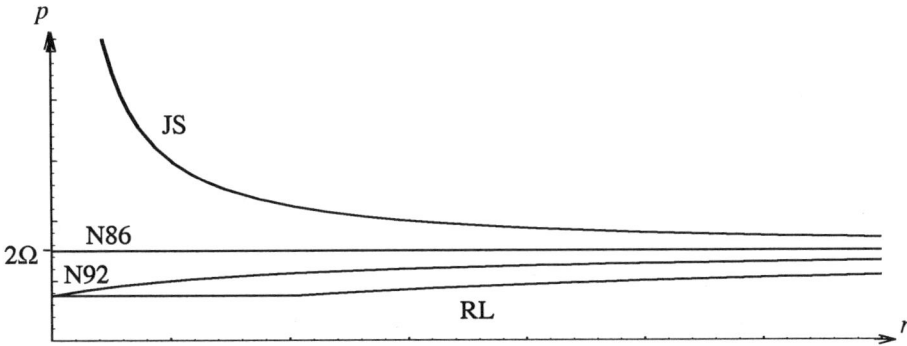

Fig. 2: Number p of views in a fan beam geometry in dependence of r, with p normalized to 1. N92: optimal number (2.5). N86: suboptimal estimate (2.6). JS: suboptimal estimate (2.7). RL: too optimistic estimate (2.8).

In order to find reconstruction algorithms which reconstruct f reliably from (2.4) we make use of part (ii) of the theorem. In [19] we obtained the following regularized inversion formula for D:

$$V * f(x) = \int_0^{2\pi} \int_{-\pi/2}^{\pi/2} v(x \cdot \theta(\beta+\alpha) - r\sin\alpha) Df(\beta,\alpha) \cos\alpha \, d\alpha \, d\beta \ .$$

Here, V and v are filters defined by their Fourier transforms

$$\begin{aligned}\hat{v}(\sigma) &= \tfrac{1}{2}(2\pi)^{-3/2}|\sigma|\hat{\phi}\left(\tfrac{|\sigma|}{\Omega}\right) \\ \hat{V}(\xi) &= \tfrac{1}{2\pi}\hat{\phi}\left(\tfrac{|\xi|}{\Omega}\right)\end{aligned}$$

with a low pass filter ϕ of bandwidth 1, and

$$\theta(\varphi) = \begin{pmatrix} \sin\varphi \\ -\cos\varphi \end{pmatrix} \ .$$

We apply the theorem to the functions

$$g_1(\beta,\alpha) = v(x\cdot\theta - r\sin\alpha),$$
$$g_2(\beta,\alpha) = Df(\beta,\alpha).$$

It follows that, with good accuracy,

$$V*f(x) = r\Delta\beta\Delta\alpha \sum_{j=0}^{p-1}\sum_{\ell=-q}^{q} v(x\cdot\theta(\beta_j+\alpha_\ell)-r\sin\alpha_\ell)Df(\beta_j,\alpha_\ell)\cos\alpha_\ell. \quad (2.9)$$

As it stands, (2.9) requires for each x $2pq = O(\Omega^2)$ operations. Since $V*f$ has to be evaluated on a lattice with step size π/Ω, the total number of operations is $O(\Omega^4)$. This is not considered feasable in clinical practice. Therefore one has to explore possibilities to reduce the complexity.

The standard way of doing this has been pointed out by Lakshminarayanan [15]. He observed that v is approximately homogeneous of degree -2. This, together with an interpolation, turns the ℓ-sum in (2.9) into a discrete convolution, while the remaining j-sum is simply a backprojection. For details see e.g. [18], chapt. V.1. This is the filtered backprojection algorithm, which is the most widely used algorithm in tomography. It needs $O(\Omega^3)$ operations, and it reflects truly the structure of Radon's 1917 inversion formula.

It is also possible to implement (2.9) in such a way that it looks like a discrete version of Cormack's 1964 inversion formula. We only have to exploit the circular symmetry of (2.9) by putting $x = t_i\theta(\beta_k)$. Then, (2.9) reads

$$V*f(x) = r\Delta\beta\Delta\alpha \sum_{\ell=-q}^{q}\cos\alpha_\ell \sum_{j=0}^{p-1} v(t_i\cos(\beta_{j-k}+\alpha_\ell)-r\sin\alpha_\ell)Df(\beta_i,\alpha_\ell).$$
$$(2.10)$$

The j-sum is now a cyclic convolution, which can be done in $O(p\log p)$ operations for each pair i, ℓ, resulting in a complexity of $O(q^2\, p\log p) = O(\Omega^3\log\Omega)$ for the whole algorithm. This is slightly more than what the filtered backprojection algorithm needs. But the implementation of (2.9) is so much simpler than the filtered backprojection algorithm that our C-program for (2.9) is actually much faster than the filtered backprojection algorithm, typically by a factor of 6.

Since the algorithm based on (2.9) starts with an angular Fourier transform we call it circular harmonic reconstruction algorithm. Such algorithms have been derived by Hansen [12] from Cormack's inversion formula for parallel projections. Hansen's algorithm has complexity $O(\Omega^3)$. If we use (2.8) for parallel projections, i.e. for $r = \infty$, then the logarithm in the complexity of $O(\Omega^3 \log \Omega)$ of (2.9) can be removed. Thus the extra factor of $\log \Omega$ is just the price we have to pay for using fan beam instead of parallel beam scanning.

The superiority of the circular harmonic algorithm over the usual filtered backprojection algorithm is demonstrated in fig. 3. The original (right) is reconstructed from 480 fan beam projections with 241 line integrals each. This corresponds to $\Omega \rho = 360$ and $\Omega r = 720$ in (2.4). The width of the central slit in the original is 0.02ρ. Since $\frac{2\pi}{\Omega} = 0.017\rho$ this is just at the resolution limit. The circular harmonic reconstruction (left) and the filtered backprojection reconstruction (middle) both give the correct position and density of the central slit, but the density of the narrower ones is not correct. This is in agreement with our resolution analysis. Comparing filtered backprojection with circular harmonic reconstruction we find that the former produces more artefacts. A closer analysis reveals that the rings emanating from the high density spot at the top are caused by the interpolation step, while the curved bar at the bottom is due to the homogeneity approximation. In any case the circular harmonic reconstruction is much more satisfactory.

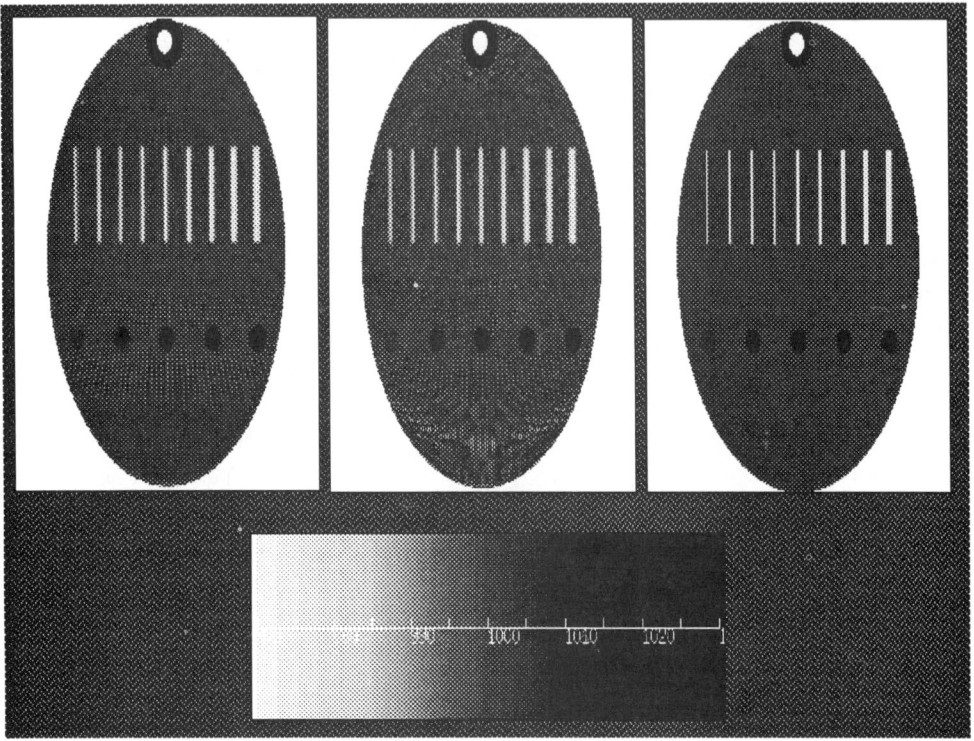

Fig. 3: Comparison of filtered backprojection (middle) with circular harmonic (left) reconstruction of the original (right).

The number of data in (2.4) is
$$\frac{2\pi}{\Delta\beta}\frac{2\arcsin\rho/r}{\Delta\alpha} = \frac{1}{\pi}\frac{4r}{r+\rho}\frac{\arcsin\rho/r}{\rho/r}\rho^2\Omega^2 . \tag{2.11}$$
It has been shown in [19] that the factor $\frac{4r}{r+\rho}$ can be dropped by using a more efficient scanning scheme. Thus the number (2.11) of data is not best possible. The efficient scanning scheme is of the form
$$\begin{aligned}\alpha = \alpha_\ell &= \ell\Delta\alpha \quad, \quad \Delta\alpha = \frac{\pi}{\Omega r}\\ \beta = \beta_{\ell j} &= j\Delta\beta + \ell(r/\rho - 1)\Delta\alpha \,, \Delta\beta = \frac{2\pi}{\Omega\rho} .\end{aligned} \tag{2.12}$$

There are several possibilities to implement (2.12) technically, see [20]. Industrial applications can be found in Desbat [5]. We note that efficient sampling for parallel scanning geometries has been studied thouroughly by Faridani [7].

In 3D, the questions of sampling, in particular efficient sampling, are almost entirely unexplored. The only results we are aware of are those of Louis and Maaß mentioned at the beginning of this section, which concern the semi-discrete case of reconstruction from finitely many complete projections. For the fully discrete case not even the simplest and apparently elementary case of a helix as source curve has been treated. In view of the fact that the number of data becomes crucial in 3D tomography this is amazing.

3 Inversion formulas for cone beam tomography

The cone beam transform of a function f in $I\!R^n$ is defined by

$$(Df)(a,\theta) = \int_0^\infty f(a+t\theta)dt \quad , \quad a \in I\!R^n \, , \quad \theta \in I\!R^n \, . \qquad (3.1)$$

In 3D transmission tomography and also in PET (with focused colimaters) one reconstructs f from $(Df)(a,\theta)$ where a runs through a curve A outside $\text{supp}(f)$ and $\theta \in S^{n-1}$. It has been shown by Hamaker et al. [11] that f is uniquely determined provided A is any infinite set and $\text{supp}(f)$ is compact. However, Finch [8] has shown that the inversion procedure is necessarily extremely ill-conditioned unless A satisfies the following condition: Every plane meeting $\text{supp}(f)$ contains at least one point of A. In other words: For each $(\theta,s) \in S^2 \times I\!R^1$ with $s \in \theta \cdot \text{supp}(f)$ there exists $a(\theta,s) \in A$ such that

$$a(\theta,s) \cdot \theta = s \, . \qquad (3.2)$$

Under this condition various authors have derived inversion formulas for D. All these formulas use a relation between D and the Radon transform (2.1) which is an outflow of a relation already obtained in [11]: Let h be a function (distribution) on $I\!R^1$, homogeneous of degree $1-n$. Then

$$\int_{S^{n-1}} (Df)(a,\omega) h(\theta \cdot \omega) d\omega = \int_{I\!R^1} Rf(\theta,s) h(a \cdot \theta - s) ds \, . \qquad (3.3)$$

For $n=3$ we may choose $h = \delta'$, obtaining

$$\frac{\partial}{\partial s} Rf(\theta, a \cdot \theta) = \int_{S^2} (Df)(a,\omega) \delta'(\theta \cdot \omega) d\omega$$

or, after some algebra,

$$\frac{\partial}{\partial s} Rf(\theta, a \cdot \theta) = - \int_{S^2 \cap \theta^\perp} \frac{\partial}{\partial \theta}(Df)(a,\omega) d\omega \, . \qquad (3.4)$$

Here, $\frac{\partial}{\partial \theta}$ means the derivative in direction θ, acting on the second argument of Df. (3.4) has been obtained by Grangeat [10]. Choosing in (3.3)

$$h(s) = \int_{-\infty}^{\infty} |\sigma| e^{-is\sigma} d\sigma ,$$

i.e.

$$h * g = H \frac{\partial}{\partial s} g$$

with H the Hilbert transform we obtain

$$H \frac{\partial}{\partial s} Rf(\theta, a \cdot \theta) = \int_{S^2} (Df)(a, \omega) h(\theta \cdot \omega) d\omega .$$

Evaluating the distribution on the right hand side this becomes the formula of Smith [26]:

$$H \frac{\partial}{\partial s} Rf(\theta, a \cdot \theta) = 2(2\pi)^{3/2} (Df)^{\wedge}(a, \theta) \qquad (3.5)$$

where $(Df)^{\wedge}$ is the Fourier transform of Df with respect to the second argument.

Finally we put $h(s) = 1/s^2$ in (3.3), obtaining

$$\int_{{I\!\!R}^1} \frac{(Rf)(\theta, s)}{(a \cdot \theta - s)^2} ds = \int_{S^2} \frac{(Df)(a, \omega)}{(\theta \cdot \omega)^2} d\omega .$$

There integrals have to be understood in the distributional sense, i.e. as the singular part. An integration by parts on the left hand side yields

$$\int_{{I\!\!R}^1} \frac{(Rf)'(\theta, s)}{a \cdot \theta - s} ds = \int_{S^2} \frac{Df(a, \omega)}{(\theta \cdot \omega)^2} d\omega$$

or, equivalently,

$$H \frac{\partial}{\partial s} Rf(\theta, a \cdot \theta) = \frac{1}{\pi} \int_{S^2} \frac{Df(a, \omega)}{(\theta \cdot \omega)^2} d\omega . \qquad (3.6)$$

This formula is due to Gelfand and Goncharov [9].

In connection with the inversion formula

$$f(x) = -\frac{1}{8\pi^2} \int_{S^2} \frac{\partial^2}{\partial s^2} Rf(\theta, x \cdot \theta) d\theta \qquad (3.7)$$

for the 3D Radon transform, (3.4) - (3.6) yield inversion formula for D if A satisfies (3.2). We work this out for (3.4). Putting $a = a(\theta, s)$ in (3.4) we obtain

$$\frac{\partial^2}{\partial s^2} Rf(\theta, s) = -\frac{\partial}{\partial s} \int_{S^2 \cap \theta^\perp} \frac{\partial}{\partial \theta}(Df)(a(\theta, s), \omega) d\omega . \qquad (3.8)$$

Inserting this in (3.7) leads to Grangeat's inversion formula

$$f(x) = \frac{1}{8\pi^2} \int_{S^2} \left[\frac{\partial}{\partial s} \int_{S^2 \cap \theta^\perp} \frac{\partial}{\partial \theta}(Df)(a(\theta, s), \omega) d\omega \right]_{s=x\cdot\theta} d\theta . \qquad (3.9)$$

In the cases (3.5) - (3.6) we have to invert the finite Hilbert transform, making these formulas less attractive than Grangeat's inversion formula (3.9).

(3.9) can be written in a different way using a parametric representation $a = a(\lambda)$ of A. Then for each $s \in \theta \cdot \text{supp}(f)$ there exists $\lambda = \lambda(\theta, s)$ such that $a(\theta, s) = a(\lambda, s)$, hence $s = a(\lambda(\theta, s)) \cdot \theta$.

Assuming $a'(\lambda(\theta, s)) \neq 0$ we may - at least locally - replace the variable s by the variable λ, and

$$\frac{\partial}{\partial \lambda} = a'(\lambda) \cdot \theta .$$

Hence (3.9) becomes

$$f(x) = \frac{1}{8\pi^2} \int_{S^2} \left[\frac{1}{a'(\lambda) \cdot \theta} \frac{\partial}{\partial \lambda} \int_{S^2 \cap \theta^\perp} \frac{\partial}{\partial \theta} Df(a(\lambda), \omega) d\omega \right]_{\lambda=\lambda(\theta, x\cdot\theta)} d\theta .$$

Now we make use of

$$(Df)^\wedge(x, \theta) = i\pi(2\pi)^{-3/2} \int_{S^2 \cap \theta^\perp} (Df)(x, \omega) d\omega + \ldots$$

where the dots stand for a function which is even in θ. This formula has been obtained by Zeng, Clack and Gullberg [28]. It can be obtained by direct computation using that $Df(x,y)$ is homogeneous of degree -1 in y. Combining the last two formulas we arrive at Tuy's formula

$$f(x) = \frac{1}{(2\pi)^{3/2}i} \int_{S^2} \left[\frac{1}{a'(\lambda)\cdot\theta} \frac{d}{d\lambda}(Df)^\wedge(a(\lambda),\theta) \right]_{\lambda=\lambda(\theta,x\cdot\theta)} d\theta, \qquad (3.10)$$

see [27].

There are some inversion procedures which seem not to fit into the framework presented here. We mention only the inversion formula of Palamodov [21] for rays tangent to a smooth surface and Finch's [8] method which, as an intermediate step, reconstructs $Df(x,\theta)$ for x in the convex hull of A.

4 A Cormack type integral equation for cone beam tomography with sources on a circle

If the source curve A is a circle around supp (f), the condition (3.2) is not satisfied. Nevertheless f is uniquely determined [11], but the reconstruction process is necessarily extremely ill-posed [8]. In spite of this ill-posedness an exact inversion formula would be useful since a regularized version of this formula could lead to a good reconstruction algorithm. We do not know such a formula. However we reduce the 3D problem $Df = g$ on $A \times S^2$ to a 1D integral equation which is very similar to Cormack's integral equation [3] in 2D tomography.

We derive the said integral equation by exploiting the symmetries of the problem. Assume that A is the circle of radius r around the origin in the x_1-x_2-plane, and that supp(f) is contained in the cylinder of radius $\rho < r$ around the x_3-axes. Then the problem $Df = g$ on $A \times S^2$ is invariant with respect to scaling in the x_3-direction and with respect to rotation around the x_3-axes. The scaling invariance is exploited by doing a Mellin transform in x_3, and the rotation invariance by a Fourier transform on A.

Let h be a function on $I\!R_+$. The Mellin transform of h is defined to be

$$(Mh)(s) = \int_0^\infty h(t) t^s \frac{dt}{t} .$$

h can be recovered from Mh by the inversion formula

$$h(t) = \frac{1}{2\pi i} \int_{\sigma-i\infty}^{\sigma+i\infty} t^{-s} (Mh)(s) ds ,$$

see [4], chapt. II.8.

For $x \in I\!R^3$ we denote by x' its orthogonal projection onto the x_1-x_2-plane. We represent f in $x_3 > 0$ as a Mellin transform with respect to x_3, i.e.

$$f(x) = \frac{1}{2\pi i} \int_{\sigma-i\infty}^{\sigma+i\infty} x_3^{-s} (Mh)(x', s) ds , \qquad (4.1)$$

$$(Mf)(x',s) = \int_0^\infty f(x',x_3) x_3^s \frac{dx_3}{x_3} . \tag{4.2}$$

Applying D to (4.1) yields for $y_3 > 0$

$$g(\theta,y) = \frac{1}{2\pi i} \int_{\sigma-i\infty}^{\sigma+i\infty} \int_0^\infty (ty_3)^{-s} (Mf)(r\theta' + ty', s) dt ds$$

$$= \frac{1}{2\pi i} \int_{\sigma-i\infty}^{\sigma+i\infty} y_3^{-s} \int_0^\infty t^{-s} (Mf)(r\theta' + ty', s) dt ds .$$

On the other hand,

$$g(\theta,y) = \frac{1}{2\pi i} \int_{\sigma+i\infty}^{\sigma-i\infty} y_3^{-s} (Mg)(\theta', y', s) ds ,$$

$$(Mg)(\theta',y',s) = \int_0^\infty g(\theta, y', t) t^s \frac{dt}{t} .$$

Comparing the two expressions for g we obtain

$$(Mg)(\theta',y',s) = \int_0^\infty t^{-s}(Mf)(r\theta' + ty', s) dt . \tag{4.3}$$

For each s, (4.3) is a generalized Radon integral equation for the 2D function $Mf(\cdot,s)$ with weight t^{-s}. Thus the Mellin transform reduces the cone beam problem to a one parameter family of generalized Radon problems in the plane.

In order to further reduce the dimension we exploit the circular symmetry. Dropping temporarily s and putting

$$\theta' = \theta(\beta), \quad y' = -\theta(\beta+\alpha), \quad \theta(\beta) = \begin{pmatrix} \cos\beta \\ \sin\beta \end{pmatrix}$$

we define the functions

$$G(\beta,\alpha) = Mg(\theta', y', s)$$
$$F(x') = Mf(x', s) .$$

(4.3) now reads

$$G(\beta, \alpha) = \int_0^\infty t^{-s} F(r\theta(\beta) - t\theta(\beta + \alpha)) dt$$

$$= \int_0^\infty t^{-s} F(U_\beta(re_1 - t\theta(\alpha))) dt \qquad (4.4)$$

where U_β is the rotation by an angle β in the mathematical positive sense, i.e.

$$U_\beta = \begin{pmatrix} \cos\beta & -\sin\beta \\ \sin\beta & \cos\beta \end{pmatrix}.$$

Now we expand F, G in Fourier series, i.e.

$$F(x) = \sum_\ell F_\ell(|x|) e^{i\ell \arg x}, \qquad (4.5)$$

$$G(\beta, \alpha) = \sum_\ell G_\ell(\alpha) e^{i\ell\beta}. \qquad (4.6)$$

Here, for $x = \begin{pmatrix} x_1 \\ x_2 \end{pmatrix}$,

$$\arg x = \arccos\left(\frac{x_1}{\sqrt{x_1^2 + x_2^2}}\right) \cdot \operatorname{sgn} x_2.$$

Inserting (4.5), (4.6) in (4.4) yields, with $u = \sqrt{r^2 + t^2 - 2rt\cos\alpha}$,

$$\sum_\ell G_\ell(\alpha) e^{i\ell\beta} = \sum_\ell e^{i\ell\beta} \int_0^\infty t^{-s} F_\ell(u) e^{-\varepsilon i\ell \arccos \frac{r-t\cos\alpha}{u}} dt$$

where $\varepsilon = \operatorname{sgn}\alpha$. It follows that

$$G_\ell(\alpha) = \int_0^\infty t^{-s} F_\ell(u) e^{-\varepsilon i\ell \arccos \frac{r-t\cos\alpha}{u}} dt. \qquad (4.7)$$

This is the Cormack type integral equation we wanted to derive. To enhance the similarity between (4.7) and Cormack's formula we replace the variable t by u. To each u corresponds 2 values of t, namely

$$t_\pm = r\cos\alpha \pm \sqrt{u^2 - r^2 \sin^2\alpha}. \qquad (4.8)$$

(4.8) becomes

$$G_\ell(\alpha) = \int_{r|\sin\alpha|}^{r} K_\ell(\alpha, u) F_\ell(u) \frac{u\,du}{\sqrt{u^2 - r^2 \sin^2 \alpha}}, \qquad (4.9)$$

$$K_\ell(\alpha, u) = \sum_{t \in \{t_+, t_-\}} t^{-s} e^{-\varepsilon i \ell \arccos \frac{r - t \cos \alpha}{u}}.$$

In the 2D case, Cormack's integral equation can be solved by the Mellin transform. This seems to be unlikely for (4.9) since we already exploited all the invariances of the problem. However, the numerical solution of this integral equation seems feasible, leading to a cone beam reconstruction algorithm of the circular harmonic type [12].

References

[1] Barber, D. - Brown, B. - Jossinet, J.: Electrical impedance tomography, Clin. Phys. Physiol. Meas. **9** suppl. A (1988).

[2] Braun, H. - Hauck, A.: Tomographic reconstruction of vector fields, IEEE Trans. Signal Processing **39**, 464-471 (1991).

[3] Cormack, A.M.: Representation of a function by its line integrals, with some radiological applications, J. Appl. Phys. **34**, 2722-2727 (1963).

[4] Courant, R. - Hilbert, D.: Methods of mathematical physics, Vol. 1, Springer 1953.

[5] Desbat, L. - Turlier, P.: Efficient reconstruction with few data in industrial tomography, Observatoire de Grenoble, CERMO, B.P. 53X, F-38041 Grenoble (1988).

[6] Devaney, A.J.: A filtered backpropagation algorithm for diffraction tomography, Ultrasonic Imaging **4**, 336-350 (1982).

[7] Faridani, A.: Reconstructing from efficiently sampled data in parallel-beam computed tomography, in: Inverse problems and imaging, G.F. Roach (ed.), Pitmans Research Notes in Mathematics Series, Vol. **245**, (1991), pp. 68-102.

[8] Finch, D.V.: Cone beam reconstruction with sources on a curve, SIAM J. Appl. Math. **45**, 665-673 (1985).

[9] Gelfand, I.M. - Goncharov, A.B.: Recovery of a compactly supported function starting from its integrals over lines intersecting a given set of points in space, Doklady **290** (1986), English translation in Soviet Math. Doklady **34**, 373-376 (1987).

[10] Grangeat, P.. Mathematical framework of cone beam 3D reconstruction via the first derivative of the Radon transform, in: Herman et al. (eds.): Mathematical methods in tomography, Springer 1991.

[11] Hamaker, C. - Smith, K.T. - Solmon, D.C. - Wagner, S.L.: The divergent beam X-ray transform, Rockey Mountain J. Math., **10**, 253-283 (1980).

[12] Hansen, E.W.: Circular harmonic image reconstruction, Applied Optics **20**, 2266-2274 (1981).

[13] Jerry, A.J.: The Shannon sampling theorem - its various extensions and applications: a tutorial review, Proc. IEEE **65**, 1565-1596 (1977).

[14] Joseph, P.M. - Schulz, R.A.: View sampling requirements in fan beam computed tomography, Med. Phys. **7**, 692-702 (1980).

[15] Lakshminarayanan, A.V.: Reconstruction from divergent ray data. Dept. Computer Science Tech. Report **TR-92**, State University of New York at Buffalo, 1975.

[16] Louis, A.K.: Orthogonal function series expansions and the null space of the Radon transform, SIAM J. Math. Anal. **15**, 621-633 (1984).

[17] Maaß, P.: The X-ray transform: singular value decomposition and resolution, Inverse Problems **3**, 729-741 (1987).

[18] Natterer, F.: The Mathematics of Computerized Tomography, Wiley-Teubner 1986.

[19] Natterer, F.: Sampling in fan beam tomography, SIAM J. Appl. Math. **53**, 358-380 (1993).

[20] Natterer, F.: Patentschrift **DE 4140631 C1**. Deutsches Patentamt, München 1993.

[21] Palamodov, V.P.: Inversion formulas for the three-dimensional ray transform, in: Herman, et al. (eds.): Mathematical Methods in Tomography, Springer 1991.

[22] Peterson, P.P. - Middleton, D.: Sampling and reconstruction of wavenumber-limited functions in N-dimensional euclidean space, Inf. Control **5**, 279-323 (1962).

[23] Rattey, P.A. - Lindgren, A.G.: Sampling the $2 - D$ Radon transform, IEEE Trans. Acoust. Speech Signal Procesing, **ASSP-29**, 994-1002 (1981).

[24] Sharafutdinov, V.A.: Problem of polarization tomography, J. Inverse and Ill-Posed Problems **1**, 53-72 (1993).

[25] Singer, J.R. - Grünbaum, F.A. - Kohn, P. - Zubelli, J.P.: Image reconstruction of the interior of bodies that diffuse radiation, Science **248**, 990-993 (1990).

[26] Smith, B.: Image reconstruction from cone-beam projections: necessary and sufficient conditions and reconstruction methods, IEEE Trans. Med. Imag. **4**, 14-25 (1985).

[27] Tuy, H.K.: An inversion formula cone beam reconstruction, SIAM J. Appl. Math. **43**, 546-552 (1983).

[28] Zeng, G.L. - Clack, R. - Gullberg, G.T.: Implementation of Tuy's cone beam inversion formula, Proceedings of the International Meeting on Fully Three - Dimensional Image Reconstruction in Radiology and Nuclear Medicine, June 23-25, 1993, Snowbird, Utah, USA.

University of Münster

Some mathematical aspects of 3D X-ray tomography

V.P. PALAMODOV

§1. Reconstruction formulae

Let $\mathbf{E}$ be a three-dimensional Euclidean space and $\mathbf{\Lambda}$ be the variety of straight lines $L \subset \mathbf{E}$. The ray transform of a function f on $\mathbf{E}$ with compact support is the family of integrals

$$(1) \qquad Rf(L) := \int_L f\, dL,$$

defined on $\mathbf{\Lambda}$, where dL is the line measure in $\mathbf{E}$. There are several inversion methods for the operator R which could be used for construction of tomography algorithms. We discuss here some properties of presumable algorithms under the following assumptions on the inversion method:

- the data (1) is used only for a three-dimensional family Σ of straight lines or rays L (called *a pencil*);
- an exact inversion is given by a *simple* formula.

A formula is called *simple* if it is a combination of finite set of derivations, integrations and algebraic operations. Several cases are known, where there exist simple formulas:

I Orlov's pencil $\Sigma = \Sigma(\mathbf{C}_\infty)$

II Kirillov-Tuy's pencil $\Sigma = \Sigma(\mathbf{C}_0)$

III pencil $\Sigma = \Sigma(\mathbf{S})$ of rays, which start with a smooth surface $\mathbf{S}$ and are tangent to this surface.

The following *completeness* condition is assumed:

for any point $x \in supp\, f$ and for any plane H through this point there exists a line $L \in \Sigma$, which passes through x and belongs to H.

1991 *Mathematics Subject Classification.* Primary: 44A12, Secondary: 92C55.

The author is acknowledging to the Center for Advanced Study at the Norwegian Academy of Science and Letters for its hospitality and support for this research.

For each of the cases I,II,III there is a simple reconstruction formula which consists of two steps: first the two-dimensional Radon transform

$$Rf(H) \equiv Rf(p,\omega) = \int_H f dH$$

or its derivative $\partial/\partial p\, Rf(p,\omega)$ is calculated. Here H means a plane with an equation $\omega \cdot x = p$. The second step is an application of the Lorentz-Radon inversion formula

(2) $$f(x) = -\frac{1}{8\pi^2}\int_\Omega \frac{\partial^2}{\partial p^2} Rf(\omega \cdot x,\omega) d\omega.$$

We call any reconstruction of this kind *back-projection* formula, because the back-projection operation for the data $\partial^2/\partial p^2\, Rf(p,\omega)$ is used on the second step.

Now we list some first step reconstruction formulae for the above cases.

I The Orlov's pencil $\Sigma(\mathbf{C}_\infty)$ is the set of lines $L(x,e)$, where e runs over a curve $\mathbf{C}_\infty$ in the unit sphere $\Omega \in \mathbf{E}$ and $L(x,e)$ means the line, which contains a point x and is parallel to a unit vector e.

The completeness condition for this pencil means that any plane H is a union of parallel lines $L(x(t),e), e \in \mathbf{C}_\infty, t \in \mathbb{R}$. Therefore we can find the Radon transform integrating the line data on the parameter t against the measure $dt := dH/dL$:

$$Rf(H) = \int Rf(L(x(t),e)\,dt.$$

II The Kirillov-Tuy's pencil $\Sigma(\mathbf{C}_0)$ is the manifold of rays with origins on a curve $\mathbf{C}_0 \subset \mathbf{E}$. Then Grangeat-Finch formula gives a derivative of the Radon transform

$$\frac{\partial}{\partial p} Rf(H) = \int_0^{2\pi} \frac{\partial}{\partial \theta} Rf(L(x,e))|_{\theta=0}\, d\varphi,$$

where $L(x,e)$ means the ray in E, which starts from a point $x \in \mathbf{C} \cap H$ and is parallel to a vector $e \in \Omega$; $\varphi =$ longitude and $\theta =$ latitude are coordinates of e on Ω with the pole ω. There are other reconstruction formulae for this pencil.

III For the pencil $\Sigma(\mathbf{S})$ there is the following reconstruction formula (A.S. Denisjuk, V.P. Palamodov [1]):

$$\frac{\partial}{\partial p} Rf(H) = \frac{1}{\delta} \int_{\mathbf{C}(H)} [-\kappa \frac{\partial}{\partial q} + \csc^2 \psi \frac{d\psi}{ds}] Rf(L(x,e))\, ds,$$

where s is the natural parameter on a curve $\mathbf{C}(H) \subset \mathbf{S} \cap H$, e is the tangent vector and κ is the curvature of this curve, ψ is the angle between H and $\mathbf{S}$ at a point x; $q = \omega \cdot e$. The curve $\mathbf{C}(H)$ is submitted to the following condition: the natural mapping $\mathbf{C}(H) \times \mathbb{R}_+ \to H$ is proper over the set $supp\, f \cap H$ and its degree δ does not vanish.

§2. Algorithms and errors

Any simple formula may be used as a starting point for a computerized tomography algorithm. The algorithm should include the following steps:
(d) discretization of integrals, in particular discretization of the back-projection operation (2).
(f) filtering of derivations and
(i) interpolation of the data if necessary.

We call it a *back-projection* algorithm and claim that any back-projection algorithm produces image errors and artifacts whose geometry should have some features which do not depend on the simple formula used for the first step.

Fix a back-projection algorithm $\mathcal{A}$. The total error $E(f) = E(\mathcal{A}, f)$ of the reconstruction of an original f is the difference

$$E(f) := g - f,$$

where g is the result of the tomographic reconstruction. It can be written as a sum of two terms

$$E(f) = E_s(f) + E_h(f),$$

where $E_s(f)$ is the part caused by the operations (d),(f),(i) only (software part) and $E_h(f)$ the part caused by the physical origins (hardware part). Namely we define the software part as follows

$$E_s(f) := \mathcal{A}(Rf(\Sigma[d])) - f,$$

where $\mathcal{A}(Rf(\Sigma[d]))$ is the reconstruction, which is given by the algorithm $\mathcal{A}$ with the data of integrals $Rf(L)$ for a finite sampling $\Sigma[d] \subset \Sigma$. Here $d \ll 1$ is the average distance between adjacent segments $L \cap supp\, f$, $L \in \Sigma[d]$. Whence, we get

$$E_h(f) = g - \mathcal{A}(Rf(\Sigma[d])).$$

This part of the total defect may be caused by several physical sources, in particular, by
(i) the effect of "partially filled volume": for a simple model this means that

$$\int \exp(-\int f\, dL)\, c\, dt \neq \exp(-\iint f\, dL\, c\, dt),$$

where the function $c = c(t)$ is a characteristics of collimator of a detector.
(ii) non-linearity of the detector characteristics, especially if the ratio noise/signal is not small enough;
(iii) polychromatism of the radiation and "beam hardening".

These effects imply together that the real data which the algorithm works up does not coincide with (and sometimes is far from) the exact values of the integral (1).

Remark Note that the software part $E_s(\cdot)$ is a *linear operator*, unlike the hardware part $E_h(f)$ which is typically a *non-linear* operator. Therefore these operators respond differently to a source of errors. The main such source is a discontinuity of the original f. This source begets an error $E_s(f)$ whose core is localized in the vicinity of the singular set of f, but the essential support of $E_h(f)$ may extend far beyond of this set.

§3. Convergence of back-projection algorithms

We call an algorithm $\mathcal{A}$ *convergent* for an original f, if the software error $E_s(\mathcal{A}, f)$ tends to zero as $d \to 0$.

CLAIM 1. *Let $\mathcal{A}$ be a back-projection algorithm that includes an appropriate filtering and interpolation and is applied to the integral data (1) available for a properly distributed sampling $\Sigma[d] \subset \Sigma$. Then the function $E_s(f)$ tends to zero uniformly as $d \to 0$ for any function $f \in C^q(\mathbf{E})$ with compact support, if q is big enough.*

We call a filter appropriate, if it has an effective window in the spectral domain of the size $\leq 1/2d$ like, for example, the 2D Shepp-Logan filter. Any properly distributed sampling should be d-dense in the phase space $T^*(\mathbf{E})$ in the following sense: for any point $(x, \xi) \in T^*(\mathbf{E})$, $x \in supp\, f$, $|\xi| = 1$ there is a line $L \in \Sigma[d]$, such that
$$dist(x, L) \leq d, \quad dist^*(\xi, L^\perp)) \leq \rho \cdot \frac{d}{r}.$$
Here r is radius of the smallest ball that contains $supp\, f$, $L^\perp$ means the plane in $T^*_x(\mathbf{E})$ that is orthogonal to L and $dist^*$ means the Euclidean distance the dual space $T^*_x(\mathbf{E}) \cong \mathbf{E}^*$. This condition is akin to the Nyqwist inequality; the optimal values of the factor ρ and an effective size of window of the filter should be found. See [2] for a discussion of similar problems for 2D back projection algorithms. To transform this Claim to a theorem the conditions on filters and interpolation should be specified. We shall call an algorithm that satisfies these conditions an *appropriate* Σ-algorithm.

For a function f with singularities the convergence of an appropriate algorithm is not certain even for an open set, where the function is smooth enough. Some simple examples of 2D computer simulated tomography show that the singular set of f spreads around a spot of error $E_s(f)$. The shape of this spot depends on the geometry of the singular set. To get some ideas about the shape of E_s we specify the class of originals. Suppose that the function f has the following simple form

(3) $$f = a\,\delta(B) \quad \text{or} \quad f = a\,\chi(V)$$

where $a \in C_0^\infty(\mathbf{E})$, $\chi(V)$ denotes the characteristic function of an open set $V \subset \mathbf{E}$ with a smooth boundary B and δ_B is the delta-function on the boundary. In fact the delta-function is a model for the delta-like density $\frac{1}{2\varepsilon}\chi(B_\varepsilon)$, where ε is small and B_ε means ε-neighborhood of B. Apparently the value of $|E_s(f)|$ can not be small near B since $\mathcal{A}(Rf)$ is an approximation of the discontinuous original f with help of continuous functions.

We give a qualitative estimate of this value in terms of local geometry of B. In particular, we shall say that the error E_s is greater at a point $x \in B$ at one side of the surface B than at another side, if the set $y \in U : |E_s(f)| \geq l\,|F(x)|$, is larger at this side for a small ball U centered at x. Here $F(x)$ is an average values of the function f at this point and $l > 0$ is a small parameter. We have $F(x) \approx 1/2\varepsilon$, if $f \approx \delta(B)$ and $F(x) \approx 1/2$ if $f = \chi(V)$ for any point $x \in B$.

CLAIM 2. *If the set V is convex, then for an appropriate Σ-algorithm $\mathcal{A}$ the error $E_s(\chi(V))$ tends to zero uniformly as $d \to 0$ on any compact set $K \subset E\backslash B$. In a neighbourhood of B the quantity $|E_s(f)|$ is smaller inside of V than outside.*

A theorem of this kind can be proved by means of technique like [3,4].

Let now V be an arbitrary domain with smooth boundary B. Denote by K the Gaussian curvature of the boundary. Recall that an *inflexional* tangent to a surface B is a tangent with zero normal curvature. A curve $A \subset B$ is called an *asymptotic curve*, if any tangent line L to A is inflexional for B. An inflexional tangent line L to B is called *simple*, if it is not an inflexion tangent for the corresponding asymptotic curve A. This means that

(4) $$dist(x, B) \sim dist(x, B \cap L)^{k+1}$$

for $x \in L$ close to $B \cap L$, where $k = 2$. We call a straight line *a double* inflexional tangent to B, if it is a simple inflexional tangent to A. This is equivalent to the relation (4) with $k = 3$.

CLAIM 3. *For any appropriate Σ-algorithm $\mathcal{A}$ and any original of the form (4) such that $K(x) < 0$ the error $E_s(f)$ is greater near a point $x \in B$, where there is a double inflexional tangent $L_x \in \Sigma$ comparing with points $y \in B$, where there is no such inflexional tangent as d tends to 0.*

It is plausible that $E_s(\chi(V)) \to 0$ outside the union of all inflexional tangents $L_x \subset \Sigma$. In spite of that the error E_s may be not small at least the shape of V can be recognized by means of an appropriate algorithm. This is no more the case, if the completeness condition is not fulfilled. A reconstruction will be not adequate for the open part B' of the boundary such that for any $x \in B'$ there is no line $L \in \Sigma$ such that $x \in L \subset T_x(B)$. This failure is a corollary of the lack of the data and does not depend on the kind of algorithm used. See [2,5,3] for discussion of the similar problem in 2D-tomography.

§4. Geometry of line space and singularity of tangent line pencils

The line space $\mathbf{\Lambda}$ possesses a geometric structure of pseudo-Minkowski space: if we consider $\mathbf{E}$ as a real twistor space, we get an exact analogy with Penrose's construction of the complex Minkowski space which starts with a complex twistor space $\mathbb{C}^3$. To explain the pseudo-Minkowski geometry we choose the following charts for $\mathbf{\Lambda}$: fix two parallel planes H_1, H_2 in $\mathbf{E}$ and two linear functions α, β on $\mathbf{E}$, which are linearly independent on these plains. Taking a line L that is not parallel to these planes, we denote by α_1, β_1 and α_2, β_2 the values of α and β in the points $L \cap H_1$ and $L \cap H_2$ correspondingly. Hence we get four coordinates $\alpha_1, \beta_1, \alpha_2, \beta_2$, defined on an open part of $\boldsymbol{\Lambda}$. Note some simple properties of these coordinates:

(i) varying the functions α, β and the plane H_1 one makes a linear affine transformation of the coordinates. A change of the planes H_1, H_2, induces a linear projective transformation of the coordinates.

(ii) For two lines L, L' the equation

$$\det \begin{vmatrix} \alpha_1 - \alpha_1' & \beta_1 - \beta_1' \\ \alpha_2 - \alpha_2' & \beta_2 - \beta_2' \end{vmatrix} = 0, \qquad \alpha_i' = \alpha_i(L'),\ \beta_i' = \beta_i(L')$$

holds if and only if these lines have a common point or are parallel. For a fixed line L this equation defines a quadratic cone in $\boldsymbol{\Lambda}$ of signature $(2, 2)$, which is called *the light cone* with the vertex L.

(iii) the set $\Lambda(x)$ of lines that contains a fixed point $x \in \mathbf{E}$ is the set of solutions of two linear affine equation on coordinates $\alpha_1, \beta_1, \alpha_2, \beta_2$. Really we may shift the plane H_2, because of (i) hence, we may suppose that $x \in H_1$. Then the set of lines through x will be given by the equations $\alpha_1 = 0, \beta_1 = 0$. Whence, $\Lambda(x)$ is a plane in $\boldsymbol{\Lambda}$.

For any plane H in $\mathbf{E}$ the set $\Lambda(H)$ of lines $L \subset H$ is as well a plane in $\boldsymbol{\Lambda}$. This implies that

(iv) For any point $x \in \mathbf{E}$ and any plane H through x the set of lines L such that $x \in L \subset H$ is a projective line $\Lambda(x, H)$ in $\boldsymbol{\Lambda}$ (called *light ray*).

Now we take in the play a smooth surface $B \subset \mathbf{E}$. The pencil $\Sigma(B)$ of lines, which are tangent to B is a threefold in $\boldsymbol{\Lambda}$, which may be singular. This pencil is an union of projective lines $\Lambda(x, T_x(B)), x \in B$, where $T(B)$ is the tangent bundle of B. It is easy to check the following

PROPOSITION 1. *If B is strictly convex, i.e. $K > 0$, then $\Sigma(B)$ is smooth.*

PROPOSITION 2. *If $K(x) < 0$ or $K(x) = 0, dK(x) \neq 0$ for a point $x \in B$ and L_x is a simple inflexion tangent to B, then the set $\Sigma_2(B) \subset \Sigma(B)$ of all simple inflexion tangent to B is locally diffeomorphic to the product $D_2 \times \mathbb{R}^2$, where D_2 is the plane cusp curve, given by the equation*

(5) $$4s_1^3 + 27s_0^2 = 0.$$

This means that there exists a diffeomorphism of germs

$$(s, t) : (\boldsymbol{\Lambda}, L_x) \to (S \times \mathbb{R}^2, (0, 0))$$

that takes $\Sigma(B)$ onto $D_2 \times \mathbb{R}^2$ and $\Sigma_2(B)$ onto $0 \times \mathbb{R}^2$, where S is a plane with the coordinates s_0, s_1.

The following equation holds

(6) $$s_0(L) = \alpha_1 + o(\alpha_1, \alpha_2, \beta_1, \beta_2),$$

if we choose for α a linear function that vanishes on the tangent plane $T_x(B)$, for β a function that vanishes on L_x, and take for H_1 a plane that contains x. Any line $\Lambda(x, T_x(B))$ meets $\Sigma_2(B)$ twice and is tangent to this surface.

PROPOSITION 3. *Suppose that $K(x) < 0$ and L_x is a double inflexional tangent to B at x. Then there exists a diffeomorphism of germs*

$$(s,t) : (\mathbf{\Lambda}, L_x) \xrightarrow{\sim} (S \times \mathbb{R}, (0,0))$$

such that

$$\Sigma(B) \xrightarrow{\sim} D_3 \times \mathbb{R}, \qquad \Sigma_3(B) \xrightarrow{\sim} \{0\} \times \mathbb{R},$$

where $\Sigma_3(B)$ is the set of all double inflexion tangents and D_3 is the discriminant surface in $S = \mathbb{R}^3$ ("swallow tail"). If we choose coordinates on $\mathbf{\Lambda}$ as in Proposition 2 and coordinates s_0, s_1, s_2 on S as below, then the equation (7) holds once more. The light ray $\Lambda(x, T_x(B))$ is tangent to the surface given by the equations $s_0 = s_1 = 0$ in $\mathbf{\Lambda}$.

The surface D_3 is given by the equation

(7) $\qquad 256 s_0^3 - 128 s_2^2 s_0^2 + 16 s_2^4 s_0 - 4 s_2^3 s_1^2 + 144 s_2 s_1^2 s_0 - 27 s_1^4 = 0,$

with the parabola $s_2 < 0, s_1 = 0, 4 s_0 = s_2^2$ cut off. See [6] for details and pictures.

Proof Choose a smooth function φ such that $\varphi = 0, d\varphi \neq 0$ on B and consider the mapping $\lambda : \mathbb{R} \times \mathbf{\Lambda} \to E$ that takes a pair (t, L) into $y = y(t, L)$, where $y(\cdot.L)$ is a smooth parameterization of lines $L \in \mathbf{\Lambda}$. The pullback $\psi := \lambda^*(\varphi)$ is a smooth function on $\mathbb{R} \times \mathbf{\Lambda}$ and satisfies the equation $\psi(t, L_x) \sim (t - t(x))^{k+1}$ where $y(t(x), L_x) = x$ and $k = 2, 3$ correspondingly. Applying the Malgrange's preparation theorem [7] we get a factorization $\psi = hq$, where h is a smooth function which does not vanishes at the point $(t(x), L_x)$ and

$$q(t, L) = t^{k+1} + s_k t^k + s_{k-1} t^{k-1} + \cdots + s_1 t + s_0$$

where $s_0, s_1, \ldots, s_k$ are smooth functions of L. Setting $t = r - \frac{s_k}{k+1}$, we get the equation $q(t, L) = p_k(r, s(L))$ where $p_k(r, s)$ is a similar polynomial with $s_k = 0$. A line L is tangent to B if and only if the function $\psi(\cdot, L)$ has a real multiple root. This is equivalent to the condition that $p_k(\cdot, s(L))$ has a multiple root, where $s = (s_0, s_1, \ldots, s_{k-1})$. The last condition means that the point $s(L)$ belongs to the corresponding discriminant set (5),(7). This proves Propositions 2 and 3.

COROLLARY 4. *In a neighbourhood of the set $\Sigma_2(B)$ there exists a smooth mapping $x_2 : \mathbf{\Lambda} \to B$ whose restriction on $\Sigma_2(B)$ coincides with the natural projection onto B.*

We define $x_2(L)$ to be the point on B, where the line $L(0, t)$ is an inflexional tangent, $t = t(L)$ is a component of the mapping given in Proposition 2 and $L = L(s, t)$ is the inverse mapping. Using Proposition 3 we define in a similar way a projection $x_3 : \mathbf{\Lambda} \to I$. Here $I \subset B$ is a smooth curve of points y, where a double inflexion tangent L_y touches B.

§5. Singularities of the ray transform

Consider the ray transform Rf of the original like (3). This function is in C^∞ outside the threefold $\Sigma(B)$, whose singularities were described in the previous section. We give here an asymptotic representation of Rf near $\Sigma(B)$ by means some special functions.

If the body V is convex, then an asymptotic of Rf near $\Sigma(B)$ is well-known for a function like (4) as well as for more general singular functions. For the sake of completeness we write it down here. Taking a line L that is close to $\Sigma(B)$ and meets V, we find a point $x \in B$ such that the plane $P(L, x)$ through L and x contains the normal vector $n(x)$ to B. We denote $x_1(L) := x$, $\sigma(L) := dist(L, x_1)$ and define $\kappa(L)$ to be the curvature of the section $P \cap B$ at x_1. Then we have the following asymptotic development for the ray transform of the delta-like original:

$$R(a\delta(B))(L) = [a(x_1(L)) + o(1)] |\kappa(x_1(L))|^{-\frac{1}{2}} \sigma(L)^{-\frac{1}{2}}.$$

For the original $f = a\chi(V)$ we get a similar formula where the function $\sigma^{-\frac{1}{2}}$ is changed by its primitive $2\sigma^{\frac{1}{2}}$.

Now we pass to the case of non-convex V, where the geometry of $\Sigma(B)$ was described by Propositions 2 and 3. Fix $k > 1$ and consider the following family of polynomials

$$p(r, s) = r^{k+1} + s_{k-1} r^{k-1} + s_{k-2} r^{k-2} + \cdots + s_1 r + s_0$$

with real coefficients $s = (s_0, s_1, \ldots s_{k-1})$. Let D_k be the set of points $s \in S = \mathbb{R}^k$ such that $p(r, s)$ has at least one real multiple root r. For $k = 2, 3$ this set was described in the previous section. For $s \in S \setminus D_k$ we define

$$v_k(s) := \sum \frac{1}{|p'(r_i(s), s)|},$$

where the sum is taken over the set of all simple real roots $r_i(s), i = 1, 2, \ldots$ of p; we put $v_k(s) = 0$, if there is no such a root. This function is real analytic on the complement to D_k.

THEOREM 1. *Under the conditions of Proposition 2 the ray transform of the function $f = a\delta(B)$ admits the following asymptotic representation in a neighborhood of $\Sigma_2(B)$:*

$$Rf(L) = [a(x_2(L)) + o(1)] g_2(x_2(L)) v_2(s(L))$$

as $L \to \Sigma_2(B)$, where $s = s(L)$ is the submersion defined in Proposition 2, $x_2(L)$ is given in Corollary 4 and $g_2(x)$ is a smooth non-zero function on B (see below).

In a neighborhood of the set $\Sigma_3(B)$ a similar equation holds:

$$Rf(L) = [a(x_3(L)) + o(1)] g_3(x_3(L)) v_3(s(L))$$

as $L \to \Sigma_3(B)$, where g_3 is a smooth non-vanishing function on the curve I.

The quantity $o(1)$ tends uniformly to zero as L tends to a compact subset of $\Sigma_2(B)$ and of $\Sigma_3(B)$ correspondingly.

To get similar formulae for an original like $\chi(V)$ we use the following continuous special functions:

$$w_2(s) := \int_0^{s_0} v_2(u, s_1)\, du, \qquad w_3(s) := \int_{s_0}^{\infty} v_3(u, s_1, s_2)\, du.$$

Note that the function $w_3(s)$ vanishes in the component of $S \backslash D_3$, where $s_0 \geq O(|s_1|^{\frac{4}{3}} + s_2^2)$, since the function v_3 does.

THEOREM 2. *Under the same hypothesis if $f = a\chi(V)$, then we have*

$$Rf(L) = [a(x_k(L)) + o(1)]\, g_k(x_k(L))\, w_k(s(L))$$

as $L \to \Sigma_k'$, where $k = 2, 3$.

We specify the functions g_2, g_3 in the following way: take a point $x \in B$ an inflexional tangent L_x at x and the plane P that is orthogonal to B at x and contains L_x. Then choose Euclidean coordinates α, γ in P with the origin in x, where α is as in Proposition 2; we can reach the equation $\|\alpha\| = 1$ keeping (6) and (7) and rescaling in S. Write down an equation $\alpha = \alpha(\gamma)$ of the curve $P \cap B$ and have

$$\alpha(0) = \alpha'(0) = \alpha''(0) = 0, \alpha'''(0) \neq 0, \text{ if } L_x \text{ is simple inflexional}$$

and

$$\alpha(0) = \alpha'(0) = \alpha''(0) = \alpha'''(0) = 0, \alpha''''(0) < 0, \text{ if } L_x \text{ is double inflexional.}$$

The negative sign of the forth derivative means that the α-axis has the outward direction with respect to the (non-strictly) convex curve $P \cap B$. Then we have

$$g_2(x) = \frac{1}{2}\, \Big|\, \frac{6}{|z'''(0)|}\, \Big|^{\frac{1}{3}}; \qquad g_3(x) = \Big|\, \frac{24}{z''''(0)}\, \Big|^{\frac{1}{4}}.$$

Remark 3. The similar statement is true as well for the case $K(x) = 0$ and any order k of contact in (4) however the mapping (s, t) may be not a diffeomorphism.

Note that the singular support of the function $v_k(s(L))$ coincides with the set $\Sigma_k(B)$ for $k = 2, 3$ since this set is a pullback of the discriminant set D_k according to Propositions 2 and 3.

For a proof of Theorem 1 and Remark 3 we return to the arguments of Propositions 2,3. Calculating line integrals we find
(8)
$$Rf(L) = \sum \frac{a(r_i(s), s)\sqrt{1 + \psi'(r_i(s), s)^2}}{|\psi'(r_i(s), s)|} = [a(x_k(L)) + o(1)] \sum \frac{1}{|\psi'(r_i(s), s)|},$$

where $s = s(L)$ and $r_i(s)$ are roots of the function $q(\cdot, s)$ and the numbers $\psi'(r_i(s), s)$ are small. We conclude form the equation $\psi = hq$ that

$$\psi'(r_i(s), s) = h(r_i(s), s))q'(r_i(s), s).$$

Combining this equation with (8), we get

$$Rf(L) = [a(x_k(L)) + o(1)]h(x)^{-1}v_k(s(L)).$$

This implies Theorem 1 if we calculate the number $h(x)$. It is easy to do comparing the asymptotics of functions Rf and v_k on the α_1-axis.

To prove Theorem 2 we note that the derivative $\partial Rf(L)/\partial \alpha_1$ has an alike asymptotics. Then we pass to primitives.

§6. Geometry of non-linear artifacts

Consider a singular original that admits the following form

$$f \approx a_B \delta_B + a_C \delta_C + a_F \delta_F,$$

where a_B, a_C, a_F are in $C_0^\infty(\mathbf{E})$ and $\delta_B, \delta_C, \delta_F$ mean respectively the delta-function on a smooth surface B, smooth curve C and on a finite set F. We mean that f is in fact a sum of "delta-like" functions

$$(9) \qquad f_\varepsilon = a_B \frac{1}{\omega_1 \varepsilon} \chi(B_\varepsilon) + a_C \frac{1}{\omega_2 \varepsilon^2} \chi(C_\varepsilon) + a_F \frac{1}{\omega_3 \varepsilon^3} \chi(F_\varepsilon) + a,$$

where G_ε means ε-neighborhood of a set $G \subset \mathbf{E}$ and ω_k is the volume of the k-dimensional unit ball. A reconstruction of a function of this type with small parameter d may have heavy artifacts, which are big far from the singularity set $B \cup C \cup F$ of the original. Artifacts of this kind are well-known for 2D case; they should be identified as images of the non-linear part $E_h(f)$ of the defect. We try to describe the geometry of $E_h(f)$ for an appropriate algorithm without specifying its details.

For this we need more geometry. First, introduce a flag space Φ, which consists of pairs (x, L), where $x \in L \in \Lambda$. This is a five-dimensional manifold which has two natural projections

$$\mathbf{E} \xleftarrow{\varepsilon} \Phi \xrightarrow{\lambda} \Lambda,$$

which send a pair (x, L) to x and L correspondingly. For any smooth surface $B \subset \mathbf{E}$ we define a threefold $\Phi(B) \subset \Phi$ that consists of pairs $(x, L), x \in B$, where L is a tangent line to B at x. Evidently $\lambda(\Phi(B)) = \Sigma(B)$. Then for any curve C in $\mathbf{E}$ we define $\Phi(C)$ to be the threefold of pairs $(x, L), x \in C \cap L$. For any finite subset $F \subset \mathbf{E}$ a surface $\Phi(F)$ is defined in a similar way. For a function like (9) we set

$$\Phi(f) := \Phi(B)) \cup \Phi(C)) \cup \Phi(F)).$$

This is a subvariety of Φ, which may have self-intersection. Consider the mapping

$$(10) \qquad \varphi : \Phi(f) \to \Lambda \supset \Sigma,$$

which is a restriction of the projection λ, Σ is a pencil. We call a line $L \in \Sigma$ a *singular* element of the pencil, if
(i) it is a critical value of φ or
(ii) it has several preimages under φ or
(iii) it is a point, where the mapping φ is not transversal to Σ.

The following lines are examples of singular elements:
any line that is tangent to B in two or more points;
each inflexional tangent to B;
any line that is tangent to B and meets the set $C \cup F$;
any line that meets $C \cup F$ two or more times.

For some cases nonlinear artifacts may appear near any singular line. To show it we choose a simple mathematical model for E_h. Set

$$g := \mathcal{A}\{Tr_\Delta(Rf(\Sigma[d]))\},$$

where Tr_Δ is the following truncation operator: $Tr_\Delta(a) = a$, if $|a| \leq \Delta$ and $Tr_\Delta(a) = sign\, a \cdot \Delta$, if $|a| \geq \Delta$, $a \in \mathbb{R}$. Hence we have

$$E_h(f) = \mathcal{A}\{Tr_\Delta(Rf(\Sigma[d])) - Rf(\Sigma[d])\}.$$

CLAIM 4. *For any appropriate Σ-algorithm, any function f_ε like (8) and any singular line L of the pencil Σ the function $E_h(f_\varepsilon)$ may tend to infinity near L as $\varepsilon \sim \Delta^{-1} \sim d \to 0$.*

We mean that the hardware error may tend to infinity near a given singular line for a certain relation between the small parameters ε, Δ^{-1} and d. See [9] for 2D case.

It may be worthwhile to take in account all the points of Σ, where the mapping φ has a peculiarity with respect to the quasi-Minkowski geometry. A plane $\Lambda(H)$ or $\Lambda(x)$ may have a non-generic intersection with the image of the mapping φ. We call such points x and planes H singular. The error $E_h(f_\varepsilon)$ may be relatively big near any singular point or plane.

We anticipate a complicated structure of $E_h(f)$ near singular points, lines and planes (cf. [9]). Apparently if we change the singular function $\delta(B)$ in (10) to the function $\chi(V)$, some artifacts on singular lines still may appear. But the analysis of $E_h(f)$ is more complicated in this case.

REFERENCES

1. V.P.Palamodov, *Inversion formula for three-dimensional ray transform* in Lecture Notes in Mathematics vol.1497 (G.T.Herman, A.K.Louis, F.Natterer, eds.), Springer-Verlag, 1990, pp. 53-62.
2. F.Natterer, *Mathematical problems of Tomography*, Wiley, New York, 1986.
3. V.P.Palamodov, *Some singular problems in tomography* in Translations of Mathematical Monographs Vol.81, AMS, 1990, pp. 123-140.
4. S.I.Gonchar, *Approximation of a function using a discrete Radon transform*, Ph.D. Thesis, Moscow State University, Moscow, 1986.
5. A.Louis, *Incomplete data problem in X-ray computerized tomography 1. Singular value decomposition of the limited angle transform*, Numer. Math. **48** (1986), 251-262.

6. T.Poston, I.Stewart, *Catastrophe Theory and its Applications*, Pitman, London, 1978.
7. B.Malgrange, *Ideals of Differentiable Functions*, Oxford University Press, 1966.
8. V.P.Palamodov, *Distributions and Harmonic Analysis* in Encyclopaedia of Mathematical Sciences Vol.72, VINITI, Moscow, 1991, pp. 5-134; English transl. Springer-Verlag, pp. 1-134.
9. V.P.Palamodov, *Nonlinear artifacts in tomography*, Dokl. Akad.Nauk SSSR **291** (1986), 333-336; English transl. in Soviet Phys.Dokl. **31(11)** (1986), 888-890.

MATHEMATICAL COLLEGE OF THE INDEPENDENT MOSCOW UNIVERSITY, MOSCOW, FOTIEVOY 18. HOME ADDRESS: 117571 MOSCOW, BAK.KOM.3-1-422.

E-mail address: palamo@tomogr.msk.su

A Note on Consistency Conditions in Three Dimensional Diffuse Tomography

S. K. PATCH

February 1, 1994

ABSTRACT. Consistency conditions amongst the data for a general three dimensional model in diffuse tomography are studied in detail for the smallest nontrivial example. These conditions appear as rank deficient submatrices of the data matrix and cause there to be far fewer independent data than unknowns. A method of smoothing noisy data for large systems is discussed as well.

(i) Introduction
(ii) Derivation of Conditions
(iii) The $2 \times 2 \times 2$ problem
(iv) Larger Systems
(v) Smoothing Noisy Data
(vi) Conclusion

1. Introduction

The word "tomography" refers to imaging an object by slices. X rays, for example, have high energy and travel straight through the body. Data analysis is linear and yields a scalar valued function. The oxymoron "diffuse tomography" refers to low energy imaging in which the paths of the radiant energy are not necessarily straight and are *unknown*. Data analysis in diffuse tomography is

---

1991 *Mathematics Subject Classification*. Primary 60, Secondary 62, 05.

The author was supported in part by AFOSR under Contract FDF-49620-92-J-0067-11792, by the Applied Mathematical Sciences Subprogram of the Office of Energy Research, Department of Energy, Under Contract Number DE-AC03-76SF00098, by the National Aeronautics and Space Administration under Grant NAG3-1143, and by the National Science Foundation under Grant DMS89-02831.

This paper is in final form, and no version of it will be submitted for publication elsewhere.

© 1994 American Mathematical Society
0075-8485/94 $1.00 + $.25 per page

highly nonlinear and yields a vector valued function. Problems in diffuse tomography are highly nonlinear because low energy is used. Clinical applications such as neonatal imaging and annual mammograms are not amenable to high energy techniques which might overexpose the patient to harmful radiation. Experimentalists in the medical arena are presently working with near infrared radiation; mathematicians have done preliminary mathematical analysis of diffuse tomographic methods in [**2, 3, 4, 5**]. In this paper we study consistency conditions amongst the boundary data for the three dimensional problem.

Consistency conditions have the unfortunate effect of reducing the amount of independent data. When working on an inverse problem, we would like to have as much information as possible. At best, we may recover as many parameters as independent data. In two dimensions, there are precisely as many data as unknowns. Consistency conditions amongst the data prevent inversion of the forward map. To glean really useful information from the data additional information about the system is required. In three dimensions, however, there are far more data than unknowns. There must be consistency conditions amongst the data, since the rank of the forward map can be at most the dimension of its domain. The question here is not whether there are consistency conditions, but whether they reduce the rank of the forward map so that it is rank deficient, like its two dimensional counterpart.

Before embarking on a study of consistency conditions amongst boundary data we must first understand the system which generates the data. Consider an $n \times n \times n$ array of voxels in $\mathbb{R}^3$ enclosing the object to be reconstructed. On each of the $6n^2$ outer faces there are two devices. One device shoots photons across the outside face into the neighboring voxel; the other device detects photons as they leave the system. For each of the $6n^2$ outside faces we collect $6n^2$ pieces of data. Within the array, photons travel in six directions: *north*, *south*, *east*, *west*, *up*, and *down*. They may change direction as long as they travel in one of the six preferred directions. They do not interact and may be absorbed within a voxel. Photons move according to a two step Markov process. The probabilities with which a photon moves to a neighboring voxel depend upon its previous, as well as present, location. In this two step formulation the state space consists of locations. We may redefine the state space so that photons move according to a one step Markov process. In the new state space a single state consists of the photon's location and direction of travel.

There are three different types of these Markov states: incoming, outgoing, and hidden. The probabilities with which photons move from one state to another are referred to as transition probabilities. The transition matrix, M, is sparse and may be written as a block matrix with nontrivial subblocks which we refer to as P_{io}, P_{ih}, P_{ho}, and P_{hh}. P_{io}, for example, contains the probabilities with which photons in incoming states move directly to outgoing states. P_{ih} contains the probabilities with which photons in incoming states move to hidden states. P_{ho} and P_{hh} are the transition matrices for photons starting in hidden states travelling to outgoing and hidden states, respectively. P_{io} and P_{hh} are always square matrices. If we order the Markov states carefully, all four of these submatrices of M have a block structure.

The data is written as a $6n^2 \times 6n^2$ data matrix, Q. $Q[i,j]$ represents the probability that a photon which enters the system at source i exits the system at detector j. Q provides no time-of-flight information. The forward map we wish to invert is a function of the transition probabilities and equals Q. Given Q, we wish to recover the transition probabilities. For a given object the transition probabilities give a discretized "image" of the object. In traditional imaging, we recover a single parameter per voxel. From this information a visual picture of the object is made. In diffuse tomography, however, we want to recover many parameters per voxel. From this information we could make several "pictures" of the object. In both classical and diffuse tomography, fine discretizations of the covering array are required to obtain detailed information about the object being imaged.

2. Derivation of Conditions

There are many rank deficient submatrices of Q. Each of these rank deficient submatrices represents travel from one "part" of the system to another "part". The "parts" of the system must be separated by a "barrier". A simple example of such a division of a system is shown in figure 2. The following is a proof of the rank deficiency of submatrices of Q representing travel from the leftmost voxels in a square system to the rightmost voxels. The same (albeit notationally messier) proof holds for barriers which are not straight. In the two dimensional case, all independent consistency conditions can be derived from rank deficient submatrices corresponding to straight barriers [7]. In three dimensions, however, rank deficient submatrices corresponding to bent barriers are crucial, generating many conditions independent of those generated by straight barriers.

There are $(n-1)$ possible vertical barriers we may use to separate an $n \times n \times n$ array of voxels into left and right parts. Assume for the moment that $1 \leq x \leq (n-1)$, $x \in \mathbb{N}$ and consider the barrier separating the leftmost $n^2 x$ voxels from the remaining voxels. Assume in this example that the leftmost incoming states are labeled 1 through $n^2 + 4xn$. Define, Q_{lr}^x to be the submatrix representing the probabilities that photons which enter the system on the left of the vertical barrier exit the system on the right of the barrier.

$$(2.1) \quad Q_{lr}^x = \begin{bmatrix} Q[1, m+1] & Q[1, m+2] & \ldots & Q[1, N] \\ Q[2, m+1] & Q[2, m+2] & \ldots & Q[2, N] \\ \vdots & \vdots & & \vdots \\ Q[m, m+1] & Q[m, m+2] & \ldots & Q[m, N] \end{bmatrix}$$

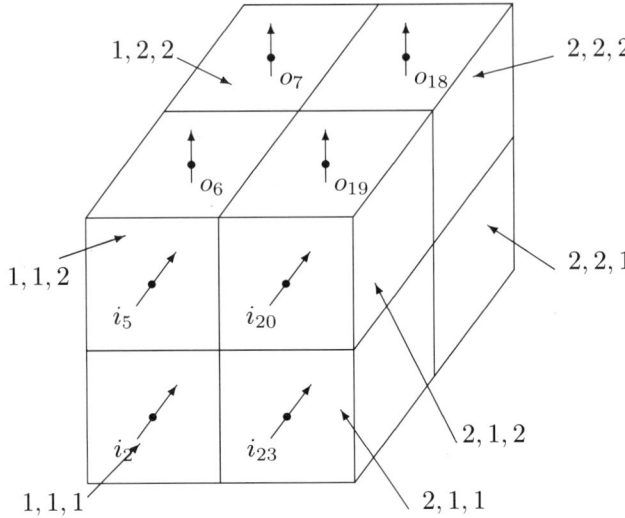

FIGURE 1. Eight voxels, seven of which are labelled above. Voxel 1,2,1 is hidden from view. Some incoming and outgoing states are labeled as well.

where $N = 36n^2$, $m = n^2 + 4nx$.

By taking advantage of the Markovian nature of the model, we may easily prove that Q_{lr}^x is rank deficient. A photon travels along a given path connecting incoming state i to hidden state j with some (unknown) probability, which we associate with the path. Define

$$p_{i,j} = \text{probability of going ``directly'' from incoming state } i \text{ to hidden state } j$$

$$s_{i,j} = \text{probability of starting in hidden state } i \text{ and ever reaching outgoing state } j$$

For the purpose of deriving the rank deficiency of Q_{lr}^x a photon is said to travel "directly" if its path from incoming state i to hidden state j involves travel among only the leftmost voxels. For the purpose of calculating $p_{i,j}$, acceptable paths are those which exit the leftmost voxels only at their last step. $p_{i,j}$ is the sum over all acceptable paths of their associated probabilities. In the $2 \times 2 \times 2$ case, two of the paths $p_{3,24}$ takes into account are shown in figure 3. One of the paths which $s_{24,21}$ represents is shown in figure 4.

Claim: rank $(Q_{lr}^x) \leq n^2$.

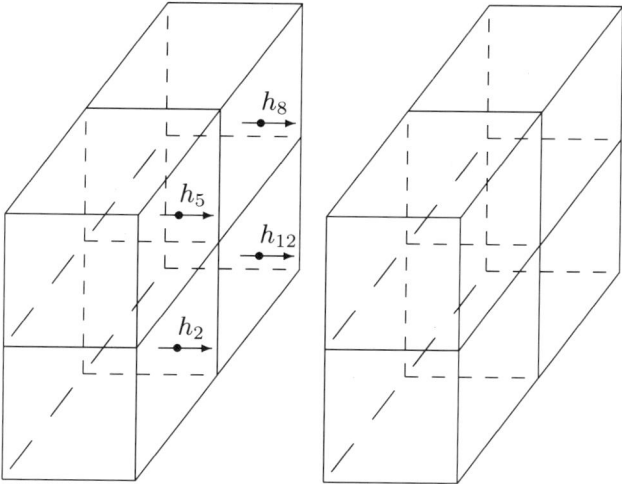

FIGURE 2. A $2 \times 2 \times 2$ system is split apart by a vertical barrier. A few hidden states are labeled above. Voxels 111, 121, 112, and 122 are the "leftmost" voxels; voxels 211, 221, 212, and 222 are "rightmost" voxels.

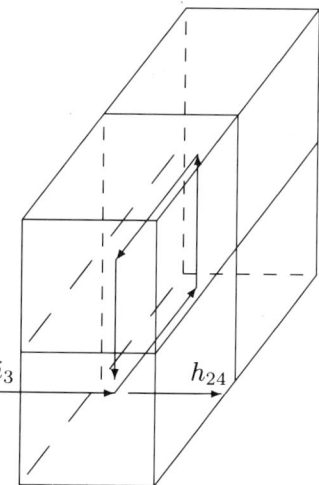

FIGURE 3. A few examples of paths which are taken into account by $p_{3,24}$. A photon may travel straight through voxel 111, or it may turn inside 111 and take a more circuitous path before exiting the leftmost voxels via hidden state h_{24}

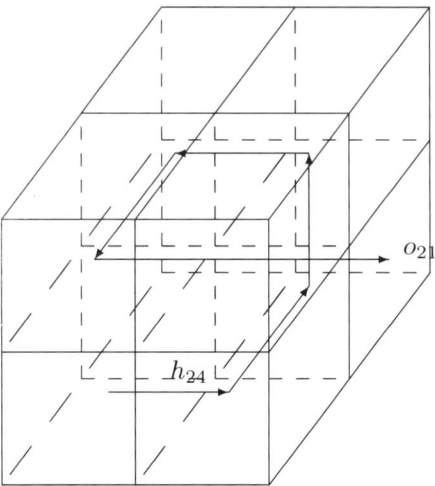

FIGURE 4. A path taken into account by $s_{24,21}$. $s_{24,21}$ is the sum over *all* paths from hidden state h_{24} to outgoing state o_{21}.

Proof: Let $h_{\alpha_1}, h_{\alpha_2}, h_{\alpha_3}, \ldots, h_{\alpha_{n^2}}$ be the hidden states by which a photon may travel east across the vertical barrier. For any $Q[i,j]$ in Q_{lr}^x,

$$Q[i,j] = \sum_{k=1}^{n^2} p_{i,\alpha_k} \, s_{\alpha_k, j}, \text{ i.e.,}$$

(2.2)
$$Q_{lr}^x = \begin{bmatrix} p_{1,\alpha_1} & p_{1,\alpha_2} & \cdots & p_{1,\alpha_{n^2}} \\ p_{2,\alpha_1} & p_{2,\alpha_2} & \cdots & p_{2,\alpha_{n^2}} \\ \vdots & \vdots & & \vdots \\ p_{m,\alpha_1} & p_{m,\alpha_2} & \cdots & p_{m,\alpha_{n^2}} \end{bmatrix} \begin{bmatrix} s_{\alpha_1, m+1} & s_{\alpha_1, m+2} & \cdots & s_{\alpha_1, N} \\ s_{\alpha_2, m+1} & s_{\alpha_2, m+2} & \cdots & s_{\alpha_2, N} \\ \vdots & \vdots & & \vdots \\ s_{\alpha_{n^2}, m+1} & s_{\alpha_{n^2}, m+2} & \cdots & s_{\alpha_{n^2}, N} \end{bmatrix}$$

Since Q_{lr}^x is the product of a $(n^2 + 4nx) \times n^2$ matrix with a $n^2 \times (5n^2 - 4nx)$ matrix the rank of Q_{lr}^x is at most n^2 for $x = 1, 2, \ldots, (n-1)$. By the same argument Q_{rl}^x, Q_{tb}^x, Q_{bt}^x, Q_{fb}^x, and Q_{bf}^x are also of rank less than or equal to n^2 for $x = 1, 2, \ldots, (n-1)$.

Naturally, this proof has an obvious two dimensional analog. The difference between the two and three dimensional cases is not in the existence proof of consistency conditions, but in its application. Notice that in both two and three dimensions all relevant barriers represent travel from part A to part B where A and B are disjoint parts of the system and A and B contain at least two corners each. (Suppose part C contains less than two corners. Then the barrier separating C from the rest of the system has at least as many faces/edges as C has outer faces/edges.) In two dimensions, straight barriers all have n edges and account for all of the independent conditions amongst the data. Bent barriers correspond to rank deficient submatrices of rank $> n$. In three dimensions, straight barriers have n^2 faces but do not account for all of the independent conditions amongst the data. In fact, there are many bent barriers which correspond to rank deficient submatrices of rank $< n^2$.

3. The $2 \times 2 \times 2$ problem

Consider the setup for the $2 \times 2 \times 2$ problem as shown in figures 1 and 2. In this section we make use of the conditions derived in section 2, to prove the following claim:

Claim: The $(6 * 2^2) \times (6 * 2^2)$ data matrix, Q, for the $2 \times 2 \times 2$ problem has at most 240 independent data.

Because of this recovery of the transiton probabilities from Q alone is impossible, since there are fewer independent data than the $6^2 * 2^3 = 288$ unknown transition probabilities. The table below shows which incoming and outgoing states correspond to which voxels:

(3.1)

States	*Voxel*
1, 2, 3	1, 1, 1
4, 5, 6	1, 1, 2
7, 8, 9	1, 2, 2
10, 11, 12	1, 2, 1
13, 14, 15	2, 2, 1
16, 17, 18	2, 2, 2
19, 20, 21	2, 1, 2
22, 23, 24	2, 1, 1

Every relevant rank deficient submatrix is a submatrix of some rows and columns of Q such that the intersection of the row numbers and column numbers is the empty set. The submatrix of Q from rows 1 through 12 and columns 13 through 24 represents the probabilities that a photon which enters the system through one of the leftmost voxels exits through one of the rightmost voxels. We call this submatrix Q^1_{lr}. The submatrix from rows 13 through 24 and columns 1 through 12 represents the probabilities that a photon which enters the system through one of the rightmost voxels exits through one of the leftmost voxels and is denoted by Q^1_{rl}. Similarly, the submatrix from rows 7 through 18 and columns 1, 2, 3, 4, 5, 6, 19, 20, 21, 22, 23, 24 represents travel from back to front and is called Q^1_{bf}, while its transpose represents travel from front to back and is called Q^1_{fb}. Finally, Q^1_{bt} is the submatrix from rows 1, 2, 3, 10, 11, 12, 13, 14, 15, 22, 23, 24 and columns $4, 5, 6, 7, 8, 9, 16, 17, 18, 19, 20, 21$ representing travel from bottom to top; Q_{tb}^1 is the transpose of Q_{bt}^1. Each of these 12×12 submatrices is generically of rank four.

There are twelve barriers which separate two voxels along an edge from the other six voxels. Each of these barriers has four faces and corresponds to a 6×18 and a 18×6 submatrix of rank four. The submatrix from the first six rows and last 18 columns, for example, represents travel from voxels 111 and 112 to the other six voxels. A barrier which separates three voxels in one "half" of the system, (four voxels on one side of a straight barrier), from the other five voxels corresponds to one 9×15 and one 15×9 submatrix of rank five. The first nine rows and last 15 columns of Q form such a submatrix representing travel from voxels 111, 112, and 122 to the other voxels. Because of these rectangular rank deficient submatrices and Q_{lr}^1, Q_{rl}^1, Q_{fb}^1, Q_{bf}^1, Q_{tb}^1, and Q_{bt}^1 there are at most 240 independent data for the $2 \times 2 \times 2$ problem. Figure 5 is a block matrix representation of the 24×24 data matrix, Q.

Notation: $I_{c_1,c_2}^{r_1,r_2}$ denotes the entries of Q in rows $r_1 \ldots r_2$ and columns $c_1 \ldots c_2$. The I indicates the origin of the data, in this case that it is independent of all consistency conditions. G means that the data is given. lr, rl, fb, and bf imply that the data was computed from given data and the fact that Q_{lr}^1, Q_{rl}^1, Q_{fb}^1, and Q_{bf}^1 respectively must be of rank four.

Assuming that all of the necessary inverses exist we can write explicit expressions for the following submatrices:

$$(3.2) \quad \begin{aligned} lr_{13,20}^{5,12} &= G_{21,24}^{5,12} \, (G_{21,24}^{1,4})^{-1} \, G_{13,20}^{1,4} \\ bf_{1,6}^{7,14} &= G_{21,24}^{7,14} \, (G_{21,24}^{15,18})^{-1} \, G_{1,6}^{15,18} \\ fb_{7,12}^{5,6} &= G_{21,24}^{5,6} \, (G_{21,24}^{15,18})^{-1} \, G_{1,6}^{15,18} \\ rl^* &= G_{1,4}^{19,24} \, (G_{1,4}^{15,18})^{-1} \, G_{5,6}^{15,18} \\ bf^* &= G_{21,24}^{13,18} \, (G_{21,24}^{9,12})^{-1} \, (G_{21,24}^{9,12} \, (G_{21,24}^{1,4})^{-1} \, G_{19,20}^{1,4}) \\ fb_{7,10}^{19,20} &= G_{1,4}^{19,20} \, (G_{1,4}^{21,24})^{-1} \, G_{7,10}^{21,24} \\ fb_{11,18}^{19,20} &= G_{1,4}^{19,20} \, (G_{1,4}^{21,24})^{-1} \, G_{7,10}^{21,24} \, (G_{7,10}^{1,4})^{-1} \, G_{11,18}^{1,4} \\ fb_{11,18}^{21,24} &= G_{7,10}^{21,24} \, (G_{7,10}^{1,4})^{-1} \, G_{11,18}^{1,4} \end{aligned}$$

Computing the rest of the data as done above forces several of the submatrices which should be rank deficient to be of their proper rank. The following chart shows which of the 6×18 submatrices which should be of rank four have already been forced to be rank four. Their transposes are also of rank four.

$$
(3.3) \quad \begin{array}{cc} Rows & Columns \\ 1-6 & 7-24 \\ 7-12 & 1-6, 13-24 \\ 13-18 & 1-12, 19-24 \\ 19-24 & 1-18 \end{array}
$$

Many other submatrices which should be rank deficient are not necessarily rank deficient. There are eight more pairs of 6×18 and 18×6 submatrices which should also be of rank four and 24 pairs of 9×15 and 15×9 submatrices which sould be of rank five.

All of the data except for the data in the blocks marked with a, b, c, d, e, f, g, and h is written in terms of the independent and the given data. To simplify notation, we now refer to all known data with the standard prefix Q. First we shall consider the 9×15 and 15×9 submatrices which should be of rank five. The subblocks

$$
(3.4) \quad \begin{bmatrix} a & Q_{7,18}^{1,3} \\ Q_{4,6}^{19,24} & Q_{7,18}^{19,24} \end{bmatrix} \quad \begin{bmatrix} a & Q_{7,12}^{1,3} \\ Q_{4,6}^{13,24} & Q_{7,12}^{13,24} \end{bmatrix}
$$

should be of rank five. Note that these submatrices overlap with Q_{fb}^1, Q_{bf}^1, Q_{rl}^1, Q_{lr}^1 and the submatrices noted in 3.3. Assuming that $\begin{bmatrix} Q_{7,10}^{1,3} \\ Q_{7,10}^{21,24} \end{bmatrix}$ and $\begin{bmatrix} Q_{4,10}^{21,24} \end{bmatrix}$ both span $\mathbb{R}^4$ it suffices for

$$
(3.5) \quad \begin{bmatrix} a & Q_{7,10}^{1,3} \\ Q_{4,6}^{21,24} & Q_{7,10}^{21,24} \end{bmatrix}
$$

to be of rank five. This means that every 6×6 minor of 3.5 must be indentically zero. There are $\binom{7}{6}^2 = 49$ different 6×6 minors of 3.5 of which only four are independent. Consider the minors obtained by omitting the fourth or fifth column and the first or second row. The Laplacian expansion along the first two rows of these minors yields a quadratic equation in four of the entries of a:

$$0 = (-1)^c \begin{vmatrix} a_c^r & a_6^r \\ a_c^3 & a_6^3 \end{vmatrix} |Q_{7,10}^{21,24}| +$$

$$\sum_{j=7}^{10} ((-1)^{c+j} \begin{vmatrix} a_c^r & Q_j^r \\ a_c^3 & Q_j^3 \end{vmatrix} |Q_{ac\sim\{c,j\}}^{21,24}| + (-1)^j \begin{vmatrix} a_6^r & Q_j^r \\ a_6^3 & Q_j^3 \end{vmatrix} |Q_{ac\sim\{6,j\}}^{21,24}|) +$$

(3.6)
$$\sum_{i=7}^{9} \sum_{j=i+1}^{10} (-1)^{i+j} \begin{vmatrix} Q_i^r & Q_j^r \\ Q_i^3 & Q_j^3 \end{vmatrix} |Q_{ac\sim\{i,j\}}^{21,24}|$$

where

$$\begin{aligned} ac &= \{c, 6, 7, 8, 9, 10\} \\ c &= 4 \ or \ 5 \\ r &= 1 \ or \ 2 \end{aligned}$$

$|Q_{ac\sim\{i,j\}}^{21,24}|$ = determinant of the minor taken from rows 21 through 24 and columns $\{c, 6, 7, 8, 9, 10\} \sim \{i, j\}$

There are eight more 9×15 and 15×9 submatrices which should be of rank five and contain the submatrix a. We shall use these submatrices to find five other minors which can be used with 3.6 to solve for the entries of a in terms of the other data. These submatrices do not overlap with rank deficient submatrices of rank four to the same extent as the submatrices in 3.4. If the rest of the submatrices which should be rank deficient of rank four were of rank four, then these 9×15 and 15×9 submatrices would also be of rank seven. In order to avoid equations which will become trivial when we force Q_{bt}^1 and Q_{tb}^1 and the rest of the 6×18 and 18×6 submatrices to be of rank four we use 6×6 minors similar to 3.6. We choose these equations so that none of the other 9×15 or 15×9 submatrices is forced to be of rank five.

Unfortunately, Bezout's theorem says there may be as many as 2^9 *different* solutions to this system of nine quadratic equations. Because Q is a transition matrix acceptable solutions must lie in $\mathbb{R}^{+^9}$, and satisfy the following condition

(3.7)
$$0 \leq \sum_{\lambda=1}^{24} Q[i, \lambda] \leq 1 \qquad i = 1, 2, \ldots, 24$$

Similar constraints hold for the subblocks b, c, d, e, f, g, and h.

If we had the good fortune that for each of the eight subblocks there were only one acceptable solution to its system of nine quadratic polynomials, then we would have been able to compute Q from only 72 independent data and 192 pieces of data which are subject to consistency conditions. We have not yet taken into account all of the conditions corresponding to the 9×15 and 15×9 submatrices which should be of rank five. They shall be considered later. First we shall force the rest of the 6×18 submatrices to be rank four. Then we shall see that in the generic case Q^1_{bt} and Q^1_{tb} and the rest of the 18×6 submatrices are also of rank four. Finally, we shall see that the remaining conditions upon the rank five submatrices are superfluous.

Consider the submatrix from rows four through nine and columns $1-3, 10-24$.

$$(3.8) \quad \begin{bmatrix} b & Q^{4,6}_{10,12} & Q^{4,6}_{13,24} \\ Q^{7,9}_{1,3} & c & Q^{7,9}_{13,24} \end{bmatrix}$$

where we already know that

$$(3.9) \quad \begin{bmatrix} b & Q^{4,6}_{19,24} \\ Q^{7,9}_{1,3} & Q^{7,9}_{19,24} \end{bmatrix} \text{ and } \begin{bmatrix} Q^{4,6}_{10,12} & Q^{4,6}_{13,18} \\ c & Q^{7,9}_{13,18} \end{bmatrix}$$

are of rank five and that $Q^{4,9}_{13,24}$ is of rank four. To force both of the matrices in 3.9 to be rank four requires one condition apiece. Assuming that both $Q^{4,9}_{13,18}$ and $Q^{4,9}_{19,24}$ are of rank four this is all that is required to force 3.8 to be rank four. The same argument holds to show that two conditions are required to force each of the submatrices indicated below to be rank four.

$$(3.10) \quad \begin{array}{cc} Rows & Columns \\ 4-9 & 1-3, 10-24 \\ 10-15 & 1-9, 16-24 \\ 16-21 & 1-15, 22-24 \\ 1-3, 22-24 & 4-21 \end{array}$$

Only four of the 6×18 submatrices which should be of rank four have not been considered. One such is from rows $4-6, 19-21$ and columns $1-3, 7-18, 22-24$.

$$(3.11) \quad \begin{bmatrix} b & Q^{4,6}_{7,18} & Q^{4,6}_{22,24} \\ Q^{19,21}_{1,3} & Q^{19,21}_{7,18} & g \end{bmatrix}$$

Unlike the 6×18 submatrices in 3.10, none of the 9×15 or 15×9 submatrices constrain 3.11 significantly. Four conditions are required, therefore, to force this generically rank six submatrix to be of rank four. The same argument holds to show that four conditions are required for each of the submatrices indicated below in order to force them to be of rank four.

	Rows	Columns
(3.12)	$4-6, 19-21$	$1-3, 7-18, 22-24$
	$1-3, 10-12$	$4-9, 13-24$
	$7-9, 16-18$	$1-6, 10-15, 19-24$
	$13-15, 22-24$	$1-12, 16-21$

When we consider the 18×6 submatrices which should be rank four we find that in the generic case they are rank four. Consider the submatrix from rows $1-3, 7-18, 22-24$ and columns $4-6, 19-21$.

$$(3.13) \qquad \begin{bmatrix} a & Q^{1,3}_{19,21} \\ Q^{7,18}_{4,6} & Q^{7,18}_{19,21} \\ Q^{22,24}_{4,6} & h \end{bmatrix}$$

Because it overlaps with Q^1_{bf} the middle twelve rows, $[Q^{7,18}_{4,6} \;\; Q^{7,18}_{19,21}]$ are of rank four. Furthermore several submatrices are of rank four by virtue of the fact that 3.13 overlaps with of some of the 6×18 rank four submatrices.

$$(3.14) \qquad \begin{bmatrix} a & Q^{1,3}_{19,21} \\ Q^{10,12}_{4,6} & Q^{10,12}_{19,21} \end{bmatrix} \quad \text{and} \quad \begin{bmatrix} Q^{13,15}_{4,6} & Q^{13,15}_{19,21} \\ Q^{22,24}_{4,6} & h \end{bmatrix}$$

are of rank four as is

$$(3.15) \qquad \begin{bmatrix} a & Q^{1,3}_{19,21} \\ Q^{22,24}_{4,6} & h \end{bmatrix}$$

Let S denote the space spanned by the rows of $[Q^{7,18}_{4,6} \;\; Q^{7,18}_{19,21}]$. Let $S^{1,3}$ denote the space spanned by the rows of $[a \;\; Q^{1,3}_{19,21}]$ and $S^{22,24}$ denote the space spanned by the rows of $[Q^{22,24}_{4,6} \;\; h]$. In the generic case $[Q^{10,12}_{4,6} \;\; Q^{10,12}_{19,21}]$ and $[Q^{13,15}_{4,6} \;\; Q^{13,15}_{19,21}]$ are both of rank three. Because the submatrices in 3.14 are of rank four,

$$(3.16) \qquad \begin{aligned} dim(S \cap S^{1,3}) &\geq 2 \\ dim(S \cap S^{22,24}) &\geq 2 \end{aligned}$$

In the generic case we expect that

$$(3.17) \qquad dim((S \cap S^{1,3}) \cup (S \cap S^{22,24})) \geq (2+2) = 4$$

or

(3.18) $$S \subseteq (S^{1,3} \bigcup S^{22,24})$$

Since $dim(S) = 4$. Because of 3.15 we know that

(3.19) $$dim(S^{1,3} \bigcup S^{22,24}) = 4$$

Therefore, $S = (S^{1,3} \bigcup S^{22,24})$ and the rank of the submatrix 3.13 is generically four. The same holds for the rest of the 18×6 submatrices which should be of rank four. A similar argument holds to show that Q^1_{bt} and Q^1_{tb} are generically of rank four.

Finally, the rest of the 9×15 and 15×9 submatrices are now generically of rank five. Consider any of the 9×15 submatrices which should be of rank five. It is the aggregate of two overlapping 6×18 submatrices of rank four. (In this paper "aggregate" refers to the submatrix of Q from the union of rows and intersection of columns of the submatrices involved.)

Assuming that the three rows in which these 6×18 submatrices overlap are of rank three then the matrix may be at most of rank five.

Although we may compute from only $72 + 192 = 264$ pieces of data the rest of the data there are $4 * 2 + 4 * 4 = 24$ conditions upon the given data. Therefore, Q is generically a function of at most $264 - 24 = 240$ independent parameters. Tests with phantom data sets have shown that the rank for the forward map is generically 240.

4. Larger Systems

As we saw in section 3, there are $240/2^3 = 30$ independent data per voxel for the $2 \times 2 \times 2$ problem. For $n = 2^k$ we could subdivide an $n \times n \times n$ system into $(2^{(k-1)})^3$ $2 \times 2 \times 2$ subsystems. Clearly, the data for the $n \times n \times n$ system is a function of the data for the $2 \times 2 \times 2$ subsystems. Therefore the data for the $n \times n \times n$ system is a function of at most $240 * (2^{(k-1)})^3 = 30 * (2^k)^3 = 30n^3$ independent parameters.

Clearly, the act of generating the data for the $n \times n \times n$ system from the $n/2 \times n/2 \times n/2$ subsystems enforces the rank deficiency of submatrices whose barriers coincide with boundaries between $n/2 \times n/2 \times n/2$ subsystems. There are many other barriers within the $n \times n \times n$ system and generating the data from subsystems' data forces some of the larger system's submatrices to be of their proper rank:

Claim: Let Q be a data matrix generated by the data matrices of two adjacent systems. Let B be a barrier in the large system such that B is the union of one barrier from each of the subsystems. Then the submatrix of Q corresponding to B is properly rank deficient.

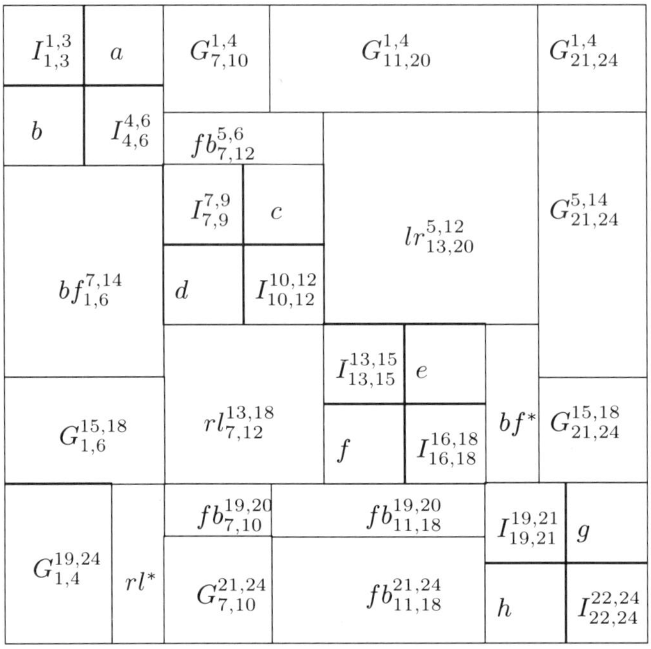

FIGURE 5. Above is a block matrix representation of the data matrix Q for a $2 \times 2 \times 2$ system. For an $n \times n \times n$ system where $n = 2^k$ for $k \in \mathbb{N}$ the dimension of the blocks in this matrix grows by a factor of $(2^{k-1})^2$ and the diagonal blocks are no longer entirely filled with independent data.

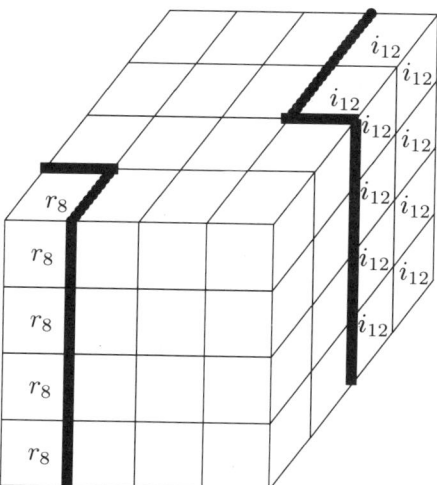

FIGURE 6. The submatrix corresponding to travel from the voxels 111, 112, 113, and 114 (marked with "r_8") is of rank eight. The submatrix corresponding to travel from the voxels 441, 442, 443, 444, 431, 432, 433, and 434, (marked with "i_{12}") is of rank twelve.

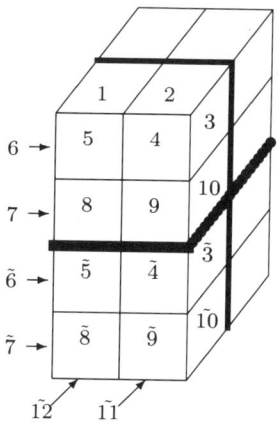

FIGURE 7. The $2 \times 2 \times 4$ system shown above has one front-back submatrix. Its barrier is outlined by the thinner bold lines. The system is composed of two $2 \times 2 \times 2$ subsystems. The first ten rows of Q_{fb}^1 correspond to incoming states 1-10 of the top subsystem; the last ten rows of Q_{fb}^1 correspond to incoming states $\tilde{3} - \tilde{12}$ of the bottom system. Each face corresponding to one of these incoming states is labeled with the number of its incoming state.

This claim is proved for a particular barrier in the the $2 \times 2 \times 4$ system shown in figure 7, but is easily generalized. The systems in figure 7 has one front-back, one back-front, one left-right, and one right-left submatrix. All of these submatrices should be of rank eight. It also has three top-bottom and three bottom-top submatrices which should be of rank four. We denote the data matrix for the entire system as Q and the data matrices for the top $2 \times 2 \times 2$ and bottom $2 \times 2 \times 2$ subsystems by QT and QB, respectively. If we were to generate Q from QT and QB then Q_{tb}^2 and Q_{bt}^2 would automatically be of rank four. There are submatrices of Q corresponding to barriers in the large system composed of barriers existing within the subsystems. Such submatrices are also properly rank deficient. For example, Q_{fb}^1 is already of rank eight. The same proof holds to show that Q_{bf}^1, Q_{lr}^1, Q_{rl}^1, Q_{bt}^1, Q_{tb}^1, Q_{bt}^3, and Q_{tb}^3 as well as several submatrices of Q corresponding to bent barriers are properly rank deficient.

Assume that the first ten rows of Q_{fb} correspond to the first ten incoming states of the top system. They may be written as

(4.1) $\qquad QT_{13,24}^{1,10}M1 + QT_{11,12}^{1,10}M21(QB_{13,24}^{1,2}M2 + QB_{1,2}^{1,2}QT_{13,24}^{11,12}M1)$

where $M21 = (I - QB_{1,2}^{1,2}QT_{11,12}^{11,12})^{-1}$ and the 12×20 transition matrices $M1$ and $M2$ are (complicated) functions of QT and QB. Similarly, the last ten rows of Q_{fb} may be written as follows:

(4.2) $\qquad QB_{13,24}^{3,12}M2 + QB_{1,1}^{3,12}M12(QT_{13,24}^{11,12}M1 + QT_{13,24}^{11,12}QB_{13,24}^{1,2}M2)$

where $M12 = (I - QT_{11,12}^{11,12}QB_{1,2}^{1,2})^{-1}$.

We may use 4.1 and 4.2 to express Q_{fb} in block matrix form. See figure 8. Q_{fb} is the product of a 20×24 matrix and a 24×20 matrix:

(4.3) $\qquad \begin{bmatrix} QT_{13,24}^{1,12}M1 \\ QB_{13,24}^{1,12}M2 \end{bmatrix}$

Also,

$$rank(QT_{13,24}^{1,12}) \leq 4 \quad and \quad rank(QB_{13,24}^{1,12}) \leq 4$$

Therefore,

$$rank(QT_{13,24}^{1,12}M1) \leq 4 \quad and \quad rank(QB_{13,24}^{1,12}M2) \leq 4$$

This means that 4.3 is of rank eight or less. Hence, $rank(Q_{fb}) \leq 8$. The same argument applies to other systems like the $4 \times 2 \times 4$ system discussed below.

Consider now a $4 \times 2 \times 4$ system. See figure 9. (Q now refers this system's data matrix.) There are many other submatrices of Q which should be rank deficient. Some of them are automatically of their proper rank because of rank deficient submatrices like those discussed above. M_c, the submatrix representing travel from the C-shaped set of voxels shown on the left, should be of rank 18 because its barrier has 18 faces. M_o, the submatrix representing travel from the O-shaped

$I_{10\times 10}$	m_1 m_2	$0_{10\times 10}$	$QB_{13,24}^{1,12} M2$
$0_{10\times 10}$	m_3 m_4	$I_{10\times 10}$	$QT_{13,24}^{1,12} M1$

FIGURE 8. A block matrix representation of Q_{fb}. Here $m_1 = QT_{11,12}^{1,10}\ M21\ QB_{1,2}^{1,2}$, $m_2 = QT_{11,12}^{1,10}\ M21$, $m_3 = QB_{1,2}^{3,12}\ M12$, and $m_4 = QB_{1,2}^{3,12}\ M21\ QT_{11,12}^{11,12}$. m_1, m_2, m_3, and m_4, are all 10×2.

set of voxels shown on the right, should be of rank 16. M_c is automatically of rank 18. It is not clear, however, that generating Q from subsystems' data forces M_o to be of rank 16.

Let s_1 be the submatrix representing travel from voxels 114, 214, 314, and 414; s_2 represent travel from voxels 114, 113, 112, and 111; s_3 represent travel from voxels 111, 211, 311, and 411; and s_4 represent travel from voxels 411, 412, 413, and 414. s_1, s_2, s_3, and s_4 are generically of rank eight.

M_c is the aggregate of s_1, s_2, and s_3. Generically, the rows common to s_1 and s_2 are of rank three and the rows common to s_2 and s_3 are also of rank three. Therefore, $rank(M_c) \leq 3*8 - 2*3 = 18$. No further conditions are required to force M_c to be of its proper rank.

Applying the same argument to M_o, the aggregate of s_1, s_2, s_3, and s_4, implies that $rank(M_o) \leq 4*8 - 4*3 = 20$. But M_o's barrier has only 16 faces, so M_o should be at most of rank 16. M_c has fewer rows and more columns than M_o. Since we should have $rank(M_c) \geq rank(M_o)$, it is clear that the columns of M_c which M_o lacks span a space that does not lie in the column space of the submatrix contained by M_c and M_o. It may be that submatrices such as M_o place additional conditions upon the entries of Q, reducing the amount of independent data so that there are fewer than 30 independent data per voxel.

5. Smoothing Noisy Data

An interesting aside for applications is the following claim. Presumably, (to a theoritician at least), it is more difficult to collect data for which the incoming and outgoing states are very near to each other. Data representing travel across the bulk of the system should be much easier to collect. Unfortunately, the toughest data to measure is preciesey the data corresponding to the $8*3^2 + 12(n-2)2^2 + 6(n-2)^2\ 1^2 = 6n^2 + 24n$ entries of P_{io} and is completely independent of all conditions. The only positive note here is that the ratio of such independent

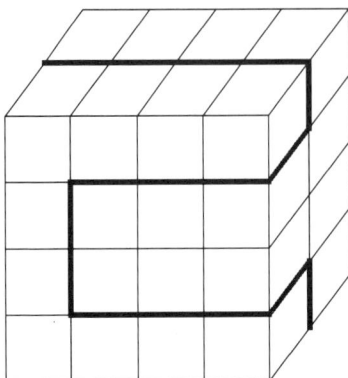 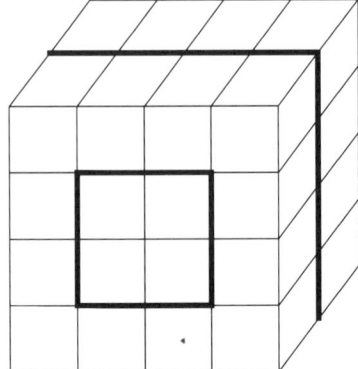

FIGURE 9. The barrier on the left corresponds to a submatrix which should be of rank eighteen; the submatrix corresponding to the barrier on the right should be of rank sixteen.

data to total data decreases to zero as n approaches infinity. Furthermore, the claim below shows that the rest of the data which is difficult to collect may be computed from data which should be easy to measure.

Claim: Data which is neither independent nor in the square rank deficient submatrices of rank n^2 may be expressed in terms of the data in the squre rank deficient submatrices of rank n^2.

Proof: Let $x \in \mathbb{N}$, $1 \leq x < n/2$ and assume that $\forall y \in \mathbb{N}$ such that $x < y < (n-x)$, Q_{lr}^y, Q_{rl}^y, Q_{bt}^y, Q_{tb}^y, Q_{fb}^y, and Q_{bf}^y are known. Consider the submatrix Q_{rl}^x. It is the rank deficient submatrix representing travel from right to left across the vertical left right barrier separating the $n^2 + 4nx$ rightmost states from the $5n^2 - 4nx$ leftmost states. Q_{rl}^x is a $(n^2 + 4nx) \times (5n^2 - 4nx)$ matrix of rank less than or equal to n^2. All but $4n$ of the columns of Q_{rl}^x overlap with $Q_{rl}^{(x+1)}$, which is known. Denote any one of the $4n$ "unknown" columns as column c, representing travel ending in an outgoing state, "o". Without loss of generality assume that o is an outgoing state by which photons exit the system through one of its topmost faces. State o is either in the front half or the back half of the system; assume without loss of generality that o lies in the front half. Only the entries of column c representing travel starting in incoming states into the upper x rows of the front half of the system are not part of the known submatrices $Q_{bt}^{n-(x+1)}$ and $Q_{bf}^{n/2}$. Hence $n/2((x+1)+x) + x(x+1) = nx + n/2 + x^2 + x$ of the entries in column c are unknown. Then $(n^2 + 4nx) - (nx + n/2 + x^2 + x)$ of

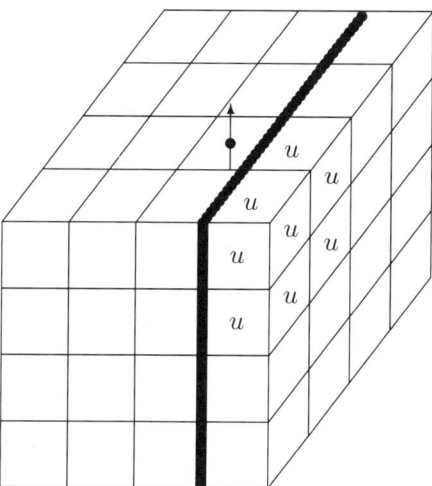

FIGURE 10. Q_{rl}^1 represents travel from the right side of the thick black barrier to the left side of the barrier. The outgoing state "o" is represented by an arrow leaving a voxel on the top of the system. Suppose that the column vector c represents travel starting on the right of the barrier and ending in state o and Q_{bt}^2 and Q_{bf}^2 are both known. Then most of column c is known. Only the entries which represent travel starting at states marked with "u" are unknown.

the data in column c are known. Since

$$\begin{aligned}(n^2 + 4nx) - (nx + n/2 + x^2 + x) &= n^2 + (3nx - n/2 - x(x+1)) \\ &> n^2 + (3nx - n/2 - n/2(x+1)) \\ &= n^2 + (3nx - n/2(x+2)) \\ &= n^2 + n(3x - (x+2)/2) \\ &= n^2 + n(5/2x - 1) \\ &> n^2\end{aligned}$$

$rank(Q_{rl}^x) \le n^2$, and more than n^2 columns of Q_{rl}^x are completely known we may compute the rest of column c. Each of the $4n$ incomplete columns of Q_{rl}^x can be completed in this way. Hence all of the (previously) unknown data in Q_{rl}^x is redundant. See figure 10 for an example. The same argument holds for Q_{lr}^x, Q_{bt}^x, Q_{tb}^x, Q_{fb}^x, and Q_{bf}^x. Similar arguments hold for Q_{rl}^z, Q_{rl}^z, Q_{bt}^z, Q_{tb}^z, Q_{fb}^z, and Q_{bf}^z where $z = (n - x)$. The assumption in the first line holds by hypothesis for $x = (n/2 - 1)$. The claim follows by induction.

6. Conclusion

We are able to smooth diffuse tomographic data because there are consistency conditions amongst the data. The forward map (from the transition probabilities to the data matrix Q) is rank deficient because of consistency conditions - even in three dimensions where there is far more data in Q than there are unknown transition probabilities. Consistency conditions amongst the data arise because photons make a random walk of sorts on a lattice. The Markovian nature of their walk was used in section 2 to derive the conditions. Photons traveling in a three dimensional lattice have far more "wiggle room" than photons traveling on a lattice in the plane. Because of this there are far more consistency conditions amongst the data in three dimensions than in two dimensions. In order to find the amount of independent data in Q, we need to determine the number of independent constraints the conditions impose upon Q. Two dimensional $n \times n$ systems generate at most $(n+1)/2n$ as much independent data as unknowns. In section 4 we saw that three dimensional $n \times n \times n$ systems generate *at most* $30n^3/36n^3 = 5/6$ as much independent data as unknowns. The author believes that this bound is far from tight and will be pleasantly surprised if three dimensional systems generate half as much independent data as unknowns. Further study is required to find a minimal set of conditions which completely describe the conditions amongst the data.

References

1. F. A. Grünbaum, "Tomography with Diffusion", *Inverse Problems in Action*, ed. P. Sabatier, pp. 16–21, Springer-Verlag, Berlin, 1990.
2. J. Singer, F. A. Grünbaum, P. Kohn and J. Zubelli, "Image reconstruction of the interior of bodies that diffuse radiation," *Science*, Vol. 248, 990–993, 1990.
3. F. A. Grünbaum, "An inverse problem in transport theory: diffuse tomography," *Invariant Imbedding and Inverse Problems*, SIAM 1993, in Honor of R. Kruger, J. Corones editor, pp.209-215.
4. F. A. Grünbaum, S. K. Patch, "Analytic inversion of a general model in diffuse tomography," Inverse Problems in Scattering and Imaging, Michael A. Fiddy, Editor, PROC S.P.I.E. Vol. 176744-54, (1992).
5. F. A. Grünbaum, S. K. Patch, "Simplification of a general model in diffuse tomography," Inverse Problems in Scattering and Imaging, PROC S.P.I.E., to appear.
6. F. A. Grünbaum, S. K. Patch, "The use of Graßmann Identities for inversion of a general model in diffuse tomography", Proceedings of the Lapland Conference on Inverse Problems, June 14-20, 1992. Saariselkä, Finland.
7. S. K. Patch, "Consistency Conditions in Diffuse Tomography", *Inverse Problems*, accepted for publication.
8. W. Feller, *An Introduction to Probability Theory and its Applications*, 2nd ed., John Wiley and Sons, Inc., New York, 1962.
9. C. Aitken, *Determinants and Matrices*, 8th ed., Oliver and Boyd Ltd., Edinburgh, 1954.

Department of Mathematics, University of California, Berkeley, CA 94720
E-mail address: patch@math.berkeley.edu

Radon Transforms on Curves in the Plane

ERIC TODD QUINTO

ABSTRACT. We prove support theorems for Radon transforms integrating on curves in the plane. We consider transforms that integrate over translations of one fixed curve and transforms that integrate over circles of varying radius. The proofs require the microlocal analysis of the Radon transforms and a microlocal Holmgren theorem.

1. Introduction and Results

Radon transforms are integral transforms. A typical Radon transform integrates functions over members of a class of submanifolds. Radon transforms on curves in the plane are applied to fields as diverse as X-ray tomography [**Na**], geophysical imaging [**Mu**], and complex analysis. Our theorems are presented with the last application in mind. Recall that the classical Morera Theorem states that, if $\int_C f dz = 0$ for all closed curves in a region, then f is holomorphic in that region. More general Morera theorems specify subclasses of curves which can be used to determine holomorphy. In [**GQ**], support theorems for Radon transforms on curves are used to determine such subclasses of curves.

Support theorems for Radon transforms on curves in arc-length measure are known in many cases including lines [**He**], circles [**Za**], rotation invariant sets of curves [**Co, Ku**], and other cases [**Mu, Ro**]. Support theorems that are valid with more general measures are in [**BQ 1987, Q 1983, Q 1993**]. The main results of this article are general support theorems for fairly arbitrary sets of

---

1991 *Mathematics Subject Classification.* Primary: 44A12, Secondary: 35S30.

Key words and phrases. Radon Transform, Support Theorem, Microlocal Analysis, Fourier Integral Operators.

The author thanks Larry Zalcman for getting him started on Morera problems, the motivation of this article and for providing some important references. He thanks Mark Agranovsky, Carlos Berenstein, and Josip Globevnik for many captivating and educational conversations. The author was partially supported by NSF grant MCS 9123862 and the Humboldt Stiftung.

This paper is in final form and no version of it will be submitted for publication elsewhere.

curves. We consider the case of translations of curves in 1.1 and the case of circles of varying radius in 1.2.

This research is based on the pioneering work of Guillemin and Sternberg [**Gu, GS**] that uses microlocal analysis to understand Radon transforms. The theory of real analytic Fourier integral operators is used to deduce analytic smoothness of a distribution f from support restrictions on $R_\mu f$ (Propositions 2.2 and 2.4). Then a theorem of Hörmander Kawai, and Kashiwara [**Hö, Ka**] about analytic singularities and support is used to deduce support restrictions on f from analytic smoothness of f (Lemma 3.2). These proofs follow naturally from the ideas in [**BQ 1987, Q 1993, Q 1980**].

We will now define the various Radon transforms and state our theorems. In §2, we will give the microlocal analysis of the transforms and in §3, we will prove the support theorems.

The Radon transforms in §1.1 and 1.2 are easily defined on domain $C_c(\mathbb{R}^2)$. However, our theorems are stated for distributions because we prove in §2 that these Radon transforms are Fourier integral operators. As shown in [**Tr**], Fourier integral operators are continuous operators on distributions.

1.1. Radon transforms on translates of curves. Let C be a real analytic curve in the plane. The set $Z = \{(x,y) \in \mathbb{R}^2 \times \mathbb{R}^2 \mid x \in y + C\}$ is called the *incidence relation* for the Radon transform (1.1) below [**He**]. Now, let $\mu(x,y)$ be a nowhere zero real analytic function on Z. Let f be a continuous function of compact support, $f \in C_c(\mathbb{R}^2)$, then the *Radon transform* of f (associated to Z and μ) is defined for $y \in \mathbb{R}^2$ by

$$(1.1) \qquad R_\mu f(y) = \int_{x \in y+C} f(x)\mu(x,y) ds(x)$$

where ds is the arc length measure on $y + C$. $R_\mu f(y)$ is simply the integral of f over the curve $y + C$ in weight μ. We exclude pathological cases in which the integral is not defined by requiring C to be either a smooth closed curve or an unbounded curve that does not oscillate too much. Our conditions will imply that C is a closed one-manifold without boundary that is imbedded in $\mathbb{R}^2$.

We include the weight μ in the definition of the Radon transforms above for several reasons. Allowing non-standard weights can help focus on properties intrinsic to the Radon transform rather than on specific symmetry properties that are valid only for special cases. This research is motivated by applications of these results to Morera theorems in complex analysis [**GQ**], and for this purpose, our theorems are needed for the non-standard measure dz.

We say that a smooth curve C is *flat to order one* at a point $w = (w_1, w_2) \in C$ if and only if the tangent line to C at w does not have higher than first order contact with C at w. If the curve is given by $x_2 = f(x_1)$ then the condition is, of course, equivalent to $f''(w_1) \neq 0$.

THEOREM 1.1. *Let C be a unbounded convex real analytic curve (that is, C divides the plane into two regions, one of which is convex). Assume C is flat to* order one at all points on C. Let $\mathcal{A} \subset \mathbb{R}^2$ be open, connected, and non-empty. Let R_μ be the Radon transform on translates of C with nowhere zero real analytic weight μ. Assume $f \in \mathcal{E}'(\mathbb{R}^2)$ with $R_\mu f(y) = 0$ for all $y \in \mathcal{A}$ and assume, for some $y_0 \in \mathcal{A}$, the curve $y_0 + C$ is disjoint from supp f. Then for all $y \in \mathcal{A}$, $y + C$ is disjoint from supp f.

The flatness assumption in Theorem 1.1 insures that C is strictly convex. The theorem is false if C is not strictly convex. The easiest example uses a line for C. Example 3.3 is more interesting. The hypothesis that there exists a $y_0 \in \mathcal{A}$ with $y_0 + C$ disjoint from supp f is also necessary, and an example is outlined after Example 3.3.

The next theorem deals with bounded curves.

THEOREM 1.2. *Let C be a smooth closed convex curve parameterized in polar coordinates by $r = r(\theta)$ where $r : [0, 2\pi] \to (0, \infty)$ is real analytic. Assume C is flat to order one at all points on C. Let $\mathcal{A} \subset \mathbb{R}^2$ be open, connected, and non-empty. Let R_μ be the Radon transform on translates of C with nowhere zero real analytic weight μ. Assume $f \in \mathcal{D}'(\mathbb{R}^2)$ with $R_\mu f(y) = 0$ for all $y \in \mathcal{A}$. Let D be the convex hull of C. Assume that, for some $y_0 \in \mathcal{A}$, the set $y_0 + D$ is disjoint from supp f. Then for all $y \in \mathcal{A}$, $y + D$ is disjoint from supp f.*

If one uses the classical measure, then R_1 is a convolution operator with a distribution in $\mathcal{E}'$ and so a simple Fourier transform argument proves this transform is injective on the domain of integrable functions. The proof of Theorem 1.2 is, morally, a microlocal version of this simple argument.

Negative results are known if the curve C is a circle. The example in [**Q 1993**] shows that the conclusion of Theorem 1.2 is false if one weakens the hypotheses about supp f to become: *for some $y_0 \in \mathcal{A}$, the curve $y_0 + C$ (not the set $y_0 + D$) is disjoint from* supp f. John has a counterexample if "$y_0 + D$" is replaced by "$y_0 + \text{int } D$" in this statement.

Positive results are also known if C is a circle. In this case and for $\mu \equiv 1$, this theorem follows from a result of Fritz John ([**Jo**, p. 115], see [**Q 1993**]). This theorem for transforms on circles with general measures is a special case of the theorem on Riemannian manifolds in [**Q 1993**]. In fact, the transform (with classical measures) on translates of two circles is injective on domain $C(\mathbb{R}^2)$, if their radii are 'well chosen' [**Za**] (see also [**BG**]).

1.2. Radon transforms on circles. The Radon transform integrating over all circles in the plane is overdetermined, since the set of all circles has dimension three, which is, of course, greater than the dimension of $\mathbb{R}^2$. Strong support theorems will be given in [**GQ**] for this general case. However, it is also appropriate to look for two dimensional subsets of circles on which uniqueness and support theorems hold. The set of translates of one fixed circle is two dimensional, and Theorem 1.2 includes this case. The two dimensional set we consider in this section is the set of all circles with centers constrained to lie on a fixed curve,

γ. This is analogous to the admissible complex of lines in space meeting a fixed curve.

We will consider only the case that γ is a circle because the arguments become rapidly more complicated otherwise.

For $\theta \in [0, 2\pi]$, define $\overline{\theta} = (\cos\theta, \sin\theta)$. Let $t > 0$, then the circle of radius t centered at the origin is parameterized by $\gamma(\theta) = t\overline{\theta}$ for $\theta \in [0, 2\pi]$. This γ will be the curve containing the centers of the circles for the Radon transform (1.2). Let the weight $\mu(x, \theta, r)$ be continuous on the incidence relation for this Radon transform, $Z_t = \{(x, \theta, r) \in \mathbb{R}^2 \times [0, 2\pi] \times (0, \infty) \mid |x - t\overline{\theta}| = r\}$. Now we define the circular Radon transform for $f \in C(\mathbb{R}^2)$ as

$$(1.2) \qquad S_t f(\theta, r) = \int_{\phi=0}^{2\pi} f(t\overline{\theta} + r\overline{\phi}) \mu(t\overline{\theta} + r\overline{\phi}, \theta, r) d\phi.$$

This is the integral of f over the circle centered at $t\overline{\theta}$ of radius r in weight μ. We suppress the μ dependence for notational convenience; the radius, t of γ is important in the following theorem.

THEOREM 1.3. *Let $t > 0$ and choose $s \in (t, \infty)$. Let $R > \sqrt{s^2 - t^2}$, and let $\mathcal{A} = [0, 2\pi] \times (0, R)$. Let S_t and S_s be the Radon transforms defined in (1.2) with possibly different nowhere zero real analytic weights. Assume $f \in \mathcal{D}'(\mathbb{R}^2)$ with $S_t f(\theta, r) = S_s f(\theta, r) = 0$ for all $(\theta, r) \in \mathcal{A}$ and assume, for some $(\theta_0, r_0) \in \mathcal{A}$ with $r_0 > \sqrt{s^2 - t^2}$, the closed disk centered at $t\overline{\theta}_0$ of radius r_0 is disjoint from supp f. Then for each $(\theta, r) \in \mathcal{A}$, the disk centered at $t\overline{\theta}$ and of radius r and the disk centered at $s\overline{\theta}$ and of radius r are both disjoint from supp f.*

The proof of this theorem in §3 really gives a stronger theorem in which $\mathcal{A}$ is more general than $[0, 2\pi] \times (0, R)$. That stronger theorem is described in Remark 3.7

The 'shadow circle'–the circle of radius s–is not just an artifact of the proof. Example 3.8 shows that Theorem 1.3 is not true if integrals are known only over circles with centers on one circle. In requiring circles with centers on two curves ($|a| = t$ and $|a| = s$), Theorem 1.3 is a little like the theorem in [**Za**]; uniqueness follows in that theorem, if one has integrals over translations of all circles of *two* 'well chosen' radii. In Theorem 1.3, however, the radii of the curves of centers, $|a| = t$ and $|a| = s$, do not need to be 'well chosen.' Little is known about this case, and one might guess that a theorem that does not contradict Example 3.8 might be true without the 'shadow circle.'

Similar theorems are true in higher dimensions and the proofs are more complicated versions of the proofs given below.

Note added in proof: The author has just learned about the following recent results related to Theorem 1.3. These results are valid for the Radon transform that integrates functions over circles with centers on a given curve, γ, in arc length measure. Mark Agranovsky informed me of the proof of the following lovely theorem: if γ is not contained in the zero set of a non-zero harmonic polynomial, then this transform is injective on the domain $C_c(\mathbb{R}^2)$. For closed, real analytic curves (and some other real analytic curves) one can prove this using Proposition 2.4 and Lemma 3.2 below. The other results are for $f \in C(\mathbb{R}^2)$ and where the set of circle-centers, γ, is a collection of concentric circles. Valery Volchkov has recently proven a neat uniqueness theorem for this Radon transform when the circle-centers lie on two concentric circles, $|z| = s$, and $|z| = t$: if the radii, s and t, are "well chosen," and integrals of a function $f \in C(\mathbb{R}^2)$ over all circles centered on $|z| = s$, and $|z| = t$ are zero, then $f \equiv 0$. Our Theorem 1.3 requires an additional hypothesis compared to Volchkov's theorem: f is zero on a disk. However, our theorem doesn't require "well chosen" radii, and it is more "local" than Volchkov's theorem in that it can be used to conclude restrictions on supp f from restrictions on the support of its Radon transform. Larry Zalcman pointed out the intriguing counterexample of a function ($f(x) = J_0(|x|)$, the radial Bessel function) which has zero integrals over all circles with centers on an infinite collection of concentric circles (with "badly chosen" radii).

2. Radon transforms as analytic Fourier integral operators

The analytic wave front set, $\mathrm{WF}_A(f)$, of a distribution $f \in \mathcal{D}'(\mathbb{R}^2)$ is defined in [**Tr**] or [**Hö**]. When describing curves in polar coordinates, we assume that 0 and 2π are identified in $[0, 2\pi]$ and that functions of θ satisfy the natural compatibility conditions at 0 and 2π.

DEFINITION 2.1. *Let C be a smooth curve in the plane and let $N^*C \subset T^*\mathbb{R}^2$ denote the conormal bundle of C. We say $x \in C$ and $x' \in C$ are C-parallel if and only if the tangent lines to C at the two points are parallel.*

Now we can state the microlocal regularity theorem for the Radon transform (1.1).

PROPOSITION 2.2. *Let C be a curve that is parameterized in polar coordinates by $r = r(\theta)$ where $r : I \to (0, \infty)$ is real analytic on the interval $I \subset [0, 2\pi]$. Assume either that $r(\theta)$ goes to ∞ at each endpoint of I or that C is a closed curve. Let R_μ be the Radon transform on translates of C, (1.1), with nowhere zero real analytic weight μ. If C is unbounded, let $f \in \mathcal{E}'(\mathbb{R}^2)$, and if C is closed, let $f \in \mathcal{D}'(\mathbb{R}^2)$. Assume $R_\mu f$ is zero in an open neighborhood of $y \in \mathbb{R}^2$. Let $(x, \xi) \in N^*(y + C) \setminus 0$, and assume that f is zero in neighborhoods of all $(y + C)$-parallel points to x. Then $(x, \xi) \notin \mathrm{WF}_A(f)$.*

These growth conditions on C imply that C is a closed submanifold without boundary that is imbedded in $\mathbb{R}^2$. In general, Radon transforms detect only $\mathrm{WF}_A(f)$ conormal to the curve being integrated over. In this case, Proposition 2.2 shows that wavefront conormal to $y + C$ above x is detected as long as there are no singularities of f at the $(y+C)$-parallel points to x to mask this wavefront.

PROOF. The key to the proof of Proposition 2.2 is an understanding of the microlocal properties of the operator R_μ. This analysis is based on the double fibration [**GGS**] and the arguments of Guillemin and Sternberg [**Gu, GS**]. Recall that the incidence relation for this Radon transform is $Z = \{(x,y) \in \mathbb{R}^2 \times \mathbb{R}^2 \mid x \in y + C\}$. The set N^*Z is the conormal bundle of Z in $T^*(X \times Y)$. The diagram needed for the proof is the microlocal analog of the double fibration:

(2.1)
$$\begin{array}{ccc} \Gamma = N^*(Z) \setminus 0 & \xrightarrow{\pi_2} & T^*(\mathbb{R}^2) \setminus 0 \\ \downarrow {\pi_1} & & \\ T^*(\mathbb{R}^2) \setminus 0 & & \end{array}$$

The maps are the natural projections onto the first or second factors.

To prove the statements about microlocal singularities in Proposition 2.2, we will show:

(2.2) covectors $(x, y; \xi, \eta) \in \Gamma$ and $(x', y; \xi', \eta) \in \Gamma$ have the same image under π_2 only if x and x' are $(y+C)$-parallel. π_2 is a local diffeomorphism.

First, we calculate N^*Z in good coordinates. For $w \in \mathbb{R}^2$ let $\arg w$ be the angle of w in polar coordinates (the angle between the positive horizontal axis and w). Although $\arg w$ is defined only mod 2π, all relevant functions are 2π periodic. Points $(x,y) \in Z$ are determined by the equation $|x-y|^2 - r^2(\arg(x-y)) = 0$, and the differential of this equation gives a basis of the fibers of N^*Z. Coordinates on Z are given by:

(2.3)
$$\begin{array}{c} I \times \mathbb{R}^2 \to Z \\ (\phi, y) \to (y + r(\phi)\overline{\phi}, y). \end{array}$$

Using these coordinates for Z gives coordinates for $N^*Z \setminus 0$ as follows:

(2.4)
$$\begin{array}{c} I \times \mathbb{R}^2 \times (\mathbb{R} \setminus 0) \to N^*Z \setminus 0 \\ (\phi, y, a) \to \big(y + r(\phi)\overline{\phi}, y; a(r(\phi)\overline{\phi} - r'(\phi)\phi^\perp)(\mathbf{dx} - \mathbf{dy})\big). \end{array}$$

Here, $(w_1, w_2)\mathbf{dx} = w_1 \mathbf{dx}_1 + w_2 \mathbf{dx}_2$ is the covector in $T^*\mathbb{R}^2$ corresponding to $(w_1, w_2) \in \mathbb{R}^2$ and $\phi^\perp = (-\sin\phi, \cos\phi)$.

Equation (2.4) shows that π_1, and π_2 do not map to the zero section since $\overline{\phi}$ and $\phi^\perp$ are independent. So, R_μ is a Fourier integral operator associated to the Lagrangian manifold, Γ [**Tr**, Theorem 2.1, p. 316] (see also [**GS**] and [**Q 1980**]). This explains why R_μ can be evaluated on distributions. R_μ is elliptic since μ is nowhere zero.

The map π_2 is equivalent to the corresponding map in coordinates (2.4):

(2.5)
$$(\phi, y, a) \xrightarrow{\tilde{\pi}_2} (y; -a(r(\phi)\overline{\phi} - r'(\phi)\phi^\perp)\mathbf{dy}).$$

First, note that the vector $(r(\phi)\overline{\phi} - r'(\phi)\phi^\perp)$ in (2.5) is perpendicular to $y + C$ at $y + r(\phi)\overline{\phi}$. So, if (ϕ, y, a) and (ϕ', y, a') map to the same point under $\tilde{\pi}_2$, (2.5) shows that $y + r(\phi)\overline{\phi}$ and $y + r(\phi')\overline{\phi'}$ are $(y+C)$-parallel. This shows the first claim of (2.2).

To show that π_2 is an local diffeomorphism, one calculates the differential of $\tilde{\pi}_2$ and discovers that π_2 is a local diffeomorphism if and only if $\forall \phi \in I$, $r^2(\phi) -$

$r(\phi)r''(\phi) + 2(r'(\phi))^2 \neq 0$. An elementary calculation shows this is equivalent to the assumption that C is flat to order one at all points on C.

Now, assume f is as in the hypotheses of Proposition 2.2. R_μ has been shown to be an analytic elliptic Fourier integral operator associated with Γ. The calculus of such operators implies the conclusion of Proposition 2.2. Let $(x,\xi) \in N^*(y+C) \setminus 0$ and assume f is zero near all $(y+C)$-parallel points to x. By (2.2), only singularities at $(y+C)$-parallel points to x can mask singularities of f above x. But, for all $(y+C)$-parallel points, x', to x, $\text{WF}_A(f)$ is empty above x'. Therefore, singularities at $(y+C)$-parallel points to x cannot mask singularities at x. Since $R_\mu f$ is zero near y, $(x,\xi) \notin \text{WF}_A f$. (Precisely, we make a C^∞ partition of unity, $1 = \psi_p + \psi_x + \psi_0$, with the following conditions: ψ_p is one near each $y+C$-parallel point to x and ψ_p is sufficiently localized around the $(y+C)$-parallel points to x so that $\psi_p f = 0$; ψ_x is one near x and sufficiently localized around x so that $g \mapsto R_\mu \psi_x g$ satisfies the Bolker Assumption locally above (x,y) (the restricted π_2 is an injective immersion). Therefore, ψ_0 is zero near x and all its $(y+C)$-parallel points, so by (2.5) and the calculus of Fourier integral operators [**SKK**, **Ka**], $R_\mu \psi_0 f$ is smooth in directions (y,η) when $(x,y;\xi,-\eta) \in \Gamma$. Therefore, as $R_\mu f = R_\mu \psi_p f = 0$ and $(y,\eta) \notin R_\mu \psi_0 f$, $(y,\eta) \notin \text{WF}_A(R_\mu \psi_x f)$. Since the operator $g \mapsto R_\mu \psi_x g$ satisfies the Bolker assumption above (x,y), $(x,\xi) \notin \text{WF}_A(f)$.) □

The regularity theorem for the Radon transform (1.2) requires some smoothness conditions on f at certain points. Let

$$(2.6) \qquad c_t(\theta, r) = \{x \in \mathbb{R}^2 \mid |x - t\overline{\theta}| = r\}$$

be the circle centered at $t\overline{\theta}$ and of radius r. This is the circle that $S_t f(\theta, r)$ integrates over.

DEFINITION 2.3. Points x and x' in $c_t(\theta, r)$ are said to be $c_t(\theta, r)$-*mirror* if and only if they are reflections about the diameter of $c_t(\theta, r)$ that is perpendicular to $\overline{\theta}$.

The diameter in Definition 2.3 is the one tangent to the circle of radius t centered at the origin–the curve of centers of the circles $c_t(\theta, r)$.

PROPOSITION 2.4. *Let $t > 0$ and let S_t be the Radon transform in (1.2) with nowhere zero real analytic weight. Let $f \in \mathcal{D}'(\mathbb{R}^2)$. Assume $S_t f$ is zero in an open neighborhood of $(\theta, r) \in [0, 2\pi] \times (0, \infty)$. Let $(x,\xi) \in N^* c_t(\theta,r) \setminus 0$, and assume that f is zero in a neighborhood of the $c_t(\theta,r)$-mirror point to x. Then $(x,\xi) \notin \text{WF}_A(f)$.*

If x is on the diameter of $c_t(\theta,r)$ perpendicular to $\overline{\theta}$, then x is its own mirror and Proposition 2.4 gives no useful conclusion about x.

PROOF. The proof will only be outlined because it is similar to the proof of Proposition 2.2. Recall that the incidence relation for S_t is $Z_t = \{(x, \theta, r) \in$

$\mathbb{R}^2 \times [0, 2\pi] \times (0, \infty) \mid x \in c_t(\theta, r)\}$. The appropriate microlocal diagram is:

$$\Gamma = N^*(Z) \setminus 0 \xrightarrow{\pi_2} T^*([0, 2\pi] \times (0, \infty)) \setminus 0$$

(2.7)
$$\downarrow \pi_1$$

$$T^*(\mathbb{R}^2) \setminus 0$$

The goal is to prove that π_2 in (2.7) satisfies:

(2.8)   covectors $(x, \theta, r; \xi, \eta) \in \Gamma$ and $(x', \theta, r; \xi', \eta) \in \Gamma$ have the same image under π_2 only if x and x' are $c_t(\theta, r)$-mirror. π_2 is a local diffeomorphism except above points (x, θ, r) where $x \in c_t(\theta, r)$ is its own mirror.

First, we calculate $N^* Z_t$ in good coordinates. Points $(x, \theta, r) \in Z_t$ are determined by the equation $|x - t\overline{\theta}|^2 - r^2 = 0$, and the differential of this equation gives a basis of the fibers of $N^* Z_t$. Coordinates for $N^* Z_t \setminus 0$ are:

$$[0, 2\pi]^2 \times (0, \infty) \times (\mathbb{R} \setminus 0) \to N^* Z_t \setminus 0$$

(2.9)
$$(\phi, \theta, r, a) \to \left(x, \theta, r; a([x - t\overline{\theta}]\mathbf{dx} - [t(x - t\overline{\theta}) \cdot \theta^\perp]\mathbf{d\theta} - r\mathbf{dr})\right)$$

where $x = r\overline{\phi} + t\overline{\theta}$.

Equation (2.9) shows that π_1 and π_2 do not map to the zero section so, R_μ is a Fourier integral operator associated to the Lagrangian manifold, Γ [**Tr,** Theorem 2.1, p. 316] (see also [**GS**] and [**Q 1980**]). This explains why R_μ can be evaluated on distributions. R_μ is elliptic since μ is nowhere zero.

The map π_2 is equivalent to the corresponding map in coordinates (2.9):

(2.10)
$$(\phi, \theta, r, a) \xrightarrow{\tilde{\pi}_2} \left(\theta, r; -a([t(r\overline{\phi} \cdot \theta^\perp)]\mathbf{d\theta} - r\mathbf{dr})\right).$$

Therefore, π_2 determines only $\overline{\phi} \cdot \theta^\perp$ so $x = t\overline{\theta} + r\overline{\phi}$ is known only up to its $c_t(\theta, r)$-mirror. This shows the first claim of (2.8). The calculation that $\tilde{\pi}_2$ is a local diffeomorphism except at self-mirror points is left to the reader, and the rest of the proof is parallel to that of Proposition 2.2. □

3. Proofs

DEFINITION 3.1. Let $f \in \mathcal{D}'(\mathbb{R}^2)$ and let C' be a smooth curve. Let $x \in$ supp $f \cap C'$. We say that *supp f is on one side of C' near x* if and only if there is a neighborhood U of x such that C' divides U into two open sets and f is zero on one of these open sets.

PROOF OF THEOREM 1.1. The curve C is convex and flat to order one at each point, so C is strictly convex. The key observation is that, since C is strictly convex and unbounded, for each $x \in C$, there is no other C-parallel point. Therefore, Proposition 2.2 and the hypotheses of Theorem 1.1 imply that

(3.1) $$\forall y \in \mathcal{A}, \ \mathrm{WF_A}(f) \cap N^*(y + C) = \emptyset.$$

Since there is a $y_0 \in \mathcal{A}$ such that $y_0 + C$ is disjoint from supp f and $\mathcal{A}$ is connected, there is a $y_1 \in \mathcal{A}$ such that $y_1 + C$ just touches supp f. Precisely, there is a point $x \in (\text{supp } f) \cap (y_1 + C)$ such that supp f is on one side of $(y_1 + C)$ near x. Now, (3.1) implies that $\text{WF}_A(f) \cap N^*(y_1 + C) = \emptyset$. However, the following theorem of Hörmander, Kawai, and Kashiwara [**Hö, Ka**] gives a contradiction.

LEMMA 3.2. *Let $h \in \mathcal{D}'(\mathbb{R}^2)$ and let C' be a smooth curve. Let $x \in \text{supp } h \cap C'$ and assume supp h is on one side of C' near x. If $(x, \xi) \in N^*C' \setminus 0$, then $(x, \xi) \in \text{WF}_A(f)$.*

This contradiction between (3.1) and Lemma 3.2 applied to $y_1 + C$ finishes the proof. □

EXAMPLE 3.3. We construct a real analytic non-convex curve for which Theorem 1.1 is false by constructing a non-zero function in the null space of the Radon transform integrating over this curve in arc-length measure. Let C be the curve $x_2 = \sin x_1$ and let f be a function that is supported in $[0, 4\pi] \times [0, 10]$ and is $(+1)$ on $[0, 2\pi] \times [0, 10]$ and (-1) on $[2\pi, 4\pi] \times [0, 10]$. Then, the integral of f over any translate of C is zero because, for each $y \in \mathbb{R}^2$, the same length of $y + C$ meets $[0, 2\pi] \times [0, 10]$ as meets $[2\pi, 4\pi] \times [0, 10]$.

A counterexample to the conclusion of Theorem 1.1 can be made for an unbounded convex curve, C, when the hypothesis of Theorem 1.1 that some $y_0 + C$ is disjoint from supp f is left out. One chooses a convex curve, C, and constructs a function like the one in Example 3.3 that is both $(+1)$ and (-1) on strips that meet C. Then, one chooses a measure on each $y + C$ that changes as y varies around zero in such a way that the integrals on both parts of $(\text{supp } f) \cap (y + C)$ cancel. For example, one can take a Gaussian weight on C and adjust the location of the maximum of the Gaussian for each y near zero so that the integrals over the strips cancel.

PROOF OF THEOREM 1.2. The proof is much like the one in [**Q 1993**] for Riemannian spheres so it will only be outlined. For each $\epsilon > 0$, let D_ϵ be the convex hull of $\cup_{|y| \leq \epsilon}(y + C)$. Let $y_0 \in \mathcal{A}$ as in the statement of Theorem 1.2 and assume the conclusion of the theorem is false. Because $\mathcal{A}$ is open and connected, as in [**Q 1993**], one can find an $\epsilon > 0$ and a $y_1 \in A$ such that:

i) If $|y - y_1| \leq \epsilon$, then $y \in \mathcal{A}$.
ii) int $(y_1 + D_\epsilon)$ is disjoint from supp f.
iii) $\partial(y_1 + D_\epsilon)$ meets supp f and $\partial(y_1 + D_\epsilon)$ is a smooth curve.

Assume $x \in \partial(y_1 + D_\epsilon) \cap (\text{supp } f)$ and let $(x, \xi) \in N^*\partial(y_1 + D_\epsilon) \setminus 0$. So, by *ii)*, *iii)*, and Lemma 3.2, $(x, \xi) \in \text{WF}_A(F)$. By *i)*, there is a $y_2 \in \mathcal{A}$ such that $(y_2 + C) \subset (y_1 + D_\epsilon)$ and $x \in (y_2 + C)$. However, since C is strictly convex the one $(y_2 + C)$-parallel point to x is in int $(y_1 + D_\epsilon)$. Therefore, Proposition 2.2 implies that $(x, \xi) \notin \text{WF}_A(f)$. This contradiction proves the theorem. □

PROOF OF THEOREM 1.3. We assume S_t, S_s, and f are as in the hypothesis of Theorem 1.3. The proof is fairly geometric and is easier to describe using some simple terminology (and for the reader to draw pictures illustrating the terms and the proof itself). Using a slight abuse of notation, we will refer to the curves of centers as $|a| = t$ and $|a| = s$. Recall that $c_t(\theta, r)$ is the circle centered at $t\bar{\theta}$ and of radius r, the circle of integration for $S_t f(\theta, r)$.

We define the *mirror diameter* of $c_t(\theta, r)$ to be the diameter tangent to $|a| = t$ at $t\bar{\theta}$. Therefore, mirror points (Definition 2.3) are reflections of each other in the mirror diameter of $c_t(\theta, r)$. Self-mirror points on $c_t(\theta, r)$ are the endpoints of the mirror diameter. The mirror diameter divides $c_t(\theta, r)$ into two open semicircles. We refer to the one closer to the origin as the *inner* open semicircle and the other one as the *outer* open semicircle.

The following lemma is one of the technical keys to the proof.

LEMMA 3.4. *Assume the distribution f is zero inside $c_t(\theta, r)$ and $S_t f$ is zero near (θ, r). Assume also that f is zero in a neighborhood of the inner (or the outer) open semicircle of $c_t(\theta, r)$. Then, f is zero in a neighborhood of the other open semicircle.*

Note that the proposition draws no inference at the self-mirror points.

PROOF. As $S_t f$ is zero near (θ, r) and f is zero in a neighborhood of the outer or inner open semicircle of $c_t(\theta, r)$, Proposition 2.2 implies that conormals to the other open semicircle are not in $\text{WF}_A f$. Now, one uses Lemma 3.2 to conclude that f is zero on a neighborhood of the other open semicircle. □

In the proofs of Theorems 1.1 and 1.2, we used the curves that defined the Radon transform to eat away at $\text{supp } f$. For this theorem, we need a bigger set than $c_t(\theta, r)$. We use a capsule shaped object,

$$(3.2) \qquad K(\theta, r) = \text{Ch}\left(c_t(\theta, r) \cup c_s(\theta, r)\right)$$

where Ch A is the convex hull of the set $A \subset \mathbb{R}^2$.

The following lemma will be needed as we eat away at supp f.

LEMMA 3.5. *Let f and S_t, S_s be as in the hypotheses of Theorem 1.3 and let $r_3 > \sqrt{s^2 - t^2}$. Assume $S_t f = S_s f = 0$ in a neighborhood of (θ_3, r_3). Assume $S_s f(\theta, r) = 0$ in a neighborhood of each (θ, p) such that $c_s(\theta, r)$ is tangent to $K(\theta_3, r_3)$ and is contained in $K(\theta_3, r_3)$. Assume f is zero on int $K(\theta_3, r_3)$. Then, f is zero on a neighborhood of $K(\theta_3, r_3)$.*

PROOF. We can use Lemma 3.4 to show $f = 0$ in neighborhoods of the outer open semicircle of $c_s(\theta_3, r_3)$ and the inner open semicircle of $c_t(\theta_3, r_3)$. This can be done because the opposite semicircles are inside $K(\theta_3, r_3)$.

Let ℓ be one of the closed line segments on $\partial K(\theta_3, r_3)$. We show that f is zero in a neighborhood of ℓ. Let x_3 be the point of intersection of ℓ and $c_s(\theta_3, r_3)$. For each point $x \in \ell \setminus \{x_3\}$, there is a circle $C = c_s(\theta_1, r_1)$ that has center on $|a| = s$, that is tangent to ℓ, and that is contained in $K(\theta_3, r_3)$. By the hypothesis of this lemma, $S_s f$ is zero near (θ_1, r_1). The point of tangency of C with ℓ is the only point on C that could possibly meet supp f. That point is not a self-mirror point since $x \neq x_3$ so $C \neq c_s(\theta_3, r_3)$. Therefore, Lemma 3.4 can be used to show f is zero in a neighborhood of this point. (*This argument works for points $x \in \ell \setminus \{x_3\}$ that are outside of $|a| = s$ because, for each such x, the circle C exists.*)

Since $r_3 > \sqrt{s^2 - t^2}$, the above argument is valid for all points on $\ell \setminus \{x_3\}$.

Now we show f is zero in a neighborhood of x_3. We will do this by constructing circles centered on $|a| = s$ that have only a part of their outer semicircles outside of $K(\theta_3, r_3)$. We will use these to eat away at supp f at x_3. The circles we use are easier to describe in local coordinates. Choose local coordinates $\overline{x} = (\overline{x}_1, \overline{x}_2)$ so that $s\overline{\theta}$ is the origin and $x_3 = (r_3, 0)$. Let the circle $|a| = s$ correspond in local coordinates to the circle γ_s of radius s and centered at $(0, -s)$. Let $\delta \in (0, s-t)$, and let C_δ be the smaller circle centered on γ_s that goes through $(r_3, -\delta)$ and $(r_3, 0)$. The center of C_δ is $\overline{a} = (\sqrt{s\delta - \delta^2/4}, -\delta/2)$.

Let r_δ be the radius of C_δ. Using estimates, one can show that for sufficiently small δ, the slope of the mirror diameter of C_δ is more negative than the slope of the segment between $\overline{a}$ and $(r_3, -\delta)$. Therefore, the mirror diameters and inner open semicircles of C_δ and all circles centered at $\overline{a}$ of radius less than r_δ are contained in $K(\theta_3, r_3)$. If δ is sufficiently small so that $S_s f$ is zero near these circles, Lemma 3.4 can be used to show that supp f is disjoint from all circles centered at $\overline{a}$ of radius less than or equal to r_δ. Thus, $x_3 \notin \text{supp } f$. (*This argument to show $x_3 \notin \text{supp } f$ works for all $r_3 > 0$.*)

This finishes the proof that supp f is disjoint from all of $K(\theta_3, r_3)$. □

Now we have the tools to prove the theorem. We start with $c_t(\theta_0, r_0)$ and its inside disjoint from supp f. We first show that $K(\theta_0, r_0)$ is disjoint from supp f.

LEMMA 3.6. *Under the hypotheses of Theorem 1.3, if $c_t(\theta_0, r_0)$ and its inside is disjoint from* supp f, *then $K(\theta_0, r_0)$ is disjoint from* supp f.

PROOF. First, note that the outer half circle of $c_t(\theta_0, r_0)$ is outside of $|a| = s$ as $r_0 > \sqrt{s^2 - t^2}$. There is a radius $r_1 > 0$ such that the self-mirror points on the circle $c_s(\theta_0, r_1)$ are on $c_t(\theta_0, r_0)$ and only the outer semicircle of this circle is outside $c_t(\theta_0, r_0)$. Therefore, we can use Lemma 3.4 to show that $c_s(\theta_0, r_1)$ is disjoint from supp f. (If not, there is a largest radius $r_2 \leq r_1$ such that supp f meets $c_s(\theta_0, r_1)$ and is locally on one side of $c_s(\theta_0, r_1)$. Apply Lemma 3.4 to this circle to show supp f is disjoint from this circle and its interior. This contradiction shows that $c_s(\theta_0, r_1)$ and its inside is disjoint from supp f.)

Let $D_t(\theta_0, r_0)$ be the closed disk that has boundary $c_t(\theta_0, r_0)$. We have just proven that $D_t(\theta_0, r_0) \cup K(\theta_0, r_1)$ is disjoint from supp f. Assume $K(\theta_0, r_0)$ is not disjoint from supp f. As we let r_1 increase to r_0, there is a first radius, r_2 such that $D_t(\theta_0, r_0) \cup K(\theta_0, r_2)$ meets supp f, and supp f is disjoint from the interior of $D_t(\theta_0, r_0) \cup K(\theta_0, r_2)$. By Lemma 3.4, supp f is disjoint from the outer open semicircle of $c_t(\theta_0, r_2)$. The boundary of $D_t(\theta_0, r_0) \cup K(\theta_0, r_2)$ is made up of semicircles and two line segments. The segments are outside of $|a| = s$ because the outer semicircle of $c_t(\theta_3, r_3)$ is outside of $|a| = s$. Since these segments are outside of $|a| = s$, the arguments in the proof of Lemma 3.5 that showed the segment ℓ is disjoint from supp f can be used here (see the italicized statements in the proof of Lemma 3.5). This shows that the entire set $D_t(\theta_0, r_0) \cup K(\theta_0, r_2)$ is disjoint from supp f, and so $r_2 = r_0$ and the lemma is proved. □

These lemmas are now used to finish the proof. By Lemma 3.6, we find that $K(\theta_0, r_0)$ is disjoint from supp f. As in [**BQ 1987**] we can find a path in $\mathcal{A}$ from (θ_0, r_0) to some (θ_3, r_3) such that $r_3 > \sqrt{s^2 - t^2}$ and $\partial K(\theta_3, r_3)$ meets supp f but int $K(\theta_3, r_3)$ does not meet supp f. Now, we can use Lemma 3.5 to draw a contradiction. This finishes the proof of the theorem. □

REMARK 3.7. Note that the proof is valid if $\mathcal{A} \subset [0, 2\pi] \times (0, \infty)$ is an open connected set such that if $(\theta_3, r_3) \in \mathcal{A}$ then so are $(\theta_3, \sqrt{s^2 - t^2})$ as well as all (θ, r) such that $c_s(\theta, r)$ is tangent to $\partial K(\theta_3, r_3)$ and $c_s(\theta, r) \subset K(\theta_3, r_3)$. This requirement is all that is needed for one to apply Lemmas 3.5 and 3.6.

EXAMPLE 3.8. Let S_2 be the Radon transform that integrates over circles centered on $|a| = 2$ in standard arc length measure. We construct a smooth non-zero function $F(x)$ with $S_2 F \equiv 0$ and with $\{x \in \mathbb{R}^2 \mid |x| \leq 1 \text{ or } |x| = 3\} \subset$ supp F but supp f is disjoint from $\{x \in \mathbb{R}^2 \mid 1 < |x| < 3\}$.

A similar construction, outlined below, shows that there is no general Morera theorem for this set of circles. The construction provides a function that is not holomorphic but that has zero integrals with respect to the analytic measure, dz, over all circles centered on the curve $|a| = 2$.

This example shows that Theorem 1.3 is not valid without a shadow curve. If $s \in (2, \infty)$ and $S_2 F \equiv 0 \equiv S_s F$, then Theorem 1.3 implies that $F \equiv 0$. As noted above, $\{x \in \mathbb{R}^2 \mid |x| = 1 \text{ or } |x| = 3\} \subset$ supp f. The reason this example is possible is that wavefront at the c_2 mirror points on $|x| = 1$ and $|x| = 3$ cancel.

CONSTRUCTION. Let $k : [0, \infty) \to \mathbb{R}$ be continuous. Then, for $r \in [0, \infty)$ we define Radon transform $S_2 k(r)$ to be $S_2[k(|x|)](\theta, r)$ for any $\theta \in [0, 2\pi]$. This is well defined independent of θ because $k(|x|)$ is a radial function and S_2 is rotation invariant since the weight $\mu \equiv 1$.

To define F, we first specify a smooth, non-negative, even function $f_1 \in C^\infty(\mathbb{R})$ with supp $f_1 = [-1, 1]$. Next we use f_1 to construct the smooth function $\overline{f}_2$ with supp $\overline{f}_2 \subset [3, 7)$ by solving an integral equation so that $-S_2 f_1(r) = S_2 \overline{f}_2(r)$ for $r \in [0, 5)$. Then $F(x) = f_1(|x|) + \overline{f}_2(|x|)$ will satisfy the conditions in the example for $|x| < 7$ and $r \in [0, 5)$. Finally we will outline how to extend the construction.

Now, $\overline{f}_2(u)$ is constructed. By the choice of f_1,

(3.3) $\qquad S_2 f_1(r)$ is smooth and supp $S_2 f_1(r) = [1, 3]$.

If $f(u)$ is a function supported in $[3, 7)$ then an exercise using the law of cosines shows for $w = r + 2 \in [3, 7)$ that

$$(3.4) \qquad S_2 f(w-2) = 4 \int_3^w \frac{u(w-2)f(u)du}{\sqrt{w-u}\sqrt{(w+u)(u^2-(w-4)^2)}}.$$

Because of (3.4), the equation

$$(3.5) \qquad -S_2 f_1(w-2) = S_2 \overline{f}_2(w-2)$$

is a first kind Abel integral equation for $\overline{f}_2(u)$. By (3.3), the function $S_2 f_1(w-2)$ is zero to infinite order at $w = 3$. Therefore, the integral equation (3.5) satisfies the hypotheses of Theorem B [**Q 1983**]. (see also [**Yo**]). So, one can solve (3.5) for the function $\overline{f}_2(u)$ for $u \in [3, 7)$. As $S_2 f_1$ is smooth, $\overline{f}_2$ is smooth on $[3, 7)$ [**Yo**]. As $r = 1 \in \text{supp}(S_2 f_1)$, $u = 3 \in \text{supp } \overline{f}_2$. Since $S_2 f_1(w-2)$ is zero to infinite order at $w = 3$, $\overline{f}_2(u)$ is zero to infinite order at $u = 3$; so, $\overline{f}_2$ can be smoothly extended to $[0, 7)$ to be zero on $[0, 3]$ and with $3 \in \text{supp } \overline{f}_2$. Now, by (3.5),

$$(3.6) \qquad S_2(f_1 + \overline{f}_2)(w-2) = 0 \text{ for } w \in [2, 7).$$

The extension is completely analogous to the argument in Example 3.2 of [**Q 1993**] so it will only be outlined. First let $\epsilon \in (0, 1/4)$. Define $f_2(u)$ to be equal to $\overline{f}_2(u)$ for $u \in [0, 7 - \epsilon/2)$ and to smoothly taper to zero and have support in $[3, 7)$. Now, solve the integral equation equivalent to (3.4), $-S_2(f_1 + f_2)(w-2) = S_2 \overline{f}_3(w-2)$ on $w \in [7 - \epsilon/2, 11 - \epsilon/2)$, for $\overline{f}_3(u)$. By the choice of f_1 and f_2, $\overline{f}_3$ is smooth, supported in $[7 - \epsilon/2, 11 - \epsilon/2)$. One defines f_3 by cutting off $\overline{f}_3$ smoothly between $11 - 3\epsilon/4$ and $11 - \epsilon/2$. One continues this process as in [**Q 1993**].

If one integrates with respect to the analytic measure, dz, then $S_2 f(\theta, r)$ is no longer radial, and the integral (3.4) changes in unessential ways. $S_2 f(\theta, r)$ becomes $ire^{i\theta}$ times an integral like (3.4) but with the addition of $[(w-2)-(w^2-u^2)/4]/(w-2)$ to the inside of the integral. The rest of the proof is essentially the same because the new integral equation is one to which Theorem B [**Q 1983**] applies. □

References

[BG] Berenstein, C. A. and Gay, R., *A local version of the two circles theorem*, Israel J. Math. **55** (1986), 267–288.

[BQ 1987] Boman, J. and Quinto, E. T., *Support theorems for real analytic Radon transforms*, Duke Math. J. **55** (1987), 943–948.

[Co] Cormack, A. M., *The Radon transform on a family of curves in the plane*, Proc. Amer. Math. Soc. **83** (1981), 325–330; *The Radon transform on a family of curves in the plane. II*, Proc. Amer. Math. Soc. **86** (1982), 293–298.

[GGS] Gelfand I. M., Graev, M. I., and Shapiro, Z. Ya., *Differential forms and integral geometry*, Functional Anal. Appl. **3** (1969), 24–40.

[GQ] Globevnik, J. and Quinto, E. T., *Morera Theorems and Microlocal Analysis*, in preparation.

[GS] Guillemin, V. and Sternberg, S., *Geometric Asymptotics*, Amer. Math. Soc., Providence, RI, 1977.
[Gu] Guillemin, V., *On some results of Gelfand in integral geometry*, Proc. Sympos. Pure Math. **43** (1985), Amer. Math. Soc., 149–155.
[He] Helgason, S., *Groups and Geometric Analysis*, Academic Press, New York, 1984.
[Hö] Hörmander, L., *The Analysis of Linear Partial Differential Operators I*, Springer, New York, 1983.
[Jo] John, F., *Plane Waves and Spherical Means*, Interscience, New York, 1966.
[Ka] Kaneko, A., *Introduction to Hyperfunctions*, Kluwer, New York, 1989.
[Ku] Kurusa, Á., *Support curves of invertible Radon transforms*, (preprint).
[Mu] Mukhometov, R. G., *The problem of recovery of a two-dimensional Riemannian metric and integral geometry*, Soviet Math. Dolk. **18** (1977), 27–31.
[Na] Natterer, F., *The Mathematics of Computerized Tomography*, Wiley, New York, 1986.
[Q 1980] Quinto, E. T., *The dependence of the generalized Radon transform on defining measures*, Trans. Amer. Math. Soc. **257** (1980), 331–346.
[Q 1983] _____, *The invertibility of rotation invariant Radon transforms*, J. Math. Anal. Appl. **91**, 510–522; Erratum, J. Math. Anal. Appl. **94**, 602–603.
[Q 1993] _____, *Pompeiu transforms on geodesic spheres in real analytic manifolds*, Israel J. Math. **84**, 353–363.
[Ro] Romanov, V. G., *Integral Geometry and Inverse Problems for Hyperbolic Equations*, Springer Tracts in Natural Philosophy, vol. 26, Springer Verlag, Berlin, New York, 1969.
[SKK] Sato, M., Kawai, T., and Kashiwara, M., *Hyperfunctions and pseudodifferential equations*, Lecture Notes in Math., vol. 287, Springer Verlag, New York, 1973, pp. 265-529.
[Tr] Treves, F., *Introduction to Pseudodifferential and Fourier integral operators*, Plenum Press, New York, 1980.
[Yo] Yosida, K., *Lectures on Differential and Integral Equations*, Interscience, New York, 1960.
[Za] Zalcman, L., *Offbeat Integral Geometry*, Amer. Math. Monthly **87** (1980), 161–175.

DEPARTMENT OF MATHEMATICS, TUFTS UNIVERSITY, MEDFORD, MA 02155 USA

E-mail address: equinto@math.tufts.edu

Inverse boundary value problems for first order perturbations of the Laplacian

GUNTHER UHLMANN

0. Introduction

The subject of *Electrical Impedance Tomography* has undergone a considerable development in the last decade in both the theoretical and applied aspects of the problem. In this non invasive inverse method one attempts to determine the electrical conductivity of a body by making current and voltage measurements at the boundary of the body. Potential applications range from medical tomography ([1], [3]) to determining cracks in aircraft ([14]), to determining defects in metals ([5]). One of the key ideas in the mathematical developments has been the construction of growing exponential solutions for the conductivity equation developed in [21, 22] building on pioneer work of Calderón ([2]). These type of solutions have in turn had applications in other inverse problems like the inverse scattering problem at a fixed energy and inverse spectral problems.

Other inverse boundary value problems arise in applications. A direct analog of the inverse conductivity problem is to determine both the electrical conductivity and permittivity of a body and its magnetic permeability by measuring the tangential components of the electrical field and the magnetic field at the boundary. A different inverse boundary value problem involves elastic measurements at the boundary. Namely one measures displacements at the boundary and the corresponding stress at the boundary. The inverse problem is to determine the Lamé parameters in the interior by making these measurements. These last two problems are modeled by systems of PDE's, Maxwell's equations in the first case and the elasticity system in the second. The solution of the identifiability problem in these two cases (see [13], [8]) involves again the construction of growing exponential solutions. Another interesting problem arising in scattering theory consists in the determination of both the electrical potential and the magnetic

---

1991 *Mathematics Subject Classification.* Primary 35R30; Secondary 35P05.
Partially supported by NSF Grant DMS–9100178 and ONR grant N00014-93-1-0295

© 1994 American Mathematical Society
0075-8485/94 $1.00 + $.25 per page

potential from boundary observations. This problem has been solved recently in [10].

The latter case, as well as Maxwell's equations and the elasticity system, can be reduced to a first order (system or scalar) perturbation of the Laplacian. The construction of exponentially growing solutions for the elasticity system in [8] applies to any first order system perturbation of the Laplacian. In this paper we survey these developments. In the first section we briefly discuss the solution of the electrical impedance tomography in dimension $n \geq 3$. In section 2 we discuss the new ideas involved in the construction of exponentially growing solutions for any first order perturbation of the Laplacian. We apply these to solve an inverse boundary value problem arising in elasticity. Finally in section 3 we discuss the case of the Schrödinger equation with a magnetic field and Maxwell's equations.

1. The inverse conductivity problem for an isotropic conductivity

Let $\Omega \subseteq \mathbb{R}^n$ be a bounded domain with smooth boundary. We denote by γ the conductivity of Ω, which we assume is in $C^\infty(\overline{\Omega})$ and strictly positive. The equation for a potential in Ω induced by a voltage f on $\partial\Omega$ is given by the solution of the Dirichlet problem

(1.1)
$$L_\gamma u = \operatorname{div}(\gamma \nabla u) = 0 \text{ in } \Omega$$
$$u|_{\partial\Omega} = f.$$

The voltage to current map or Dirichlet to Neumann map (DN) is defined by

(1.2)
$$\Lambda_\gamma(f) = \left(\gamma \frac{\partial u}{\partial \nu}\right)\bigg|_{\partial\Omega}$$

with u solution of (1.1) and ν denotes the unit outer normal to $\partial\Omega$.

The inverse problem is to determine γ from Λ_γ. There has been considerable progress in the study of this problem (see the survey [23] for theoretical developments up to 1991). In this section we sketch the proof of the following identifiability result proven in [22].

1.3 THEOREM. *Let $n \geq 3$. Let γ_1, γ_2 be smooth, positive functions in $\overline{\Omega}$ such that $\Lambda_{\gamma_1} = \Lambda_{\gamma_2}$. Then $\gamma_1 = \gamma_2$ in $\overline{\Omega}$.*

SKETCH OF PROOF. First one reduces the problem to study the Schrödinger equation at zero energy.

Let γ be a smooth positive conductivity. We define
$$w = \gamma^{\frac{1}{2}} u$$
with u solution of
$$L_\gamma u = 0.$$
Then w satisfies

(1.4)
$$(\Delta - q)w = 0 \text{ in } \Omega$$

with

(1.5) $$q = \frac{\Delta\sqrt{\gamma}}{\sqrt{\gamma}}.$$

Now if 0 is not a Dirichlet eigenvalue for $\Delta - q$ (which is the case if q is of the form (1.5)) we can define be DN map by

(1.6) $$\Lambda_q(f) = \frac{\partial w}{\partial \nu}\bigg|_{\partial\Omega}$$

where w solves

(1.7) $$(\Delta - q)w = 0 \text{ in } \Omega$$
$$w|_{\partial\Omega} = f.$$

It is easy to see the following relationship between Λ_q and Λ_γ with q and γ as in (1.5)

(1.8) $$\Lambda_q(f) = \gamma^{\frac{1}{2}}\Lambda_\gamma(\gamma^{-\frac{1}{2}}f) + \frac{1}{2}(\gamma^{-1}\frac{\partial\gamma}{\partial\nu})|_{\partial\Omega}f.$$

The theorem then follows from the following two results.

1.9 THEOREM. $(n \geq 3)$ Suppose $\Lambda_{q_1} = \Lambda_{q_2}$, for $q_i \in L^\infty(\Omega)$ with 0 not an eigenvalue of $\Delta - q_i, i = 1, 2$. Then

$$q_1 = q_2.$$

1.10 THEOREM. (Kohn & Vogelius). Let $\gamma_i \in C^\infty(\overline{\Omega})$. Assume $\Lambda_{\gamma_1} = \Lambda_{\gamma_2}$. Then

$$\partial^\alpha \gamma_1|_{\partial\Omega} = \partial^\alpha \gamma_2|_{\partial\Omega} \; \forall \; \alpha.$$

Theorem (1.10) was proven by Kohn and Vogelius ([6]) by cleverly choosing boundary data. An alternative proof that applies in more general situations was given in [7]. See also section 3 where a sketch of proof of a similar result is given for the Schrödinger equation in the presence of a magnetic field.

SKETCH OF PROOF OF THEOREM 1.9. The key result is the existence of exponentially growing solutions.

1.11 LEMMA. Let $q \in L^\infty(\mathbb{R}^n)$ with compact support. Let $\rho \in \mathbb{C}^n$ with $\rho \cdot \rho = 0$. Then there exists $R > 0$ such that if $|\rho| \geq R$ then there are solutions of $(\Delta - q)u = 0$ in $\mathbb{R}^n$ of the form

(1.12) $$u = e^{x\cdot\rho}(1 + \psi_q(x, \rho))$$

with $\|\psi_q\|_{L^2(\Omega)} \to 0$ as $|\rho| \to \infty$.

There is more detailed information in the original construction of [22] but this is all we need to prove Theorem (1.9).

Let $q_i \in L^\infty(\Omega)$ as in the statement of Theorem (1.9). We define $q_i = 0$ in $\mathbb{R}^n - \Omega$. Let $\rho_i, i = 1, 2$ as in Lemma (1.11) with

$$\rho_1 = \eta + i(k + l) \tag{1.13}$$
$$\rho_2 = -\eta + i(k - l)$$

with $\eta, k, l \in \mathbb{R}^n$ satisfying

$$\langle \eta, k \rangle = \langle k, l \rangle = \langle \eta, l \rangle = 0$$
$$|\eta|^2 = |k|^2 + |l|^2$$

and $|l| \geq R_i$, $i = 1, 2$ with R_i as in Lemma (1.11). We take

$$u_i = e^{x \cdot \rho_i}(1 + \psi_{q_i}(x, \rho_i)), \quad i = 1, 2. \tag{1.14}$$

The next important ingredient is the following identity.

1.15 LEMMA. *Let $q_i \in L^\infty(\Omega)$, $i = 1, 2$ such that 0 is not a Dirichlet eigenvalue of $\Delta - q_i$. Assume $\Lambda_{q_1} = \Lambda_{q_2}$ then*

$$\int_\Omega (q_1 - q_2) u_1 u_2 = 0 \tag{1.16}$$

for every solution u_i of $(\Delta - q_i) u_i = 0$ in $\mathbb{R}^n$.

Now we plug (1.14) into (1.16). We obtain

$$\int_\Omega e^{2i\langle x, k \rangle}(q_1 - q_2)(x) dx = -\int_\Omega e^{2i\langle x, k \rangle}(q_1 - q_2)(\psi_{q_1} + \psi_{q_2} + \psi_{q_1}\psi_{q_2}) dx. \tag{1.17}$$

By taking the limit as $|l| \to \infty$ of (1.17) we obtain

$$\widehat{(q_1 - q_2)\chi_\Omega}(-2k) = 0 \quad \forall \, k \in \mathbb{R}^n$$

proving that $q_1 = q_2$ in Ω. $\square$

2. An inverse boundary value problem for the elasticity system

Let $\Omega \subseteq \mathbb{R}^n$ be a bounded open set with smooth boundary. We consider Ω as an elastic, isotropic, inhomogeneous medium with Lamé parameters λ, μ. The generalized Hooke's law states that under the assumption of no body forces acting on Ω, the displacement u satisfies

$$(Lu)_i = (L_{\lambda,\mu} u)_i = \sum_{j,k,l=1}^n \frac{\partial}{\partial x_j} C_{ijkl} \frac{\partial}{\partial x_l} u_k = 0 \text{ in } \Omega, \quad i = 1, \ldots, n \tag{2.1}$$

$$u|_{\partial \Omega} = f$$

where

$$C_{ijkl} = \lambda \delta_{ij} \delta_{kl} + \mu(\delta_{ik}\delta_{ij} + \delta_{il}\delta_{jk}) \quad (1 \leq i, j, k, l \leq n), \tag{2.2}$$

with δ_{ij} the Kronecker delta and $(Lu)_i$ denotes the i-th component of Lu.

$C = (C_{ijkl})$ is the <u>elastic tensor</u>. The boundary value problem(2.1) has a unique solution under the strong convexity condition

(2.3) $$\mu > 0, n\lambda + 2\mu > 0 \text{ in } \bar{\Omega}.$$

There are two other tensors that one defines in linear elasticity. The <u>linear strain</u> tensor is defined by

(2.4) $$\varepsilon(u) = \frac{1}{2}(\nabla u + (\nabla u)^T)$$

with u solution of (2.1) and $(\nabla u)^T$ denotes the transpose of the Jacobian matrix ∇u. The <u>stress</u> tensor is defined by

(2.5) $$\sigma(u) = C\epsilon(u)$$

with C the elastic tensor.

In terms of cartesian coordinates we have that the strain tensor and the stress tensor are given respectively by

(2.6) $$\varepsilon_{ij}(u) = \frac{1}{2}\left(\frac{\partial u_i}{\partial x_j} + \frac{\partial u_j}{\partial x_i}\right), i,j = 1,\ldots,n$$

and

(2.7) $$\sigma_{ij}(u) = \sum_{k,l=1}^{n} C_{ijkl}\varepsilon_{kl}(u), \quad i,j = 1,\ldots,n.$$

The Dirichlet to Neumann map (DN) is defined in this case by

(2.8) $$(\Lambda_{\lambda,u}(f))_i = \sum_{l,k,l=1}^{n} \nu_j C_{ijkl} \frac{\partial u_k}{\partial x_l}\bigg|_{\partial\Omega}$$

where $\nu = (\nu_1, \ldots, \nu_n)$ is the unit outer normal to $\partial\Omega$ and u is the solution of (2.1). Physically the DN map sends the displacement at the boundary to the corresponding normal component of the stress at the boundary. In this paper we sketch the proof of the following global identifiability result proven in [8].

2.9 THEOREM. *Let* $n \geq 3$. *Let* $(\lambda_i, \mu_i) \in C^\infty(\bar{\Omega}) \times C^\infty(\bar{\Omega}), i = 1,2$ *satisfy the strong convexity condition (2.3). Assume*

$$\Lambda_{(\lambda_1,\mu_1)} = \Lambda_{(\lambda_2,\mu_2)}.$$

Then

$$(\lambda_1, \mu_1) = (\lambda_2, \mu_2) \text{ in } \bar{\Omega}.$$

SKETCH OF PROOF. The proof follows the outline of the proof of Theorem 1.9. The main difficulty is to construct solutions analogous to (1.12) for the Schrödinger equation. We first point out the analogous Lemma to (1.15) which is proven by a simple application of Green's theorem.

2.10 LEMMA. *Let (λ_i, μ_i) be as in Theorem 2.9. Assume*
$$\Lambda_{(\lambda_1,\mu_1)} = \Lambda_{(\lambda_2,\mu_2)}.$$
Then

(2.11) $$\int_\Omega \{(\lambda_1 - \lambda_2)\operatorname{div} u^{(1)} \cdot \operatorname{div} u^{(2)} + 2(\mu_1 - \mu_2)\varepsilon(u^{(1)}) \cdot \varepsilon(u^{(2)})\}dx = 0$$

where $u^{(i)}$ is a solution of

(2.12) $$L_{(\lambda_i,\mu_i)}u^{(i)} = 0 \text{ in } \Omega.$$

The boundary determination of the Lamé parameters was proven in [9].

2.13 THEOREM. *Let (λ_i, μ_i) as in Theorem (2.9). Assume*
$$\Lambda_{(\lambda_1,\mu_1)} = \Lambda_{(\lambda_2,\mu_2)}.$$
Then
$$\partial^\alpha \lambda_1|_{\partial\Omega} = \partial^\alpha \lambda_2|_{\partial\Omega}, \ \partial^\alpha \mu_1|_{\partial\Omega} = \partial^\alpha \mu_2|_{\partial\Omega} \qquad \forall\, \alpha.$$

We cannot reduce the elasticity system to a Schrödinger equation. We reduce it, though, to a first order system perturbation of the Laplacian. We first show that we can reduce the elasticity system to a third order perturbation of the biharmonic operator.

2.14 PROPOSITION. *Let $(\lambda, \mu) \in C^\infty(\bar\Omega) \times C^\infty(\bar\Omega)$ satisfying (2.3). Let*

(2.15) $$Pu = -(\lambda + \mu)\nabla \operatorname{div} u + (\lambda + 2\mu)\Delta u + (\operatorname{div} u)\alpha$$

where α is given by

(2.16) $$(\lambda + \mu)\alpha - \{(\lambda + 3\mu)\nabla(\lambda + \mu) + 2(\lambda + \mu)\nabla\mu\} = 0.$$

Then we have

(2.17) $$(\mu(\lambda + 2\mu))^{-1} L_{\lambda,\mu} P = \Delta^2 + M^{(1)}(x, D)\Delta + M^{(2)}(x, D)$$

where $M^{(j)}$ is a differential system of order j, $j = 1, 2$.

Then the construction of exponentially growing solutions for $L_{\lambda,\mu}$ is reduced to constructing these type of solutions for

(2.18) $$M(x, D) = \Delta^2 + M^{(1)}(x, D)\Delta + M^{(2)}(x, D).$$

Let $Z = \{\rho \in \mathbb{C}^n; \rho \cdot \rho = 0, |\rho| \geq 1\}$.

We construct solutions of

(2.19) $$M(x, D)u = 0 \text{ in } \mathbb{R}^n$$

(by extending $\lambda, \mu \in C^\infty(\mathbb{R}^n)$ with $\lambda = \mu = 1$ outside a large enough ball) of the form

(2.20) $$u = e^{x \cdot \rho} H(x, \rho) \text{ with } \rho \in Z.$$

To this effect we consider the operators.

(2.21) $$\Delta_\rho = e^{-x\cdot\rho}\Delta(e^{x\cdot\rho}), \quad M_\rho = e^{-x\cdot\rho}M(e^{x\cdot\rho})$$

$M(x,D)$ as in (2.19) is just the solution of

(2.22) $$M_\rho H(x,\rho) = 0.$$

We remark at this point that $\Delta_\rho, M_\rho \in L^2(\mathbb{R}^n, Z)$ where $L^m(\mathbb{R}^n, Z)$ denotes the class of pseudodifferential operators depending on a complex parameter ρ, introduced in [15]. Namely $A \in L^m(\mathbb{R}^n, Z)$ if we can write

(2.23) $$Af(x) = \int e^{i\langle x,\xi\rangle} a_\rho(x,\xi)\widehat{f}(\xi)d\xi$$

for $f \in C_0^\infty(\mathbb{R}^n)$, where $a_\rho \in S^m(\mathbb{R}^n, Z)$, i.e.

(2.24) $$\sup_{x\in K}|\partial_x^\alpha \partial_\xi^\beta a_\rho(x,\xi)| \leq C_{\alpha,\beta,K}(1+|\xi|+|\rho|)^{m-|\beta|}$$

for every compact set $K \subset\subset \mathbb{R}^n$.

We shall only consider properly supported operators. We recall $A \in L_\rho^m(\mathbb{R}^n, Z)$ is properly supported if there exists a closed set $H \subset \mathbb{R}^n \times \mathbb{R}^n$ such that the support of the Schwartz kernel of A_ρ is contained in H for all $\rho \in Z$ and the projections of H on each factor are proper.

We now reduce the problem to consider first order perturbations of the Laplacian. Let

(2.25) $$\widetilde{M}_\rho^{(j)} = M_\rho^{(j)}\Delta_\rho^{-2}, j=1,2 \quad \widetilde{\Delta}_\rho = \Delta_\rho \Lambda_\rho^{-1}$$

where

(2.26) $$\Lambda_\rho f(x) = \frac{1}{(2\pi)^n}\int_{\mathbb{R}^n} e^{ix\cdot\xi}(|\xi|^2+|\rho|^2)^{\frac{1}{2}}\widehat{f}(\xi)d\xi.$$

We consider then the matrix operator

(2.27) $$\widetilde{M}_\rho = \widetilde{\Delta}_\rho^2 + \widetilde{M}_\rho^{(1)}(x,D)\Delta_\rho + \widetilde{M}_\rho^{(2)}(x,D)$$

with $\widetilde{M}_\rho^{(j)} \in L^0(\mathbb{R}^n, Z), j=1,2$.

By setting $\Delta_\rho u = w$, we consider the enlarged $2n \times 2n$ system

(2.27) $$N_\rho = \widetilde{\Delta}_\rho + \widetilde{N}_\rho(x,D)$$

where

(2.28) $$\widetilde{N}_\rho(x,D) = \begin{pmatrix} \left(N_\rho^{(0)}\right)_{11} & \left(N_\rho^{(0)}\right)_{12} \\ \left(N_\rho^{0}\right)_{21} & \left(N_\rho^{(0)}\right)_{22} \end{pmatrix}$$

and

$$(N_\rho^{(0)})_{11} = 0, (N_\rho^{(0)})_{12} = -I, (N_\rho^{(0)})_{21} = \widetilde{M}_\rho^{(1)}(x,D), (N_\rho^{(0)})_{22} = \widetilde{M}_\rho^{(2)}(x,D).$$

The next lemma says that one can essentially construct solutions of $N_\rho w_\rho = 0$ by constructing solutions of $\Delta_\rho u_\rho = 0$.

2.29 LEMMA. *Let $N_\rho(x, D)$ be as in (2.27). Let $N \in \mathbb{Z}^+$. Then there exist $A_\rho, B_\rho \in L^0(\mathbb{R}^n, Z)$ such that*

$$(2.30) \qquad N_\rho A_\rho = B_\rho \widetilde{\Delta}_\rho \mod L^{-N}(\mathbb{R}^n, Z).$$

Moreover if $\rho = s\rho_0 + O(\frac{1}{s})$, $s \in \mathbb{R}$, $\rho_0 \in \mathbb{C}^n$ with $|\rho_0| = 1$ we can choose A_ρ, B_ρ so that

(i) *A_ρ, B_ρ is invertible for large $|s|$ and*

$$\|B_\rho^{-1}\|_{L^2(\mathbb{R}^n), L^2(\mathbb{R}^n)} \leq C$$

with C independent of s,

(ii) *Let $f \in C^\infty(\mathbb{R}^n)$ such that $\langle x \rangle^k f \in B^\infty(\mathbb{R}^n)$. Then $\{s^{-1}(\Lambda_\rho^{-2} A_\rho f(x) - |\rho|^{-2} G_{\widehat{\rho}} f(x)\}_{s \geq 1}$ are bounded in $C^\infty(\mathbb{R}^n)$, where $G_{\widehat{\rho}}$ is an invertible matrix which can be computed explicitly and $\widehat{\rho} = \frac{\rho}{|\rho|}$.*

Now we sketch the procedure to construct solutions of

$$(2.31) \qquad N_\rho u_\rho = 0 \text{ in } \Omega_0$$

where Ω_0 is any compact neighborhood in $\mathbb{R}^n$. We construct u_ρ in the form

$$(2.32) \qquad u_\rho = A_\rho v_\rho$$

with A_ρ as in (2.30) and v_ρ solution of

$$(2.33) \qquad (B_\rho \widetilde{\Delta}_\rho + R_{-N}) v_\rho = 0$$

in any compact neighborhood $\widetilde{\Omega}_0$ and $R_{-N} \in L^{-N}(\mathbb{R}^n, Z)$ with $N \geq 1$. We construct $v_\rho = \sum_{j=0}^{\infty} v_\rho^{(j)}$ with $v_\rho^{(j)}$ solution of

$$(2.34) \qquad B_\rho \widetilde{\Delta}_\rho v_\rho^{(j)} = -R_{-N} v_\rho^{(j-1)}$$

with $v_\rho^{(0)}$ any solution of $\widetilde{\Delta}_\rho v_\rho^{(0)} = 0$. Equation (2.34) has a solution with $v_\rho \in L^2(K)$ with K any compact set. This is a consequence of the fact that B_ρ is invertible, $\|R_{-N}\|_{H^k, H^{k+N}} \leq C_k(1 + |\rho|)^{-N}$ for any $k \in \mathbb{R}$ and finally the estimates for Δ_ρ proven in [22]. In this fashion we construct solutions of the form (2.19) for the elasticity system. The next step is to plug these solutions into (2.11) by choosing "enough" of them. We refer here to [8] for the details of this. □

3. Two other inverse boundary value problems.

A. Maxwell's equations.

One obtains the conductivity equation (1.1) if one neglects the time variation of the electromagnetic field in Maxwell's equations. In [16] it was proposed to study an inverse boundary value problem for the full set of Maxwell's equations. In that paper it was also proven that the linearization of this problem is injective at constant electromagnetic parameters. We now formulate the mathematical problem.

Let $\Omega \subseteq \mathbb{R}^3$ be a bounded domain with smooth boundary. The electromagnetic field (e, h) satisfies the frequency domain Maxwell's equation which are given by

$$(3.1) \qquad \operatorname{rot} e = i\omega\mu h, \quad \operatorname{rot} h = -i\omega\varepsilon + \sigma \text{ in } \Omega$$

where $\omega > 0$ is the time-harmonic frequency of the field $\varepsilon > 0$ denotes the electrical permittivity, $\mu > 0$ the magnetic permeability and $\sigma \geq 0$ the conductivity. We assume that all the functions are smooth. The direct analog to the Dirichlet to Neumann map as shown in [16] is given by

$$\Lambda_{\varepsilon,\mu,\sigma} : \nu \wedge e|_{\partial\Omega} \to \nu \wedge h|_{\partial\Omega}$$

where e, h satisfies (3.1). A global identifiability result was proven in this case in [13]. The main idea in this work comes already in [4] in which a global identifiability result was proven for the inverse scattering problem at a fixed energy for electromagnetic waves under the assumption of a constant magnetic permeability. A local result close to constant electromagnetic parameters was proven in [19] for the inverse boundary value problem. The local assumption was used in [19] to construct exponentially growing solutions. Since one can reduce Maxwell's equations to a first order perturbation of the Laplacian (see Lemma 0.13 in [19]) one can give an alternative proof of the result in [13] using Lemma (2.29) and the methods in [19]. We describe this method in more detail in the next example.

B. The Schrödinger equation in the presence of a magnetic field.

The Schrödinger equation in the presence of a magnetic field is given by

$$(3.2) \qquad H_{\vec{A},q} = \sum_{j=1}^{n}\left(i\frac{\partial}{\partial x_j} + A_j(x)\right)^2 + q, \quad i = \sqrt{-1}$$

where $\vec{A} = (A_1, A_2, \ldots, A_n) \in C^1(\bar{\Omega})$ is the magnetic potential and $q \in L^\infty(\Omega)$ is the electric potential. The magnetic potential is $\operatorname{rot}(\vec{A})$. We assume that both $\vec{A}$ and q are real-valued. In this case $H_{\vec{A},q}$ are self-adjoint. Let $\Omega \subseteq \mathbb{R}^n$ be a bounded open set with smooth boundary. Assume 0 is not a Dirichlet eigenvalue for $H_{\vec{A},q}$. Then the Dirichlet problem

(3.3)
$$H_{\vec{A},q} u = 0 \text{ in } \Omega$$
$$u|_{\partial\Omega} = f \in H^{\frac{1}{2}}(\partial\Omega)$$

has a unique solution $u \in H^1(\Omega)$. The Dirichlet to Neumann map (DN) is defined by

(3.4)
$$\Lambda_{\vec{A},q}(f) = \frac{\partial u}{\partial \nu} + i(\vec{A} \cdot \nu)u$$

where u is a solution of (3.3).

This inverse scattering problem was considered in [12]. In the case $\vec{A} = 0$ the inverse scattering problem at a fixed energy was solved in [11]. Sun ([18]) studied the inverse boundary value problem. In this case $\Lambda_{\vec{A},q}$ is invariant under a gauge transformation of the magnetic potential. Namely,

(3.5)
$$\Lambda_{\vec{A}+\nabla g,q} = \Lambda_{\vec{A},q}$$

where $g \in C^1(\bar{\Omega})$ with $\text{supp} g \subseteq \Omega$.

The natural question is whether (3.5) is the only obstruction to uniqueness. Sun proved in $n \geq 3$ that this is the case under the assumption that $\vec{A} \in C^2(\Omega)$, $\text{supp}\vec{A} \subseteq \Omega$, $q \in L^\infty(\Omega)$ and $\|\text{rot}(\vec{A})\|_{L^\infty(\Omega)}$ is small.

Using a combination of ideas used to prove this result and the intertwining property (2.30) to construct exponentially growing solutions led to the following result in the C^∞ category.

3.6 THEOREM. *(Nakamura-Sun-Uhlmann).* Let $\vec{A}_j, q_j \in C^\infty(\bar{\Omega}), j = 1, 2$. Assume
$$\Lambda_{\vec{A}_1,q_1} = \Lambda_{\vec{A}_2,q_2}.$$
Then $\text{rot}(\vec{A}_1) = \text{rot}(\vec{A}_2)$.

SKETCH OF PROOF. The first step of the proof is to show that one can determine the boundary values of $\vec{A}$ and q.

3.7 THEOREM. Let $\vec{A}_j, q_j$ as in Theorem (3.6), $j = 1, 2$. Assume $\Lambda_{\vec{A}_1,q_1} = \Lambda_{\vec{A}_2,q_2}$. Then
$$\partial^\alpha \vec{A}_1\big|_{\partial\Omega} = \partial^\alpha \vec{A}_2\big|_{\partial\Omega} \quad \forall \alpha$$
$$\partial^\alpha q_1|_{\partial\Omega} = \partial^\alpha q_2|_{\partial\Omega} \quad \forall \alpha.$$

SKETCH OF PROOF OF THEOREM (3.7). . The proof proceeds as in [7] . Namely we write

(3.8)
$$H_{\vec{A},q} = -\Delta + \sum_{j=1}^n iA_j(x)D_{x_j} + G(x)$$

where

(3.9) $$G = \vec{A}^2 - \nabla \cdot \vec{A} + q.$$

In boundary normal coordinates $x = (x^n, x')$ we write

(3.10) $$-\Delta = D_{x^n}^2 + iE(x)D_{x^n} + Q(x, D_{x'})$$

with $Q(x, D_{x'})$ a second order operator in $D_{x'}$, depending smoothly on x^n and E is a smooth function.

Then we can factorize with B a first order pseudodifferential operator

(3.11) $$H_{\vec{A},q} = (D_{x^n} + iE(x) + \widetilde{A}_n(x) + B(x, D_{x'}))(D_{x^n} - iB(x, D_{x'}))$$

modulo smoothing. Here $\widetilde{A}_j, j = 1, ..., n$, denotes the components of $\vec{A}$ in boundary normal coordinates.

The point is that

(3.12) $$\Lambda_{\vec{A},q} = B(x, D'_x) + i(\vec{A} \cdot \nu)$$

and $B(x, D_{x'})$ satisfies the Ricatti-type equation

(3.13) $$i[D_{x^n}, B] - E(x)B + i\widetilde{A}_n B + B^2 - Q - \sum_{i=1}^{n-1} \widetilde{A}_i D_{x^i} - G = 0$$

modulo smoothing. We remark here that similar Ricatti equations were derived in [16] and [20] in the development of the layer stripping algorithm.

Now one proceeds as in [7] to show that the full symbol of B determines $\partial_{x_n}^k A_j, \partial_{x_n}^{k-1} q \ \forall \ k, j = 1, \ldots, n$. □

The next step is the construction of growing exponential solutions. We look for solutions of $H_{\vec{A},q}\mu = 0$ in Ω of the form

(3.14) $$u(x, \rho) = e^{x \cdot \rho + \phi(x, \widehat{\rho})}(1 + \psi(x, \rho))$$

so that $\psi(x, \rho) = 0(|\rho|^{-1})$ uniformly in Ω where $\widehat{\rho} = \frac{\rho}{|\rho|}$. In order to do this ϕ and ψ must satisfy

(3.15) $$\rho \cdot \nabla \phi = -i\rho \cdot \vec{A},$$

(3.16) $$\Delta \psi + 2(\rho + \nabla \phi + i\vec{A}) \cdot \nabla \psi - g\psi = g$$

where

(3.17) $$g = \vec{A}^2 - i\nabla \cdot \vec{A} + q - 2i\vec{A} \cdot \nabla \phi - \nabla \phi \cdot \nabla \phi - \Delta \phi$$

The solution of (3.15) is constructed ([18]) in the form

(3.18) $$\phi(x, \widehat{\rho}) = (2\pi)^{-n} \int_{\mathbb{R}^n} e^{-ix \cdot \xi} \left(\frac{\rho \cdot \widehat{(\vec{A})}(\xi)}{\rho \cdot \xi} \right) d\xi.$$

The equation (3.16) can be rewritten in the form

(3.19) $$\Delta_\rho \psi + \vec{B} \cdot \nabla \psi - h\psi = h$$

where

(3.20) $$\Delta_\rho = e^{-x\rho}\Delta(e^{x\rho}) = \Delta + 2\rho \cdot \nabla$$
$$\vec{B} = 2(\nabla\phi + i\vec{A})\psi, \quad h = g\psi$$

Multiplying by Λ_ρ^{-1} we obtain

(3.21) $$(\widetilde{\Delta}_\rho + N_\rho)\psi = h_\rho$$

where
$$h_\rho = \Lambda_\rho^{-1} h, \quad N_\rho = \Lambda_\rho^{-1}(\vec{B} \cdot \nabla h) \in L^0(\mathbb{R}^n, Z).$$

Now we use the intertwining property to construct solutions proceeding as in section 2. The last step in the proof is to plug the solutions constructed in the following identity, which is valid if $\Lambda_{\vec{A}_1, q_1} = \Lambda_{\vec{A}_2, q_2}$

(3.22) $$i\int_\Omega (\vec{A}_1 - \vec{A}_2) \cdot (u_1\nabla\overline{u}_2 - u_2\nabla\overline{u}_1) + \int_\Omega (\vec{A}_1^2 - \vec{A}_2^2 + q_1 - q_2)u_1\overline{u}_2 = 0$$

with u_j solution of $H_{\vec{A}_j, q_j} u_j = 0$ in $\Omega, j = 1, 2$.

Let k, γ_1, γ_2 be three mutually orthogonal vectors in $\mathbb{R}^n$ with $|\gamma_1| = |\gamma_2| = 1$. Let $\zeta, \xi \in \mathbb{C}^n$ be given by $\zeta = \gamma_1 + i\gamma_2$, $\rho = s\zeta + g(s,k)\gamma_1$, where s is a positive real parameter and

$$g(s, k) = 2^{-1}|k|^2((|k|^2 + 4s^2)^{\frac{1}{2}} + 4s)^{-1}.$$

We define

(3.23) $$\rho_1 = \frac{ik}{2} + \rho, \quad \overline{\rho}_2 = \frac{ik}{2} - \rho.$$

One can check that $\rho_1 \cdot \rho_1 = \rho_2 \cdot \rho_2 = 0$. We now construct

(3.24) $$u_j(x, \rho_j) = e^{\rho_j \cdot x + \phi_j(x, \widehat{\rho}_j)}(1 + \omega_j(x, \rho_j))$$

solution of $H_{\vec{A}_j, q_j} u_j = 0$, $j = 1, 2$. Substituting (3.24) into (3.22) and letting s tend to ∞, we get

(3.25) $$\int_\Omega e^{ix \cdot k + \psi_1^* + \overline{\psi}_2^*} \zeta \cdot (\vec{A}_1 - \vec{A}_2) dx = 0$$

where $\psi_j^*(x, \zeta) = \psi_j(x, \widehat{\zeta})$, $j = 1, 2$.

Formula (3.25) is all we need to deduce that

(3.26) $$\text{rot}(\vec{A}_1) = \text{rot}(\vec{A}_2).$$

See Section 4.1 in [18] for details. Formula (3.26) implies that there exist $p \in C^1$ supported in Ω so that

(3.27) $$\vec{A}_1 - \vec{A}_2 = \nabla p \text{ in } \Omega.$$

To prove $q_1 = q_2$, we first recall that $\Lambda_{\vec{A},q}$ is invariant under gauge transformations. This fact together with (3.27) implies that $\Lambda_{\vec{A}_2,q_2} = \Lambda_{\vec{A}_2+\nabla p,q_2} = \Lambda_{\vec{A}_1,q_2}$. On the other hand, $\Lambda_{\vec{A}_1,q_1} = \Lambda_{\vec{A}_2,q_2}$. So we have

$$\Lambda_{\vec{A}_1,q_1} = \Lambda_{\vec{A}_1,q_2}.$$

This means that we may assume $\vec{A}_1 = \vec{A}_2$ when we prove $q_1 = q_2$. Letting $\vec{A}_1 = \vec{A}_2$ in (3.22) we get

(3.28) $$\int_\Omega (q_1 - q_2) u_1 \bar{u}_2 dx = 0.$$

Now substituting (3.24) into (3.28) and letting s tend to ∞ we get

$$\int_\Omega e^{ikx + \phi_1^* + \bar{\phi}_2^*} (q_1 - q_2) dx = 0,$$

from which the result follows immediately. $\square$

References

1. Barber D.C. and Brown, D.H., *Progress in Electrical Impedance Tomoghraphy*, Inverse Problems in Partial Differential equations, edited by D. Colton, R. Ewing and W. Rundell, 1990, pp. 151–164.
2. Calderón A., *On an inverse boundary value problem*, Soc. Brasileira de Matemática (1980), 65–73.
3. Cheney M. and Isaacson, D. Current problems in impedance imaging, Inverse Problems in Partial Differential Equations, edited by D. Colton, E. Ewing and W. Rundell, 1990, pp. 141–149.
4. Colton, D. and Päivärinta, L., *The uniqueness of a solution to an inverse scattering problem for electromagnetic waves*, Arch. Rat. Mech. Anal. **119** (1992), 59–70.
5. Eggleston, R.J., Schawabe R.J., Isaacson, D. and Coffin, L.F., *The application of electric current computed tomography to defect imaging in metals*, GE Research & Development Center, Physical Metalurgy Laboratory, 89CRD158, 1989.
6. Kohn, R. and Vogelius, M., *Determining conductivity by boundary measurements*, Comm. Pure Appl. Math. **38** (1985), 643–667.
7. Lee, J. and Uhlmann, G., *Determining anisotropic real-analytic conductivities by boundary measurements*, Comm. Pure Appl. Math. **42** (1989), 1097–1112.
8. Nakamura, G. and Uhlmann, G., *Global uniqueness for an inverse boundary value problem arising in elasticity*, Inventiones Math. (to appear).
9. _____, *Inverse problems at the boundary for an elastic medium*, SIAM J. Math. Anal. (to appear).
10. Nakamura, G., Sun Z. and Uhlmann, G., *Global identifiability for an inverse problem for the Schrödinger equation in a magnetic field*, preprint.
11. Novikov, R., *Multidimensional inverse spectral problems for the equation* $-\Delta \psi + (v(x) - Eu(x))\psi = 0$, Functional Analysis and its Applications **22** (1988), 263–272.
12. Novikov R. and Henkin G., $\bar{\partial}$- *equation in the multidimensional inverse scattering problem*, Russian Math. Surveys **42** (1987), 109–180.

13. Ola O., Päivärinta L. and Somersalo E., *An inverse boundary value problem in electrodynamics*, Duke Math. J. **70** (1993), 617–653.
14. Santosa F. and Vogelius M., *A computational algorithm to determine cracks from electrostatic boundary measurements*, Int. J. Eng. Sci. **29** (1991), 917–1387.
15. Shubin, M. A., *Pseudodifferential operators and spectral theory*, Springer Series in Soviet Mathematics, Springer-Verlag, 1987.
16. Somersalo, E., Isaacson, D. and Cheney, M., *A linearized inverse boundary value problem for Maxwell's equations*, Journal of Computational and Appl. Math. **42** (1992), 123–136.
17. _____, *Layer stripping: a direct numerical method for impedance imaging*, Inverse problems **7** (1991), 899–926.
18. Sun, Z., *An inverse boundary value problem for Schrödinger operator with vector potentials*, Trans. of AMS **338** (1993), no. 2, 953–969.
19. Sun, Z. and Uhlmann, G., *An inverse boundary value problem for Maxwell's equations*, Archive Rational Mech. Anal. **119** (1992), 71–93.
20. Sylvester, J., *A convergent layer stripping algorithm for a radially symmetric impedance tomography problem*, Comm. P.D.E. **17** (1992), 1955–1994.
21. Sylvester, J. and Uhlmann, G., *A uniqueness theorem for an inverse boundary value problem in electrical prospection* Comm. Pure Appl. Math. **39** (1986), 91–112.
22. _____, *A global uniqueness theorem for an inverse boundary value problem*, Annals of Math. **125** (1987), 153–169.
23. Uhlmann, G., *Inverse boundary value problems and applications*, Astérisque **207** (1992), 153–211.

DEPARTMENT OF MATHEMATICS, UNIVERSITY OF WASHINGTON, SEATTLE, WA 98195

E-mail address: gunther@math.washington.edu

Multidimensional analogue of the Erdélyi lemma and the Radon transform

ALEXANDER I. ZASLAVSKY

ABSTRACT. We consider functions $f(x)$ with compact support $D \subset \mathbb{R}^n$ such that ∂D is a union of smooth hypersurfaces in general position and $f(x)$ has singularities of the type $x_+^\mu \log^m x_+$ on each of these hypersurfaces. For such functions $f(x)$ we study the singularities of their Radon transforms and as a consequence we describe the asymptotics at infinity of their Fourier transforms in almost all directions.

Introduction

The well known Erdélyi lemma [**F**] describes the asymptotics of the Fourier transform of functions $f(x)$ defined on the real axis and having singularities of the kind $(x - x_0)_\pm^\mu \log^m(x - x_0)_\pm \phi(x)$, where $\phi(x)$ is smooth enough, $\mu > -1$. According to this lemma, the contribution of each such singularity to the asymptotics of the Fourier transform $\tilde{f}(t)$ as $t \to +\infty$ is

$$t^{-\mu-1} \log^m t \left(e^{ix_0 t} \phi(x_0)(-1)^m e^{\pm \frac{i\pi(\mu+1)}{2}} \Gamma(\mu+1) + o(1) \right).$$

The primary goal of the present paper is to generalize this result to the multidimensional case. On the one hand, this generalizes the results on the asymptotics of the Fourier transform of the characteristic function $\chi_D(x)$ of a bounded domain $D \subset \mathbb{R}^n$, see [**Hl**], [**GGV**], [**Hö**], [**RZ4**]. On the other hand, this is related to the description of the asymptotics of the Fourier transform of densities supported by hypersurfaces, see [**S**], [**BNW**]. The classical Erdélyi lemma has many applications [**E**], [**F**], so we hope its multidimensional analogue may be also useful, cf. [**LRZ**], where a special case of Theorem 2 of the present paper

---

1991 *Mathematics Subject Classification.* 44A12, 42B10.

Key words and phrases. Radon transform, asymptotics of the Fourier transform, singularities, distributions.

This paper is in final form and no version of it will be submitted for publication elsewhere

is applied to the theory of multiple Fourier series, namely, to prove estimates for the Lebesgue constants.

The geometry of the support D of the function $f(x)$ in question plays a crucial role, just as it is the case with the characteristic functions. Here, developing the ideas of [**RZ4**], we consider the case when the boundary ∂D is the union of smooth hypersurfaces in general position (see Theorem 1 below for exact smoothness assumptions). The function $f(x)$ is allowed to have singularities of the above type on each of the components of the boundary, in general with different exponents μ and m for different components.

In Theorem 2 below the asymptotics of the Fourier transform $\tilde{f}(t\alpha_1, \ldots, t\alpha_n)$ of $f(x_1, \ldots, x_n)$ as $t \to +\infty$, are described for almost all directions $(\alpha_1, \ldots, \alpha_n)$. In fact, even in the case of a smooth boundary ∂D and $f(x) = \chi_D(x)$ it is possible to give uniform asymptotics in all directions only under additional assumption, namely, that the Gaussian curvature of ∂D does not vanish, [**GGV**], [**RZ4**]. We define the set of directions for which our result is valid by some conditions similar to the nonvanishing of the Gaussian curvature. On the other hand, there are many interesting results about the asymptotics of the Fourier transform of the characteristic function in the case of smooth boundary, or density carried by a smooth hypersurface, in the exceptional directions, [**AVGZ**], [**BNW**].

We prove Theorem 2 as a consequence of the description of singularities of the Radon transform of functions $f(x)$ of the type described above. This generalizes the results of [**RZ1, RZ2**] about the singularities of the Radon transforms of characteristic functions of sets in $\mathbb{R}^n$ (see also [**RZ3**] for related results for the X-ray transform which is similar to the Radon transform but where the integration is over low-dimensional planes, contrary to hyperplanes in the case of the Radon transform). This result is formulated in Theorem 1. In the case of smooth boundary a less precise result can be found in [**P**, p.118, see also p.99]. It is interesting that the exponent of the logarithm in the resulting expression is not uniquely determined by the exponents m of the logarithms of the factors of the integrand; the formula involves geometry as well. In the case of the Fourier transform this is not the case, the exponent of the logarithm in the asymptotics always equals the sum of the exponents of the logarithms of the relevant factors of the integrand, see Theorem 2. We prove Theorem 1 considering divergent integrals and using the theory of distributions. Note that Theorem 1 is an analogue in the real space of a result of Pham [**Ph**].

If the exponent μ is less or equal than -1, the function $f(x)$ becomes non-integrable, and one can consider the corresponding distribution and its Fourier transform, the same in the multidimensional case. It is possible, using the methods of this paper, to describe the asymptotics of the Fourier transform of such distributions as well.

1. Singularities of Radon transforms

1.1. Notations. Let $D \subset \mathbb{R}^n$ be a domain with compact closure whose boundary $S = \partial D$ may be represented in the form $S = \bigcup_{j \in \mathcal{J}} S_j$, where $\mathcal{J}$ is a finite set of indices, and S_j are C^k-smooth hypersurfaces in $\mathbb{R}^n$ in general position. (The value $k \geq 1$ will be specified later. We note here only that all the results remain true in the C^∞ and real analytic framework.) The general position assumption implies, in particular, that the intersections $S_{\mathcal{J}'} = \bigcap_{j \in \mathcal{J}'} S_j$, $\mathcal{J}' \subseteq \mathcal{J}$, if nonvoid, are C^k-smooth varieties.

We consider functions whose support is the closure of D, and assume that inside D they are C^k-smooth and have the form

$$f(x) = \prod_{j \in \mathcal{J}} \rho_j(x)^{\mu_j} \log^{m_j} \rho_j(x) \cdot \phi(x), \tag{1}$$

where $\phi(x) \in C^k(\mathbb{R}^n)$, $\phi|_{\partial D} \neq 0$, and

$$\rho_j(x) = \begin{cases} \operatorname{dist}(x, S_j), & \text{if } x \in D, \\ 0, & \text{if } x \notin D. \end{cases}$$

As the example $D = \{x \in \mathbb{R}^n \mid |x| < 1\}$ shows, ρ_j may not be smooth functions in the whole of D. Therefore, the product in (1) is defined as follows: the factor $\rho_j(x)^{\mu_j} \log^{m_j} \rho(x)$ does not appear in it as long as x is far from S_j, so formula (1) must hold locally in D. The following lemma shows that (1) indeed defines a C^k-function in $U \cap D \setminus \partial D$, where U is a neighbourhood of ∂D.

LEMMA 1. *Let V be a C^k-hypersurface in $\mathbb{R}^n$, $k \geq 1$, and $\rho(x)$ a function defined in a neighbourhood U of V which is positive on one side of V, negative on the other side and $|\rho(x)| = \operatorname{dist}(x, V)$. Then there exists a neighbourhood $U' \subset U$ of V such that $\rho(x) \in C^k(U')$.*

For the proof see [**Gi**, appendix B].

Consider the Radon transform

$$R(f; \alpha) = \int_\alpha f(x) \lambda. \tag{2}$$

Here α is a hyperplane in $\mathbb{R}^n$, and λ is the Lebesgue measure on α. Integral (2) is convergent provided

$$\mu_j + 1 > 0, \quad j \in \mathcal{J}. \tag{3}$$

Condition (3) is assumed throughout.

Recall that a hyperplane in $\mathbb{R}^n$ may be considered as a point of $\mathbb{RP}_n$, so (2) defines $R(f; \alpha)$ on the whole of $\mathbb{RP}_n$ except for infinite hyperplanes. Note, however, that one may extend it continuously to the points α of $\mathbb{RP}_n$ corresponding to infinite hyperplanes by setting $R(f; \alpha) = 0$ (recall that the support of f is compact).

To a smooth variety $V \subset \mathbb{R}^n$ (or, more generally, $V \subset \mathbb{RP}_n$) one may associate the dual variety $\hat{V} \subset \mathbb{RP}_n$ defined as the closure of the set of hyperplanes not transversal to V at some point. Recall that the dual of $\hat{V}$ is the closure of V itself (see [**Zs**] and references cited there).

Without loss of generality one can assume that V is defined by a system of equations

(4) $$x_i = g_i(x_{m+1}, \ldots, x_n), \quad i = 1, \ldots, m,$$

where $m = \operatorname{codim} V$. The hyperplane $\alpha = \left\{ x \in \mathbb{R}^n \,\middle|\, \alpha_0 + \sum_{i=1}^{i=n} \alpha_i x_i = 0 \right\}$ is not transversal to V at a point $\bar{x} \in V \cap \alpha$ iff

(5) $$\alpha_j - \sum_{i=1}^{m} \alpha_i \frac{\partial g_i(\bar{x})}{\partial x_j} = 0, \quad j = m+1, \ldots, n.$$

For such α and $\bar{x}$ we denote I the inertia index of the Hessian of the function $z = \sum_{i=1}^{n} \alpha_j x_j$ on V at the point x, and $\mathfrak{J}$ the determinant of the Hessian of this function:

(6) $$\mathfrak{J} = \bar{\alpha}_n^{-n+m} \det \left(\left(\sum_{i=1}^{m} \bar{\alpha}_i \frac{\partial^2 g_i(\bar{x}_{m+1}, \ldots, \bar{x}_n)}{\partial x_j \partial x_k} \right)_{j,k=m+1,\ldots,n} \right).$$

Set $Q(S) = \bigcup_{\mathcal{J}' \subseteq \mathcal{J}} \hat{S}_{\mathcal{J}'}$. By [**RZ2**, lemma 1], the Radon transform $R(f; \alpha)$ is a smooth function for $\alpha \in \mathbb{RP}_n \setminus Q(S)$. As we shall see, the behaviour of $R(f; \alpha)$ is different at different components of $Q(S)$.

Take $\mathcal{J}' \subseteq \mathcal{J}$ such that $S_{\mathcal{J}'}$ is nonempty and $\hat{S}_{\mathcal{J}'}$ has codimension one (see [**Zs**] for the discussion of the codimension of the dual variety). Let $\mathcal{J}'$ consist of m elements; without loss of generality we may assume that $\mathcal{J}' = \{1, \ldots, m\}$. Suppose that the hypersurfaces S_j are given by the equations $\mathfrak{g}_j(x) = 0$, $j = 1, \ldots, m$, $\operatorname{grad} \mathfrak{g}_j(x) \neq 0$; let $\alpha \in \mathbb{RP}_n$ be a hypersurface not transversal to $S_{\mathcal{J}'}$ at the point $\bar{x}$. We denote

(7) $$\tilde{\mathfrak{g}}_1' = \left(\frac{\partial \mathfrak{g}_i(\bar{x})}{\partial x_k} \right)_{i,k=1,\ldots,m}, \quad \tilde{\mathfrak{g}}_2' = \left(\frac{\partial \mathfrak{g}_i(\bar{x})}{\partial x_k} \right)_{i,k=2,\ldots,m},$$

and by ζ_i, $i = 1, \ldots, m$, we denote the components of the vector

(8) $$\zeta = \bar{\alpha}_n^{-1} (\bar{\alpha}_1, \ldots, \bar{\alpha}_m) \cdot (\tilde{\mathfrak{g}}_1')^{-1}.$$

The role of the numbers $\operatorname{sgn} \zeta_j$ appearing below may be explained as follows. Consider the coordinate system $u_1, \ldots, u_n$, where for $j = 1, \ldots, m$ we have $u_j = \mathfrak{g}_j(x)$, so the domain D is the positive quadrant $u_j \geq 0$, $i = 1, \ldots, m$. We can associate with ζ the covector $\sum_{j=1}^{m} \zeta_j du_j$, and it is just the covector $\sum_{j=1}^{n} \bar{\alpha}_j dx_j$ in this system of coordinates, so the signs of the components ζ_j define to which of the quadrants does the covector ζ belong.

Now we set

(9) $$\Xi = |\mathfrak{J}|^{-1/2} \det(\tilde{\mathfrak{g}}_2')^{-1} |(\bar{\alpha}_1, \ldots, \bar{\alpha}_n)| |\bar{\alpha}_1|^{-1} \prod_{i=2}^{m} |\zeta_i|^{-1}.$$

We assume throughout that $\sum_{a \in \varnothing} = 0$, $\prod_{a \in \varnothing} = 1$, so if $m = 1$, then the second and the last factors in the right hand side are missing. Note that the notations are slightly different from those used in [**RZ2**], and this explains the difference in the signs in Theorem 1 below and Theorem 1 of op. cit.

Let $\bar{a}$ be a simple point of $\hat{S}_{\mathcal{J}'}$. We may assume that $\bar{\alpha}_1 \neq 0$. Denote $\bar{x} \in S_{\mathcal{J}'}$ the point at which the hyperplane $\bar{a}$ is not transversal to $S_{\mathcal{J}'}$; since the dual of $\hat{S}_{\mathcal{J}'}$ is $S_{\mathcal{J}'}$ and codim $\hat{S}_{\mathcal{J}'} = 1$, for a generic $\bar{\alpha} \in \hat{S}_{\mathcal{J}'}$ the point $\bar{x}$ is uniquely defined, so Ξ makes sense. For a generic $\bar{\alpha}$ the components ζ_j of the vector ζ do not vanish; denote a, $0 \leq a \leq m$, the number of positive components among ζ_i. Without loss of generality we may assume that $\zeta_i > 0$, $i = 1, \ldots, a$, and $\zeta_i < 0$, $i = a+1, \ldots, m$. We introduce the following notations:
$$\mathfrak{m}_+ = \frac{n - I - m}{2} + \sum_{j=1}^{a}(\mu_j + 1), \quad \mathfrak{m}_- = \frac{I}{2} + \sum_{j=a+1}^{m}(\mu_j + 1), \quad \mathbf{m}_+ = \sum_{j=1}^{a} m_j, \quad \mathbf{m}_- = \sum_{j=a+1}^{m} m_j.$$

1.2. Formulation of the result. The following result describes the behaviour of the Radon transform of $f(x)$ around the codimension one component $\hat{S}_{\mathcal{J}'}$ of $Q(S)$. According to this theorem, the Radon transform on each side of this hypersurface behaves like

$$y_{\pm}^{\mathfrak{m}_+ + \mathfrak{m}_- - 1} \log^{\mathbf{m}} y_{\pm} \times \text{coefficient} + \text{lower order terms,}$$

where y is essentially the distance from α to $\hat{S}_{\mathcal{J}'}$, and $\mathbf{m} = \mathbf{m}_+ + \mathbf{m}_-$ or $\mathbf{m} = \mathbf{m}_+ + \mathbf{m}_- \pm 1$, depending on the geometry of $S_{\mathcal{J}'}$ and α. For $y \in \mathbb{R}$ we denote $y_{\pm} = \max(0, \pm y)$.

Renumbering the variables if necessary we may assume that for a regular point $\bar{\alpha} \in \hat{S}_{\mathcal{J}'}$ we have $\bar{\alpha}_n \neq 0$ and that $\hat{S}_{\mathcal{J}'}$ is defined by an equation $y(\alpha) = \alpha_n^{-1}\alpha_0 - h(\alpha_n^{-1}\alpha_1, \ldots, \alpha_n^{-1}\alpha_{n-1}) = 0$, $h \in C^k$. Though we shall not need it below, we remark that the functions $h(\alpha_n^{-1}\alpha_1, \ldots, \alpha_n^{-1}\alpha_{n-1})$, on the one hand, and $z = \alpha_n^{-1}(\alpha_0 + \sum_{j=1}^{n} \alpha_j x_j)$, considered as the function on $S_{\mathcal{J}'}$, on the other hand, are connected via the generalized Legendre transform, see [**Zs**], [**RZ2**].

THEOREM 1. *Let $k \geq \max(2, \mathfrak{m}_+ + \mathfrak{m}_-)$. Then for generic $\bar{\alpha} \in \hat{S}_{\mathcal{J}'}$ there exist a neighbourhood U of $\bar{\alpha}$ and functions $r_j^{\pm}(\alpha)$, $r(\alpha) \in C^k(U)$, $j = 0, \ldots, \mathbf{m}_+ + \mathbf{m}_- + 1$, such that for $\alpha \in U$ we have:*

(i) if $\mathfrak{m}_+ \notin \mathbb{Z}$, $\mathfrak{m}_- \notin \mathbb{Z}$, $\mathfrak{m}_+ + \mathfrak{m}_- \notin \mathbb{Z}$, then

$$R(f; \alpha) = y_+^{\mathfrak{m}_+ + \mathfrak{m}_- - 1} \sum_{j=0}^{\mathbf{m}_+ + \mathbf{m}_-} r_j^+(\alpha) \log^{\mathbf{m}_+ + \mathbf{m}_- - j} y_+ +$$

$$y_-^{\mathfrak{m}_+ + \mathfrak{m}_- - 1} \sum_{j=0}^{\mathbf{m}_+ + \mathbf{m}_-} r_j^-(\alpha) \log^{\mathbf{m}_+ + \mathbf{m}_- - j} y_- + r(\alpha),$$

$$r_0^\pm(\bar\alpha) = \frac{\phi(\bar x)\Xi \sin \pi \mathfrak{m}_\pm (2\pi)^{\frac{n-m}{2}} \prod_{j=1}^m \Gamma(\mu_j+1)}{\sin\pi(\mathfrak{m}_+ + \mathfrak{m}_-)\Gamma(\mathfrak{m}_- + \mathfrak{m}_+)};$$

(ii) if $\mathfrak{m}_+ + \mathfrak{m}_- \notin \mathbb{Z}$, $\mathfrak{m}_+ \in \mathbb{Z}$, $\mathbf{m}_+ > 0$, then

$$R(f;\alpha) = y_+^{\mathbf{m}_+ + \mathbf{m}_- - 1} \sum_{j=0}^{\mathbf{m}_+ + \mathbf{m}_- - 1} r_j^+(\alpha) \log^{\mathbf{m}_+ + \mathbf{m}_- - 1 - j} y_+ +$$

$$y_-^{\mathbf{m}_+ + \mathbf{m}_- - 1} \sum_{j=0}^{\mathbf{m}_+ + \mathbf{m}_-} r_j^-(\alpha) \log^{\mathbf{m}_+ + \mathbf{m}_- - j} y_- + r(\alpha),$$

$$r_0^+(\bar\alpha) = \frac{\phi(\bar x)\Xi \pi \mathbf{m}_+ (2\pi)^{\frac{n-m}{2}} \prod_{j=1}^m \Gamma(\mu_j+1)}{\sin\pi(\mathfrak{m}_- + \mathfrak{m}_+)\Gamma(\mathfrak{m}_- + \mathfrak{m}_+)},$$

and $r_0^-(\bar\alpha)$ is as above. If $\mathfrak{m}_+ + \mathfrak{m}_- \notin \mathbb{Z}$, $\mathfrak{m}_- \in \mathbb{Z}$, $\mathbf{m}_- > 0$, then the same formulae hold with indices plus and minus interchanged;

(iii) if $\mathfrak{m}_+ \notin \mathbb{Z}$, $\mathfrak{m}_+ + \mathfrak{m}_- \in \mathbb{Z}$, then

$$R(f;\alpha) = y_+^{\mathbf{m}_+ + \mathbf{m}_- - 1} \sum_{j=0}^{\mathbf{m}_+ + \mathbf{m}_- + 1} r_j^+(\alpha) \log^{\mathbf{m}_+ + \mathbf{m}_+ + 1 - j} y_+ +$$

$$y_-^{\mathbf{m}_+ + \mathbf{m}_- - 1} \sum_{j=0}^{\mathbf{m}_+ + \mathbf{m}_- + 1} r_j^-(\alpha) \log^{\mathbf{m}_+ + \mathbf{m}_+ + 1 - j} y_- + r(\alpha),$$

$$r_0^\pm(\bar\alpha) = - \frac{\phi(\bar x)\Xi \sin \pi \mathfrak{m}_\pm (2\pi)^{\frac{n-m}{2}} \prod_{j=1}^m \Gamma(\mu_j+1)}{\pi(\mathbf{m}_+ + \mathbf{m}_- + 1)\Gamma(\mathfrak{m}_- + \mathfrak{m}_+)};$$

in addition, if $\mathbf{m}_+ + \mathbf{m}_- > 0$, then

$$r_1^\pm(\bar\alpha) = r_0^\pm(\bar\alpha) \frac{\mathbf{m}_+ + \mathbf{m}_- + 1}{\mathbf{m}_+ + \mathbf{m}_-} \left(\sum_1^m m_j \Psi(\mu_j + 1) - (\mathbf{m}_+ + \mathbf{m}_-)\Psi(\mathfrak{m}_+ + \mathfrak{m}_-) + \pi \mathbf{m}_\pm \cot \pi \mathfrak{m}_\pm \right),$$

and if $\mathbf{m}_+ + \mathbf{m}_- = 0$, then

$$r_1^\pm(\bar\alpha) = -r_0^\pm(\bar\alpha)(\mathbf{m}_+ + \mathbf{m}_- + 1)\left(\Psi(\mathfrak{m}_+ + \mathfrak{m}_-) - \frac{\pi}{2}\cot \pi \mathfrak{m}_\pm \right);$$

(iv) if $\mathfrak{m}_+ \in \mathbb{Z}$, $\mathfrak{m}_+ + \mathfrak{m}_- \in \mathbb{Z}$, $\mathfrak{m}_+ > 0$, then

$$R(f;\alpha) = y_+^{\mathfrak{m}_+ + \mathfrak{m}_- - 1} \sum_{j=0}^{\mathfrak{m}_+ + \mathfrak{m}_-} r_j^+(\alpha) \log^{\mathfrak{m}_+ + \mathfrak{m}_- - j} y_+ +$$

$$y_-^{\mathfrak{m}_+ + \mathfrak{m}_-} \sum_{j=0}^{\mathfrak{m}_+ + \mathfrak{m}_-} r_j^-(\alpha) \log^{\mathfrak{m}_+ + \mathfrak{m}_- - j} y_- + r(\alpha),$$

$$r_0^\pm(\bar\alpha) = -\frac{\phi(\bar x)\Xi(2\pi)^{\frac{n-m}{2}} \mathfrak{m}_\pm \prod_{j=1}^m \Gamma(\mu_j + 1)}{(\mathfrak{m}_- + \mathfrak{m}_+)\Gamma(\mathfrak{m}_- + \mathfrak{m}_+)};$$

(v) if $\mathfrak{m}_\pm \in \mathbb{Z}$, $\mathfrak{m}_\pm = 0$, then $R(f;\alpha)|_{y \in \mathbb{R}_\pm}$ extends to an element of $C^k(U)$. If $\mathfrak{m}_+, \mathfrak{m}_- \in \mathbb{Z}$, $\mathfrak{m}_+ = \mathfrak{m}_- = 0$, then

$$R(f;\alpha) = r^+ y_+^{\mathfrak{m}_+ + \mathfrak{m}_- - 1} + r(\alpha),$$

$$r^+ = \frac{\phi(\bar x)(-1)^{\mathfrak{m}_-}\Xi(2\pi)^{\frac{n-m}{2}} \prod_{j=1}^m \Gamma(\mu_j + 1)}{\Gamma(\mathfrak{m}_- + \mathfrak{m}_+)}.$$

REMARK 1. One can write down all the coefficients $r_j^\pm$, not just the first, the resulting formulae being cumbersome. The reason for writing explicitly the second coefficient in the case *(iii)* is that we shall need this formula for the proof of Theorem 2.

REMARK 2. We have defined y and z using nonhomogeneous coordinates in $\mathbb{RP}_n$ with the normalization $\alpha_n = 1$. Instead we can take $\alpha_k = 1$, $1 \leq k < n$. In the region $\{\alpha \in \mathbb{RP}_n | \alpha_k/\alpha_n > 0\}$ this will lead only to changing $\bar\alpha_n$ to $\bar\alpha_k$ in (6) and (8). However, in the region $\alpha_k/\alpha_n < 0$ using α_k instead of α_n will lead to changing the sign of y and z, so, besides (6) and (8), in all the formulae of Theorem 1 we shall have also to interchange $r_j^+(\alpha)$ and $r_j^-(\alpha)$, $\mathfrak{m}_+$ and $\mathfrak{m}_-$, $\mathfrak{m}_+$ and $\mathfrak{m}_-$.

REMARK 3. The above assertions in general do not hold for all $\bar\alpha \in \hat S_{\mathcal{J}'}$. As we shall see in the proof of Theorem 1, condition sufficient for $\bar\alpha \in \hat S_{\mathcal{J}'}$ to be one of those for which Theorem 1 does hold is the following: the function $\bar\alpha_0 + \sum_{j=1}^n \bar\alpha_j x_j$ considered as the function on $S_{\mathcal{J}'}$ has a single critical point $\bar x$ with critical value zero, and $\bar x$ is a Morse-type critical point.

REMARK 4. In case *(v)* the behaviour of the Radon transform of $f(x)$ may be described also by the formula symmetric to that given above:

$$R(f;\alpha) = r^- y_-^{\mathfrak{m}_+ + \mathfrak{m}_- - 1} + r(\alpha),$$

$$r^- = \frac{\phi(\bar x)(-1)^{\mathfrak{m}_+}\Xi(2\pi)^{\frac{n-m}{2}} \prod_{j=1}^m \Gamma(\mu_j + 1)}{\Gamma(\mathfrak{m}_- + \mathfrak{m}_+)}.$$

1.3. An auxiliary result. In the following lemma we consider the behaviour of the integral

$$\text{(10)} \quad \int\cdots\int_{U\cap\{\sum_{l=1}^{a} w_l - \sum_{l=a+1}^{a+b} w_l = z\}} \prod_{l=1}^{a+b}(w_l)_+^{\mu_l} \log^{m_l}(w_l)_+ f(w_1,\ldots,w_{a+b},z)dw_2\ldots dw_{a+b}$$

as $z \to 0$. Here a, b, m_l are integers, $a, b \geq 1$, $m_l \geq 0$, μ_l are real numbers, $\mu_l > -1$, $l = 1, \ldots, a+b$; U is the neighbourhood of the origin given by $|z| < \epsilon$, $|u_l| < \epsilon_l$, $l = 1, \ldots, a+b$, such that

$$\text{(11)} \quad \epsilon_l > \sum_{j=1}^{l-1} \epsilon_j, \quad l = 2, \ldots, a+b.$$

It is assumed that $f(w_1, \ldots, w_{a+b}, z) \in C^k(U)$, with k specified later. We introduce the following notations: $\mathcal{M}_+ = \sum_{j=1}^{a}(\mu_j + 1)$, $\mathcal{M}_- = \sum_{j=a+1}^{a+b}(\mu_j + 1)$, $M_+ = \sum_{j=1}^{a} m_j$, $M_- = \sum_{j=a+1}^{a+b} m_j$. Our aim is to prove that the integral (10) for $z \to \pm 0$ has the asymptotic expansion

$$z_\pm^\beta \sum_{c=0}^{B} \log^{B-c} z_\pm f_c^\pm(z) + g(z),$$

where $f_c^\pm(z), g(z)$ are in C^k, $\beta = \mathcal{M}_+ + \mathcal{M}_- - 1$, $B = M_+ + M_-$ for generic exponents and $B = M_+ + M_- \pm 1$ for special values of exponents in (10).

LEMMA 2. *Let* $f(w_1, \ldots, w_{a+b}, z) \in C^k(U)$, $k \geq \mathcal{M}_+ + \mathcal{M}_-$. *Then there exist functions* $f_c^\pm(z), g(z) \in C^k(V)$, V *being a small enough neighbourhood of zero, such that:*

(i) *If all the numbers* $\mathcal{M}_+, \mathcal{M}_-$ *and* $\mathcal{M}_+ + \mathcal{M}_-$ *are not integers, then for* $z \to \pm 0$ *integral (10) equals*

$$\text{(12)} \quad z_\pm^{\mathcal{M}_+ + \mathcal{M}_- - 1} \sum_{c=0}^{M_+ + M_-} \log^{M_+ + M_- - c} z_\pm f_c^\pm(z) + g(z),$$

where $f_c^\pm(z), g(z) \in C^k(V)$ *and*

$$\text{(12')} \quad f_0^\pm(0) = \frac{\sin \pi \mathcal{M}_\pm \prod_{j=1}^{a+b} \Gamma(\mu_j + 1)}{\sin \pi(\mathcal{M}_+ + \mathcal{M}_-)\Gamma(\mathcal{M}_+ + \mathcal{M}_-)} f(0, \ldots, 0, 0).$$

(ii) If $\mathcal{M}_+ \in \mathbb{Z}$, $\mathcal{M}_- \notin \mathbb{Z}$, $M_+ > 0$, then for $z \to -0$ integral (10) is given by formulae (12) – (12′), and for $z \to +0$ we have instead

(13)
$$z_+^{\mathcal{M}_+ + \mathcal{M}_- - 1} \sum_{c=0}^{M_+ + M_- - 1} \log^{M_+ + M_- - 1 - c} z_+ \, f_c^{\pm}(z) + g(z),$$

(13′)
$$f_0^+(0) = \frac{\pi M_+ \prod_{j=1}^{a+b} \Gamma(\mu_j + 1)}{\sin \pi (\mathcal{M}_+ + \mathcal{M}_-) \Gamma(\mathcal{M}_+ + \mathcal{M}_-)} f(0, \ldots, 0, 0).$$

If $\mathcal{M}_- \in \mathbb{Z}$, $\mathcal{M}_+ \notin \mathbb{Z}$, $M_- > 0$, the same statement holds with indices plus and minus interchanged.

(iii) If $\mathcal{M}_\pm \notin \mathbb{Z}$, $\mathcal{M}_+ + \mathcal{M}_- \in \mathbb{Z}$, then for $z \to \pm 0$ formulae (12) – (12′) are replaced by

(14)
$$z_\pm^{\mathcal{M}_+ + \mathcal{M}_- - 1} \sum_{c=0}^{M_+ + M_- + 1} \log^{M_+ + M_- + 1 - c} z_\pm \, f_c^{\pm}(z) + g(z),$$

(14′)
$$f_0^\pm(0) = -\frac{\sin \pi \mathcal{M}_\pm \prod_{j=1}^{a+b} \Gamma(\mu_j + 1)}{\pi (M_+ + M_- + 1) \Gamma(\mathcal{M}_+ + \mathcal{M}_-)} f(0, \ldots, 0, 0).$$

Here $f_c^\pm(z), g(z) \in C^k(V)$ as above. Also, in this case we have

(14″)
$$f_1^\pm(0) = f_0^\pm(0) \frac{M_+ + M_- + 1}{M_+ + M_-} (-\Psi(\mathcal{M}_+ + \mathcal{M}_-)(M_+ + M_-) + \sum_{1}^{a+b} m_j \Psi(\mu_j + 1) + \pi M_\pm \cot \mathcal{M}_+),$$

if $M_+ + M_- > 0$. If $M_+ + M_- = 0$, i.e., $m_1 = \cdots = m_{a+b} = 0$, then

(14‴)
$$f_1^\pm(0) = -f_0^\pm(0)(M_+ + M_- + 1)(\Psi(\mathcal{M}_+ + \mathcal{M}_-) - \frac{\pi}{2} M_\pm \cot \mathcal{M}_+).$$

(iv) If $\mathcal{M}_+, \mathcal{M}_- \in \mathbb{Z}$, $M_+, M_- > 0$, then for $z \to \pm 0$ integral (10) is given by (12) with $f_c^\pm(z), g(z) \in C^k(V)$ and

(15)
$$f_0^\pm(0) = -\frac{M_\pm \prod_{j=1}^{a+b} \Gamma(\mu_j + 1)}{(M_+ + M_-) \Gamma(\mathcal{M}_+ + \mathcal{M}_-)} f(0, \ldots, 0, 0).$$

(v) If $\mathcal{M}_\pm \in \mathbb{Z}$ and $M_\pm = 0$, then integral (10) for $z \in V \cap \mathbb{R}_+$ extends to an element of $C^k(V)$. If $\mathcal{M}_+, \mathcal{M}_- \in \mathbb{Z}$ and $M_+ = M_- = 0$, then integral

(10) in V may be represented by the formula

(16) $$f^+ z_+^{\mathcal{M}_+ + \mathcal{M}_- - 1} + g(z),$$

(16′) $$f^+ = \frac{(-1)^{\mathcal{M}_-} \prod_{j=1}^{a+b} \Gamma(\mu_j + 1)}{\Gamma(\mathcal{M}_+ + \mathcal{M}_-)} f(0, \ldots, 0, 0).$$

REMARK 5. It follows from (16) – (16′) that integral (10) in case (v) may be written in the form $f^- z_-^{\mathcal{M}_+ + \mathcal{M}_- - 1} + g(z)$ with

$$f^- = \frac{(-1)^{\mathcal{M}_+} \prod_{j=1}^{a+b} \Gamma(\mu_j + 1)}{\Gamma(\mathcal{M}_+ + \mathcal{M}_-)} f(0, \ldots, 0, 0).$$

PROOF OF LEMMA 2. Write (10) in the form

$$\int \cdots \int_{U \cap \{\sum_{l=1}^{a} w_l - \sum_{l=a+1}^{a+b} w_l = z\}} \prod_{l=1}^{a+b} (w_l)_+^{\mu_l} \log^{m_l}(w_l)_+ \, dw_2 \ldots dw_{a+b} \times$$

$$\sum_{|\omega|=0}^{k} \frac{\partial^{|\omega|} f(0, \ldots, 0, z)}{\partial^\omega w} \frac{w^\omega}{\omega!} +$$

$$\int \cdots \int_{U \cap \{\sum_{l=1}^{a} w_l - \sum_{l=a+1}^{a+b} w_l = z\}} \prod_{l=1}^{a+b} (w_l)_+^{\mu_l} \log^{m_l}(w_l)_+ \, dw_2 \ldots dw_{a+b} f_k(w_1, \ldots, w_{a+b}, z) dx,$$

where $f_k(w_1, \ldots, w_{a+b}, z) = o(|w|^k)$. The last integral in the right hand side is a C^k-function of z by the Lebesgue convergence theorem. As for the first integrals, we make the following observation:

$$\int \cdots \int_{U \cap \{\sum_{l=1}^{a} w_l - \sum_{l=a+1}^{a+b} w_l = z\}} \prod_{l=1}^{a+b} (w_l)_+^{\mu_l} \log^{m_l}(w_l)_+ \, dw_2 \ldots dw_{a+b} =$$

$$\text{V.P.} \int_0^{+\infty} w_2^{\mu_2} \log^{m_2} w_2 \, dw_2 \cdots \int_0^{+\infty} w_{a+b}^{\mu_{a+b}} \log^{m_{a+b}} w_{a+b} \, dw_{a+b} \times$$

$$\left(z + \sum_{l=2}^{a} w_l - \sum_{l=a+1}^{a+b} w_l\right)_+^{\mu_1} \log^{m_1}\left(z + \sum_{l=2}^{a} w_l - \sum_{l=a+1}^{a+b} w_l\right)_+^{\mu_1} + h(z),$$

with $h(z)$ analytic in a neighbourhood of the origin, and the finite part in the sense of Hadamard (V.P.) of the above multiple integral divergent at infinity is defined by the applying repeatedly the formula [**GSh**, chapter 1, section 3.8]:

$$\text{V.P.}\int_0^\infty x^\mu \log^m x\,(x+z)^\nu \log^n(z+x)dx = \int_0^1 x^\mu \log^m x\,(x+z)^\nu \log^n(z+x)dx +$$

$$\text{V.P.}\int_1^\infty x^{\mu+\nu} \log^m x \left(1+\frac{z}{x}\right)^\nu \sum_{p=0}^n \binom{p}{n} \log^p x \log^{n-p}\left(1+\frac{z}{x}\right) dx =$$

$$\int_0^1 x^\mu \log^m x\,(x+z)^\nu \log^n(z+x)dx +$$

$$\sum_{p=0}^n \binom{p}{n} \int_1^\infty x^{\mu+\nu} \log^{m+p} x \left(\left(1+\frac{z}{x}\right)^\nu \log^{n+p}\left(1+\frac{z}{x}\right) - T_{[\mu+\nu]+1,p}(z,x)\right) dx.$$

Here $T_{[\mu+\nu]+1,p}(z,x)$ is the Maclaurin polynomial of degree $[\mu+\nu]+1$ of the function $(1+u)^\nu \log^{n+p}(1+u)$ of degree with $u = z/x$. The above finite part of the divergent integral is in fact a convolution and can be calculated via the Fourier transform $\mathfrak{F}$:

$$\text{V.P.}\int_0^{+\infty} w_2^{\mu_2} \log^{m_2} w_2\, dw_2 \cdots \int_0^{+\infty} w_{a+b}^{\mu_{a+b}} \log^{m_{a+b}} w_{a+b}\, dw_{a+b}$$

$$\left(z + \sum_{l=2}^a w_l - \sum_{l=a+1}^{a+b} w_l\right)_+^{\mu_1} \log^{m_1}\left(z + \sum_{l=2}^a w_l - \sum_{l=a+1}^{a+b} w_l\right)_+^{\mu_1} =$$

$$\left(\left(w_+^{\mu_1} \log^{m_1} w_+\right) * \cdots * \left(w_+^{\mu_a} \log^{m_a} w_+\right) * \right.$$
$$\left.\left(w_-^{\mu_{a+1}} \log^{m_{a+1}} w_-\right) * \cdots * \left(w_-^{\mu_{a+b}} \log^{m_{a+b}} w_-\right)\right)(z) =$$

(17) $$\mathfrak{F}^{-1}\left(\prod_{l=1}^a \mathfrak{F}\left(w_+^{\mu_l} \log^{m_l} w_+\right)(\zeta) \cdot \prod_{l=a+1}^{a+b} \mathfrak{F}\left(w_-^{\mu_l} \log^{m_l} w_-\right)(\zeta)\right)(z).$$

We shall explain below how the convolution and the product in the right hand side of (17) must be understood.

The Fourier transform of the distribution $w_\pm^\lambda \log^l w_\pm$ can be calculated by differentiating the known formula [**GSh**]

$$\mathfrak{F}x_\pm^\lambda(\zeta) = \Gamma(\lambda+1)e^{\pm\frac{i\pi(\lambda+1)}{2}}(\zeta \pm i0)^{-1-\lambda}, \quad \lambda \neq -1,-2,\ldots,$$

with respect to λ, so for λ not a negative integer we get

$$\mathfrak{F}w_\pm^\lambda \log^l w_\pm(\zeta) = \sum_{j=1}^{l+1} a_{\lambda,l,j}(\zeta \pm i0)^{-1-\lambda} \log^{l+1-j}(\zeta \pm i0),$$

(18) $$a_{\lambda,l,0}^\pm = 0, \quad a_{\lambda,l,1}^\pm = (-1)^l e^{\pm\frac{i\pi(\lambda+1)}{2}} \Gamma(\lambda+1),$$

(18′) $$a_{\lambda,l,2}^\pm = (-1)^{l-1} l e^{\pm\frac{i\pi(\lambda+1)}{2}} \Gamma(\lambda+1)\left(\pm\frac{i\pi}{2} + \Psi(\lambda+1)\right).$$

See [**GSh**] for the definition of the distributions $x_\pm^\lambda \log^l x_\pm$, $(x \pm i0)^\lambda \log^l(x \pm i0)$.

In order to cope with the case $\lambda = -L$, $L \in \mathbb{Z}$, $L > 0$, recall that the distribution $x_\pm^{-L} \log^l x_\pm$ can be defined by the formula [**GSh**]

$$x_\pm^{-L} \log^l x_\pm = \frac{1}{l+1} \lim_{\lambda' \to -L} \frac{\partial^{l+1}}{(\partial \lambda')^{l+1}} \left((\lambda' + L) x_\pm^{\lambda'} \right),$$

therefore, using the formula $x\Gamma(x) = \Gamma(x+1)$, we can calculate in this case the coefficient of the leading term of the Fourier transform expansion:

$$(19) \quad a_{\lambda,l,0}^\pm = \frac{(-1)^{l+1}}{l+1} e^{\pm \frac{i\pi(-L+1)}{2}} \lim_{\lambda' \to -L} \left((\lambda'+L)\Gamma(\lambda'+1) \right) =$$

$$\frac{(-1)^{l+1}(\mp i)^{L-1}}{l+1} \lim_{\lambda' \to -L} \frac{\Gamma(\lambda'+L+1)}{(\lambda'+1)\ldots(\lambda'+L-1)} = \frac{(-1)^{l+1}(\pm i)^{\lambda+1}}{\Gamma(-\lambda)(l+1)}.$$

In the same fashion we calculate the second coefficient:

$$a_{\lambda,l,1}^\pm = (-1)^l e^{\pm \frac{i\pi(-L+1)}{2}} \times$$

$$\left(\pm \frac{i\pi}{2} \lim_{\lambda' \to -L} \left((\lambda'+L)\Gamma(\lambda'+1) \right) + \lim_{\lambda' \to -L} \frac{d((\lambda'+L)\Gamma(\lambda'+1))}{d\lambda'} \right) =$$

$$\frac{(-1)^l(\mp i)^{L-1}}{(L-1)!} \left(\pm \frac{i\pi(-1)^{L-1}}{2 \cdot (L-1)!} + \lim_{\lambda' \to -L} \frac{d}{d\lambda'} \frac{\Gamma(\lambda'+L+1)}{(\lambda'+1)\ldots(\lambda'+L-1)} \right) =$$

$$\frac{(-1)^l(\pm i)^{\lambda+1}}{\Gamma(-\lambda)} \left(\frac{\pm i\pi}{2} + \Gamma'(1) + \sum_{k=1}^{-\lambda-1} \frac{1}{k} \right).$$

Using the formula $\Psi(k) = -\mathbf{C} + \sum_{j=1}^{k-1} \frac{1}{j}$, where $\mathbf{C} = -\Gamma'(1)$ is the Euler constant (see [**GrR**]), yields

$$(19') \quad a_{\lambda,l,1}^\pm = \frac{(-1)^l(\pm i)^{\lambda+1}}{\Gamma(-\lambda)} \left(\pm \frac{i\pi}{2} + \Psi(-\lambda) \right).$$

Recall the well known formula (see, e.g., [**GrR**]):

$$(20) \quad \Gamma(\alpha)\Gamma(1-\alpha) = \frac{\pi}{\sin \pi \alpha},$$

where $\alpha \notin \mathbb{Z}$; later we shall need also its straightforward consequence

$$(21) \quad \Psi(\alpha) - \Psi(1-\alpha) = -\pi \cot \pi\alpha.$$

Now, assumption (3) implies that the right hand side of (17) can be represented in the form

$$\mathfrak{F}^{-1} \left(\sum_{j=0}^{M_+} b_j^+ (\zeta+i0)^{-\mathcal{M}_+} \log^{M_+ - j}(\zeta+i0) \times \right.$$

$$\left. \sum_{j=0}^{M_-} b_j^- (\zeta-i0)^{-\mathcal{M}_-} \log^{M_- - j}(\zeta-i0) \right)(z).$$

For $\zeta \neq 0$ (and in the case of noninteger $\mathcal{M}_\pm$ for all ζ) the product between the parentheses can be written as

$$\sum_{j=0}^{M_-+M_+} c_j^+ \zeta_+^{-\mathcal{M}_--\mathcal{M}_+} \log z_+^{M_-+M_+-j} + \sum_{j=0}^{M_-+M_+} c_j^- \zeta_-^{-\mathcal{M}_--\mathcal{M}_+} \log z_-^{M_-+M_+-j},$$

$$c_0^\pm = (-1)^{M_++M_-} e^{\pm \frac{i\pi(\mathcal{M}_+-\mathcal{M}_-)}{2}} \prod_{l=1}^{a+b} \Gamma(\mu_l+1),$$

$$c_1^\pm = -c_0^\pm \left(\pm \frac{i\pi(M_+-M_-)}{2} + \sum_{l=1}^{a+b} m_l \Psi(\mu_l+1) \right).$$

Since we are interested in the singularities of the inverse Fourier transform of the above product, we shall not investigate the behaviour of this product in a neighbourhood of the point $\zeta = 0$. Instead we apply (18) – (19'), (20) – (21), to get formulae (12) – (12'), (14) – (14''). However, if $\mathcal{M}_\pm \in \mathbb{Z}$, then formulae (12') and (14') give zero, so this case must be considered separately.

First let $\mathcal{M}_+ \in \mathbb{Z}$, $M_+ = 0$. The argument with the Fourier transform allows us to represent integral (10), modulo a C^k-function, in the form

$$\int_{-1}^{0} (z-w)_+^{\mathcal{M}_+-1} w_-^{\mathcal{M}_--1} \sum_{j=0}^{M_-} h_j \log^{M_--j} w_- \, dw,$$

and we may differentiate with respect to z under the sign of the integral for $z > 0$ and for $z = 0$, since for $z \geq 0$, $w \leq 0$ we have $(z-w)_+ = z-w$. Thus, in this case integral (10) for $z > 0$ is a restriction of a function from $C^k(V)$.

Now, let $\mathcal{M}_+ \in \mathbb{Z}$, $M_+ > 0$. Remark that the following identities hold:

$(w_+^{\mu_1} \log^{m_1} w_+ * w_-^{\mu_2} \log^{m_2} w_-)(z) =$
$\quad ((w+i0)^{\mu_1} \log^{m_1}(w+i0) * w_-^{\mu_2} \log^{m_2} w_-)(z), \quad z > 0;$
$(w_+^{\mu_1} \log^{m_1} w_+ * w_-^{\mu_2} \log^{m_2} w_-)(z) =$
$\left(w_+^{\mu_1} \log^{m_1} w_+ * \sum_{j=0}^{m_2} \binom{j}{m_2} (-i\pi)^j (w+i0)^{\mu_2} \log^{m_2-j}(w+i0) \right)(z), \quad z < 0.$

It follows from (18) that

$$\mathfrak{F}(w \pm i0)^\lambda \log^l(w \pm i0)\,(\zeta) = \sum_{j=0}^{l-1} d_j^\pm \zeta_\mp^{-1-\lambda} \log^{l-1-j} \zeta_\mp,$$

$$d_0^\pm = 2\pi l(-1)^{l-1} e^{\pm \frac{i\pi\lambda}{2}}.$$

Therefore, for $z > 0$ we can write (17) in the different form:

$$\mathfrak{F}^{-1}\left(\mathfrak{F}\left(\sum_{j=0}^{\mathcal{M}_+-1} e_j^+(w+i0)^{\mathcal{M}_+-1}\log^{\mathcal{M}_+-1-j}(w+i0)\right)\right. \times$$

$$\left.\mathfrak{F}\left(\sum_{j=0}^{\mathcal{M}_-} e_j^- w_-^{\mathcal{M}_--1}\log^{\mathcal{M}_--j} w_-\right)\right)(z) =$$

$$\mathfrak{F}^{-1}\left(\sum_{j=0}^{\mathcal{M}_++\mathcal{M}_--1} e_j \zeta_-^{-\mathcal{M}_+-\mathcal{M}_-}\log^{\mathcal{M}_++\mathcal{M}_--1-j}\zeta_-\right)(z),$$

$$e_0 = 2\pi \mathcal{M}_+(-1)^{\mathcal{M}_++\mathcal{M}_--1} e^{\frac{i\pi(\mathcal{M}_++\mathcal{M}_--1)}{2}} \prod_{l=1}^{a+b}\Gamma(\mu_l+1).$$

Now for $z > 0$ (18) – (19′) and (20) yield (13) – (13′) and (15) – (15′). The same argument applies to the case $z < 0$.

Finally, consider the case $\mathcal{M}_+, \mathcal{M}_- \in \mathbb{Z}$, $\mathcal{M}_+ = \mathcal{M}_- = 0$. The same argument as above transforms integral (10), modulo a C^k-function, into

$$h_0 \cdot \left(w_+^{\mathcal{M}_+-1} * w_-^{\mathcal{M}_--1}\right)(z)$$

$$= \text{smooth function} + \begin{cases} 0, & z < 0; \\ \int_0^z w^{\mathcal{M}_+-1}(z-w)^{\mathcal{M}_--1}dw \cdot h_0(-1)^{\mathcal{M}_-}, & z \geq 0. \end{cases}$$

Here $h_0 = f(0,\ldots,0,0)\prod_{l=1}^{a+b}\Gamma(\mu_l+1) \cdot (\Gamma(\mathcal{M}_+)\Gamma(\mathcal{M}_-))^{-1}$. The last integral equals $z^{\mathcal{M}_++\mathcal{M}_--1}\Gamma(\mathcal{M}_+)\Gamma(\mathcal{M}_-)(\Gamma(\mathcal{M}_++\mathcal{M}_-))^{-1}$. This proves (16) – (16′) and completes the proof of the lemma. □

1.4. Proof of Theorem 1. The argument is similar to that of [**RZ2**]. It suffices to take a curve γ in $\mathbb{RP}_n$ which intersects the hypersurface $Q(S)$ transversally at the point $\bar{\alpha}$ and to show that $R(f;\alpha)$ has the necessary behaviour along this curve. We may choose this curve to be $\gamma = \{\alpha | \alpha_i = \bar{\alpha}, \ i = 1,\ldots,n\}$, α_0 is a parameter on γ. To see that γ is transversal to $Q(S)$, one can use the fact that the hyperplane tangent to $Q(S)$ at the point $\bar{\alpha}$ is given by the equation

$$\sum_{i=1}^n \bar{x}\alpha_i + \alpha_0 = 0.$$

(Here $\bar{x}$ is the point on $\partial D \cap \bar{\alpha}$ such that the hyperplane α is not transversal to some stratum $S_{\mathcal{J}'}$ containing $\bar{x}$, at the point $\bar{x}$). This follows from the fact that the dual of $\hat{S}_{\mathcal{J}'}$ is $S_{\mathcal{J}'}$ (or from the involutivity property of the Legendre transform and its generalization, see [**RZ2**], [**Zs**]). Now, comparing this equation with the definition of γ we see that they have just one common point, so indeed γ is transversal to $Q(S)$.

Without loss of generality one may assume that $\mathcal{J}' = \{1,\ldots,m\}$, $m \leq n$. Let $\mathfrak{g}_j(x) \in C^k$ be such that $S_j = \{x | \mathfrak{g}_j(x) = 0\}$, $j \in \mathcal{J}'$, grad $\mathfrak{g}_j(x) \neq 0$, and

$D = \{x | \mathfrak{g}_j(x) \geq 0, \ j \in \mathcal{J}\}$. After renumbering the coordinates $x_1, \ldots, x_n$ if necessary, we may assume that $S_{\mathcal{J}'}$ is given by (4), so $x_{m+1}, \ldots, x_n$ are local coordinates on $S_{\mathcal{J}'}$. It follows from the Morse lemma that for almost all $\alpha \in \hat{S}_{\mathcal{J}'}$ the function $z = \alpha_n^{-1}(\alpha_0 + \sum_{i=1}^n \alpha_i x_i)$ has only Morse type critical points on $S_{\mathcal{J}'}$ (see [**RZ2**, Lemma 2]), so we may assume that this is the case with $\bar{\alpha}$. Note that if we consider z as the function of α on γ with $x = \bar{x}$, then we have $z = \bar{\alpha}_n^{-1}(\alpha_0 - \bar{\alpha}_0) = y(\alpha)|_\gamma$, and z can be used instead of α_0 and $y(\alpha)$ as a parameter on γ in a neighbourhood of the point $\bar{\alpha}$.

Set $u_i = \mathfrak{g}_i(x)$, $i = 1, \ldots, m$. The collection $u_1, \ldots, u_m$ can be completed to a coordinate system $u_1, \ldots, u_m, u_{m+1}, \ldots, u_n$ in a neighbourhood of $S_{\mathcal{J}'}$. By Morse's lemma [**M**] one may choose the coordinates $u_{m+1}, \ldots, u_n$ so that for $u_1 = \cdots = u_m = 0$ we have

$$z = \sum_{j=m+1}^{n-I} u_j^2 - \sum_{j=n-I+1}^{n} u_j^2,$$

where I is the inertia index of the Hessian of z in $S_{\mathcal{J}'}$. Then we have

$$\left| \det \left(\frac{\partial u_j}{\partial x_k} \right)_{j,k=m+1,\ldots,n} \right| = 2^{\frac{m-n}{2}} |\mathfrak{J}|^{\frac{1}{2}},$$

where $\mathfrak{J}$ is defined by (6). The partial derivatives of z with respect to the variables u_i, $i = 1, \ldots, m$, do not vanish for generic $\bar{\alpha}$. Namely, they are calculated as follows:

$$\left(\frac{\partial z}{\partial u_i} \right)_{i=1,\ldots,m} = \left(\sum_{k=1}^{m} \frac{\partial z}{\partial x_k} \frac{\partial x_k}{\partial u_i} \right)_{i=1,\ldots,m} = \bar{\alpha}_n^{-1}(\bar{\alpha}_1, \ldots, \bar{\alpha}_m) \cdot (\tilde{\mathfrak{g}}'_1)^{-1},$$

see (7) – (8). Then one has $\dfrac{\partial z}{\partial u_i} = \zeta_i$, $i = 1, \ldots, m$.

Since $\bar{\alpha} \in \hat{S}_{\mathcal{J}'}$ is generic, we may assume that $\zeta_j \neq 0$, $j = 1, \ldots, m$. After scaling the coordinates $u_j \to u'_j = u_j |\zeta_j|$, $j = 1, \ldots, m$, we obtain the equation for z in the new coordinates

$$(22) \qquad z = \sum_{j=1}^{m} \operatorname{sgn}(\zeta_j) u'_j + \sum_{j=m+1}^{n-I} u_j^2 - \sum_{j=n-I+1}^{n} u_j^2.$$

Recall that a denotes the number of positive components of the vector ζ, and that the coordinates are numbered in such a way that $\operatorname{sgn} \zeta_j = 1$, $j = 1, \ldots, a$, and $\operatorname{sgn} \zeta_j = -1$, $j = a+1, \ldots, m$. Thus, the integration domain in (2) may be locally described by the inequalities

$$(23) \qquad u'_i \geq 0, \quad i = 1, \ldots, m$$

or, according to (22), by the inequalities

$$
(24) \quad \begin{cases} u_i' \geq 0, & i = 2, \ldots, m; \\ \operatorname{sgn}(\zeta_1) \left(z - \sum_{i=2}^{m} \operatorname{sgn}(\zeta_i) u_i' - \sum_{j=m+1}^{n-I} u_j^2 + \sum_{j=n-I+1}^{n} u_j^2 \right) \geq 0. \end{cases}
$$

By [**RZ2**, Lemma 1], the integral over the complement of an appropriate neighbourhood $U_{\bar{x}}$ of $\bar{x}$ is in C^k in a neighbourhood of $\bar{\alpha}$. Thus one may study only the integral over $U_{\bar{x}}$, call it $R_1(f; \bar{\alpha}, p)$. One may assume that $U_{\bar{x}}$ is defined by (23) and

$$
(25) \quad \begin{cases} |u_j'| < \epsilon_j, & j = 1, \ldots, m; \\ \sum_{j=m+1}^{n-I} u_j^2 < \epsilon_{m+1}, \\ \sum_{j=n-I+1}^{n} u_j^2 < \epsilon_{m+2}, \end{cases}
$$

where ϵ_j satisfy (11) with $a + b = m + 2$. Change of the x_i coordinates to u_i coordinates transforms $\phi(x)\lambda$ in (2) into an expression $\psi(u,z) du_2 \ldots du_n$, where $\psi(u,z)$ is in C^k. The measure λ in (1) may be written as $\lambda = \dfrac{|(\alpha_1, \ldots, \alpha_n)|}{|\alpha_1|} dx_2 \ldots dx_n$, so the formulas for the Jacobians of the transformations $x_2, \ldots, x_n \to u_2, \ldots, u_n$ and $u_2, \ldots, u_m \to u_2', \ldots, u_m'$ yield $\psi(0,0) = 2^{\frac{n-m}{2}} \phi(\bar{x}) \Xi$, see (9). After dropping the primes we may write $R_1(f; \alpha)$ as

$$
(26) \quad R_1(f; \bar{\alpha}) = \int \cdots \int du_2 \ldots du_n \prod_{j=1}^{m} (u_j)_+^{\mu_j} \log^{m_j}(u_j)_+ \psi(u, z),
$$

integration region is the intersection of U with the plane

$$
\sum_{j=1}^{a} u_j - \sum_{j=a+1}^{m} u_j + \sum_{j=m+1}^{n-m-I} u_j^2 - \sum_{j=n-m-I+1}^{n} u_j^2 = z.
$$

Consider first the case $0 < I < n - m$. Introduce spherical coordinates in the variables u_j, $j = m+1, \ldots, n-I$ and u_j, $j = n-I+1, \ldots, n$:

$$
\rho_1 = \left(\sum_{j=m+1}^{n-I} u_j^2 \right)^{1/2}, \quad \rho_1 \in [0, \epsilon],
$$

$$
\rho_2 = \left(\sum_{j=n-I+1}^{n} u_j^2 \right)^{1/2}, \quad \rho_2 \in [0, \epsilon],
$$

$$
\omega_j = \rho_1^{-1} u_j, \quad j = m+1, \ldots, n-I, \quad (\omega_{m+1}, \ldots, \omega_{n-I}) \in S^{n-I-m-1},
$$
$$
\omega_j = \rho_2^{-1} u_j, \quad j = n-I+1, \ldots, n, \quad (\omega_{n-I+1}, \ldots, \omega_n) \in S^{I-1},
$$

where $S^{N-1} \subset \mathbb{R}^N$ is the unit sphere. Note that the function

$$\psi_1(u_1,\ldots,u_m,\rho_1,\rho_2,z) = \int_{S^{n-I-m-1}\times S^{I-1}} \psi(u_1,\ldots,u_m,\rho_1\omega_1,\rho_2\omega_2,z)d\omega_1 d\omega_2$$

is in C^k with respect to the variables ρ_1, ρ_2 and z and an even function of ρ_1, ρ_2. Indeed, if in the preceding integral we change the variables $\omega_1 = -\omega_1'$, then $\psi_1(u_1,\ldots,u_m,\rho_1,\rho_2,z)$ transforms into $\psi_1(u_1,\ldots,u_m,-\rho_1,\rho_2,z)$. Hence there exists a function $\psi_2(u_1,\ldots,u_m,v_1,v_2,z)$, $\psi_2 \in C^k$, such that

$$\psi_1(u_1,\ldots,u_m,\rho_1,\rho_2,z) = \psi_2(u_1,\ldots,u_m,\rho_1^2,\rho_2^2,z).$$

Using the formula $\Omega_N = \dfrac{2\pi^{\frac{N}{2}}}{\Gamma(N/2)}$ for the area of the unit sphere $S^{N-1} \subset \mathbb{R}^N$ yields

$$\psi_2(0,\ldots,0,0,0,0) = \psi_1(0,\ldots,0,0,0,0)\frac{4\pi^{\frac{n-m}{2}}}{\Gamma\left(\dfrac{I}{2}\right)\Gamma\left(\dfrac{n-m-I}{2}\right)}.$$

Changing the variables $\rho_j \to v_j = \rho_j^2$, $j = 1,2$, brings integral (26) to the form

$$(27) \quad \int\cdots\int du_2\ldots du_m dv_1 dv_2 (v_1)_+^{\frac{n-I-m-2}{2}} (v_2)_+^{\frac{I-2}{2}} \prod_{j=1}^m (u_j)_+^{\mu_j} \log^{m_j}(u_j)_+ \times$$

$$\frac{\psi_2(u_1,\ldots,u_m,v_1,v_2,z)}{4},$$

integration region is the intersection of U with the plane

$$\sum_{j=1}^a u_j - \sum_{j=a+1}^m u_j + v_1 - v_2 = z,$$

U is defined by the inequalities $|u_j| < \epsilon_j$, $j = 1,\ldots,m$, $|v_j| < \epsilon_{m+j}$, $j = 1,2$. Now the result follows from Lemma 2.

In the exceptional case $I = 0$ (resp. $I = n-m$) one uses the same argument, but introduces spherical coordinates in only one group of the variables. One obtains in this case an expression similar to the right hand side of (27) where v_1 (resp. v_2) are missing, and

$$\psi_2(0,\ldots,0,0,0,0) = \psi_1(0,\ldots,0,0,0,0)\frac{2\pi^{\frac{n-m}{2}}}{\Gamma\left(\dfrac{n-m}{2}\right)}.$$

Then we proceed as above. $\square$

2. The Erdélyi lemma

The following well known formula is called the Fourier slice theorem:

$$(28) \qquad \tilde{f}(t\alpha_1, \ldots, t\alpha_n) = \int_{-\infty}^{\infty} e^{it\alpha_0} R(f; \alpha) \, d\alpha_0.$$

Here $\sum_{j=1}^{n} \alpha_j^2 = 1$, $f(x_1, \ldots, x_n)$ is, for example, integrable and compactly supported in $\mathbb{R}^n$, and $\tilde{f}(t\alpha_1, \ldots, t\alpha_n)$ stands for the n-dimensional Fourier transform of $f(x)$. Using (28), Theorem 1, and the classical one-dimensional Erdélyi lemma, we obtain the multidimensional analogue of the latter. We shall see that, contrary to the case of the Radon transform, the exponent of the logarithm in the case of the Fourier transform is always $\mathbf{m}_+ + \mathbf{m}_-$ and does not depend on the geometry of $S_{\mathcal{J}'}$ and α, as well as the coefficient of the leading term.

To be precise, in the next theorem we consider functions $f(x)$ of type (1) under the same smoothness conditions as in Theorem 1. We obtain the asymptotics of the Fourier transform $\tilde{f}(t\alpha_1, \ldots, t\alpha_n)$ as $t \to +\infty$ for $\alpha \in A$, where A is a subset of the unit sphere $S^{n-1} \subset \mathbb{R}^n$ such that the complement $S^{n-1} \smallsetminus A$ has Lebesgue measure zero. When ∂D is a smooth hypersurface, i.e., $\mathcal{J}$ consists of a single element, A can be defined as follows: $\alpha \in A$ iff for every $x \in \partial D$ such that the normal to ∂D is parallel to α, the Gaussian curvature of ∂D at the point x does not vanish. In general the definition is analogous.

DEFINITION. *A point $\alpha \in S^{n-1}$ does not belong to A, if there exist $\mathcal{J}' \subseteq \mathcal{J}$ such that the function $\alpha \cdot x$ has a degenerate critical point on $S_{\mathcal{J}'}$.*

Recall that if $V \subset \mathbb{R}^n$ is a smooth manifold, $f : \mathbb{R}^n \to \mathbb{R}^1$ is a smooth function, then $x \in V$ is a critical point of f if $df(x)$ belongs to $(T_V^* \mathbb{R}^n)_x$ – the conormal of $\mathbb{R}^n$ to V at the point x, i.e., the conormal of the tangent space $T_x V \subseteq T_x \mathbb{R}^n$. The point x is a degenerate critical point of f if the Hessian of f at the point x is a degenerate quadratic form on the tangent space $T_x V$, see [**AVGZ**].

LEMMA 3. *The complement $S^{n-1} \smallsetminus A$ has Lebesgue measure zero.*

PROOF. The argument is a modification of that of [**M**]. For each $\mathcal{J}' \subset \mathcal{J}$ consider the manifold

$$\mathcal{R}_{\mathcal{J}'} = \{(\alpha_0, \ldots, \alpha_n, x) \mid (\alpha_1, \ldots, \alpha_n) \in T_{S_{\mathcal{J}'}}^* \mathbb{R}^n, \quad \alpha_0 \in \mathbb{R},$$
$$x \in S_{\mathcal{J}'}, \quad \alpha_0 + \sum_{j=1}^{n} \alpha_j x_j = 0\},$$

and a map $\sigma_{\mathcal{J}'} : \mathcal{R}_{\mathcal{J}'} \to \mathbb{R}^n$, $\sigma_{\mathcal{J}'}(\alpha_0, \ldots, \alpha_n, x) = (\alpha_1, \ldots, \alpha_n)$. Since the statement is local, we may assume that V is given by (4). Then $\alpha_1, \ldots, \alpha_m$,

$x_{m+1}, \ldots, x_n$ are local coordinates in $\mathcal{R}_{\mathcal{J}'}$, and $\sigma_{\mathcal{J}'}$ is given by

$$\sigma_{\mathcal{J}'}(\alpha_1, \ldots, \alpha_m, x_{m+1}, \ldots, x_n) = \left(\alpha_1, \ldots, \alpha_m, \left(\sum_{j=1}^{m} \alpha_j \frac{\partial g_p(x_{m+1}, \ldots, x_n)}{\partial x_j} \right)_{p=m+1,\ldots,n} \right).$$

Then (x, α) is a critical point of $\sigma_{\mathcal{J}'}$ if and only if the determinant of the Jacobian matrix of $\sigma_{\mathcal{J}'}$ vanishes, and the latter matrix is just Hessian of the function $\sum_{j=1}^{m} \alpha_j x_j$ on $S_{\mathcal{J}'}$ with the above local coordinates. Thus, $(\alpha_1, \ldots, \alpha_n) \in A$ if and only if $(\alpha_1, \ldots, \alpha_n)$ is not a critical value of $\sigma_{\mathcal{J}'}$ for all $\mathcal{J}' \subseteq \mathcal{J}'$. Now the statement follows from the Sard lemma. $\square$

For $(\alpha_1, \ldots, \alpha_n) \in A$ we shall denote $\mathcal{F}(\alpha_1, \ldots, \alpha_n)$ the set of $x \in \partial D$ such that the hyperplane $\{x' \in \mathbb{R}^n \mid \sum_{j=1}^{n} \alpha_j (x'_j - x_j) = 0\}$ is not transversal to the largest stratum $S_{\mathcal{J}'}$ containing x. Using the partition of the unity, we transform the asymptotics into the sum of contributions of $x \in \mathcal{F}(\alpha_1, \ldots, \alpha_n)$, so it suffices to consider only one contribution. In this case we assume without loss of generality that $\mathcal{J}' = \{1, \ldots, m\}$. We use the notations introduced in Section 1.1, in particular (9).

THEOREM 2. *For every direction $(\alpha_1, \ldots, \alpha_n) \in A$, the contribution of a point $x \in \mathcal{F}(\alpha_1, \ldots, \alpha_n)$ to the asymptotics of $\tilde{f}(t\alpha_1, \ldots, t\alpha_n)$ as $t \to +\infty$ is*

$$t^{-\mathbf{m}_+ - \mathbf{m}_-} \sum_{j=0}^{\mathbf{m}_+ + \mathbf{m}_-} q_j \log^{\mathbf{m}_+ + \mathbf{m}_- - j} t \left(\exp\left\{ it \sum_{l=1}^{n} \alpha_l x_l \right\} + o(1) \right),$$

and the coefficient of the leading term is

$$q_0 = \phi(\bar{x})(-1)^{\mathbf{m}_+ + \mathbf{m}_-} e^{\frac{i\pi}{2}(\mathbf{m}_+ - \mathbf{m}_- - I)} \Xi |\alpha_n|^{-\mathbf{m}_+ - \mathbf{m}_- + 1}(2\pi)^{\frac{n-m}{2}} \prod_{j=1}^{m} \Gamma(\mu_j + 1).$$

The statement follows from Theorem 1, Remark 3, the classical Erdélyi lemma, and (28).

References

[AVGZ] V. I. Arnold, A. N. Varchenko, S. M. Gussein-Zade, *Singularities of differentiable maps*, vol. 1, 2, Birkhäuser, Boston, 1985.

[BNW] J. Bruna, A. Nagel, S. Wainger, *Convex hypersurfaces and Fourier transforms*, Ann. Math. **127** (1988), 333 – 365.

[E] A. Erdélyi, *Asymptotic expansions*, Dover, New York, 1956.

[F] M. V. Fedoriuk, *Metod perevala (Saddlepoint method)*, Nauka, Moscow, 1977. (Russian)

[GGV] I. M. Gelfand, M. I. Graev, N. Ya. Vilenkin, *Generalized functions*, vol. 5: Integral geometry and problems of representation theory, Acad. Press, New York, 1966.

[GSh] I. M. Gelfand, G. E. Shilov, *Generalized functions*, vol. 1: Properties and operations, Acad. Press, New York, 1964.

[Gi] E. Giusti, *Minimal surfaces and functions of bounded variation*, Birkhäuser, Boston, 1984.

[GrR]   I. S. Gradshtein, I. M. Ryzhik, *Tables of integral, series and products*, Acad. Press, New York, 1965.
[Hl]   E. Hlawka, *Über Integrale auf konvexen korpen I*, Monatsh. Math. **54** (1950), 1–36.
[Hö]   L. Hörmander, *The analysis of linear partial differential operators*, vol. 1, Springer Verlag, Berlin, 1983.
[LRZ]   E. R. Liflyand, A. G. Ramm, A. I. Zaslavsky, *Estimates from below for Lebesgue constants*, submitted for publication.
[M]   J. Milnor, *Morse theory*, Princeton Univ. Press, Princeton, 1963.
[P]   V. P. Palamodov, *Generalized functions and harmonic analysis*, Sovremennyie problemy matematiki. Fundamental'nyie napravleniya, vol. 73, VINITI, Moscow, 1991, pp. 5 – 134. (Russian)
[Ph]   F. Pham, *Introduction à l'étude topologique des singularités de Landau*, Gauthier-Villars, Paris, 1967.
[RZ1]   A. G. Ramm, A. I. Zaslavsky, *Singularities of the Radon transform*, Bull. Amer. Math. Soc., **25** (1993), no. 1, 109–115.
[RZ2]   _____, *Reconstructing singularities of a function from its Radon transform*, Math. Comp. Modelling (to appear).
[RZ3]   _____, *X-ray transform, the Legendre transform, and envelopes*, J. Math. Anal. Appl. (to appear).
[RZ4]   _____, *Asymptotic behavior of the Fourier transform of piecewise-smooth functions*, C. R. Acad. Sci. Paris **316** (1993), no. 6, 541 – 546.
[S]   E. M. Stein, *Oscillatory integrals in Fourier analysis*, Beijing lectures on harmonic analysis (E. M. Stein, ed.), Princeton Univ. Press, Princeton, 1986, pp. 307–357.
[Zs]   A. I. Zaslavsky, *Dual varieties and Legendre transforms*, J. Math. Anal. Appl. (to appear).

DEPARTMENT OF MATHEMATICS, TECHNION, HAIFA 32000 ISRAEL

E-mail address: mar9315@technion.technion.ac.il

On the Willmore Deficit of convex surfaces

JIAZU ZHOU

ABSTRACT. We discuss the Willmore deficit, i.e., the total square mean curvature deficit $WDef(\Sigma, H) = \int_\Sigma H^2\, d\sigma - 4\pi$ of a convex surface Σ. We give geometric lower bounds for the Willmore deficit that are closely related to several classical results.

§ 1. Introduction

Let $x : \Sigma \longrightarrow \mathbb{R}^3$ be an immersion of a closed surface Σ of dimension 2 in a 3-dimensional Euclidean space $\mathbb{R}^3$. Then the mean curvature H of Σ satisfies the following inequality

(*) $$\int_\Sigma H^2\, d\sigma \geq 4\pi,$$

where $d\sigma$ denotes the volume element of Σ, the equality holds only in the case of a sphere. Many proofs for this inequality have been given by Chen, Weiner, Willmore and others [16,18,20,21].

The Willmore deficit of Σ is

(**) $$\mathrm{WDef}(\Sigma, H) = \int_\Sigma H^2\, d\sigma - 4\pi,$$

which is also called the total square mean curvature deficit of the surface Σ. We will provide some geometric estimates for the Willmore deficit by methods of integral geometry. Those lower bounds deficit obtained can be expressed by a function of volume Σ bounds, surface area and mean width of Σ. For some convex bodies the deficits are computable.

We refer to [5,6,12,17] for investigation of the following inclusion problem involving two domains D_i and D_j in a 3-dimensional Euclidean space $\mathbb{R}^3$. Let

---

1991 *Mathematics Subject Classification.* Primary 52A22, 53C15; Secondary 51M16.

Key words and phrases. Kinematic formula, kinematic measure inequality, Willmore deficit, domain, convex body, mean curvature, total square mean curvature, quermassintegrale.

The paper is in final form and no version of it will be submitted for publication elsewhere

G_3 be the group of rigid motions of $\mathbb{R}^3$ and let $\tilde{m}$ be the normalized kinematic measure. Then

(1) $\quad \tilde{m}\{g \in G_3 : gD_j \subset D_i \text{ or } gD_j \supset D_i\}$
$\qquad = m\{g \in G_3 : D_i \cap gD_j \neq \emptyset\} - m\{g \in G_3 : \partial D_i \cap g\partial D_j \neq \emptyset\}.$

By integral geometric methods it is possible to estimate the measure $m\{g \in G_3 : D_i \cap gD_j \neq \emptyset\}$ from below and the measure $m\{g \in G_3 : \partial D_i \cap g\partial D_j \neq \emptyset\}$ from above in terms of geometric invariants of D_i and D_j. This results in an inequality of the form

(2) $\quad \tilde{m}\{g \in G_3 : gD_j \subset D_i \text{ or } gD_j \supset D_i\} \geq f(A_i^1, \cdots, A_i^h; A_j^1, \cdots, A_j^h),$

where A_k^l ($k = i, j$) can be volume, surface area, total mean curvature of the boundary ∂D_k, or other geometric invariant of D_k.

As one would expect, the inequality of type (2) contains a great deal of geometric information. For example, one can then state the following containment conclusion: If $f(A_i^1, \cdots, A_i^h; A_j^1, \cdots, A_j^h) > 0$, then there is a rigid motion g such that either gD_j is contained in D_i or contains D_i. Hadwiger [**1,14,15**] first gave a criterion for D_i to contain gD_j, a rigid motion of D_j, when D_i and D_j are planar domains. Recently, this criterion is generalized to domains (or convex bodies) of higher dimensional Euclidean (see [**5,6,7,8,12,13,17**]).

As applications of the inequality of the form (2), we are going to find some geometric inequalities, by which, we hope to obtain our main results. That is, we obtain some geometric lower bounds for the Willmore deficit that seem to be new and are related to some classical results. This can be achieved by letting $D_i = D_j = D$. Then the set of $g \in G_3$ that satisfies $gD \subset D$ has measure zero and so formula (2) gives $f(A_i^1, \cdots, A_i^h; A_j^1, \cdots, A_j^h) \leq 0$. In the case of the plane X^ϵ of constant curvature ϵ, it gives the isoperimetric inequality [**22**]. All ideas and methods in this paper are mostly based on those of [**6,12,13,17**].

§2. The Willmore deficit of convex surfaces.

Let Σ be a closed surface in the 3-dimensional Euclidean space $\mathbb{R}^3$, which is always assumed to be connected and C^2-smooth. Denote by F, V, H the surface area, the volume *sigma* bounds, the mean curvature, respectively. If Σ is a convex surface, let W be the quermassintegrale of the convex body Σ bounds. We have the following results:

THEOREM 1. *Let Σ be a convex closed surface in the 3-dimensional Euclidean space $\mathbb{R}^3$. Then we have*

(3) $\qquad WDef(\Sigma, H) \geq \dfrac{8}{3F}\left(\dfrac{4V}{F} + \dfrac{3W}{\pi}\right)^2 - \dfrac{6W^2}{F}.$

THEOREM 2. *Let Σ be as Theorem 1. Denote by R the radius of the circumscribed ball of Σ. Then we have*

(4) $$WDef(\Sigma, H) \geq \frac{2}{3\pi F R}(4\pi V + 3FW) - \frac{6W^2}{F}.$$

THEOREM 3. *Let Σ be as Theorem 1. Then we have*

(5) $$WDef(\Sigma, H) \geq \frac{3\pi^2}{F^3}(4\pi V - WF)^2.$$

THEOREM 4. *Let Σ be as in Theorem 1. then*

(6) $$WDef(\Sigma, H) \geq \frac{9W^2}{F} - 4\pi.$$

To prove our theorems, let us investigate the total square mean curvature of closed surfaces first.

§3. Total square mean curvature of surfaces.

Let S be a closed surface of class C^2 in a 3-dimensional Euclidean space $\mathbb{R}^3$. Denote by H the mean curvature of S. The total mean curvature and the total square mean curvature are, respectively, defined by

(7) $$\tilde{H} = \int_S H\, d\sigma, \quad \tilde{H}^{(2)} = \int_S H^2\, d\sigma$$

where $d\sigma$ is the volume element of S.

Let S_i and S_j be two closed surfaces of class C^2 in $\mathbb{R}^3$. Assume that S_i is fixed and gS_j is moving under the rigid motion g. Let dg be the kinematic density for $\mathbb{R}^3$, so normalized that the measure of all positions about a point is $8\pi^2$. Let κ_{C_g} denote the curvature of the intersection curve $C_g = S_i \cap gS_j$. Denote by F_k the surface area, and by $\tilde{H}_k$ and $\tilde{H}_k^{(2)}$ ($k=i,j$) the total mean curvature and the total square mean curvature of S_k, respectively. Then we have C-S. Chen's formula (see [4,17])*

(8) $$\int_{G_3\{S_i\cap gS_j\neq\emptyset\}}\left(\int_{S_i\cap gS_j}\kappa_{C_g}^2\, ds\right)dg$$
$$=2\pi^3(3\tilde{H}_i^{(2)} - 2\pi\chi(S_i))F_j + 2\pi^3(3\tilde{H}_j^{(2)} - 2\pi\chi(S_j))F_i,$$

where ds is the arc-element of the intersection curve $C_g = S_i \cap gS_j$, H_k, $\chi(S_k)$ are, respectively, the mean curvature and the Euler-Poincaré characteristic of S_k.

From now on, we suppose that all the domains discussed have C^2-smooth boundaries. We assume that D_i and D_j are connected and simply connected and

---

*By using the Gauss-Bonnet formula, we can rewrite Chen's formula in the present form.

such that for all $g \in G_3$, the group of rigid motions in $\mathbb{R}^3$, the Euler-Poincaré characteristic $\chi(D_i \cap gD_j)$ is at most N_0, a finite integer.

By Blaschke and Chen's formulas, we have some different estimates of the kinematic measure of one domain D_i moving into another domain D_j under the group G_3 of rigid motions in $\mathbb{R}^3$ as follows [**12,17**]:

$$
\begin{aligned}
(9)\quad &\tilde{m}\{g \in G_3 : gD_j \subseteq D_i \quad \text{or} \quad gD_j \supseteq D_i\} \\
&= \int_{G_3\{D_i \cap gD_j \neq \emptyset\}} dg - \int_{G_3\{\partial D_i \cap g\partial D_j \neq \emptyset\}} dg \\
&\geq \frac{1}{N_0}[8\pi^2(V_i + V_j) + 2\pi(F_i\tilde{H}_j + F_j\tilde{H}_i)] \\
&\quad - \pi^2\{F_iF_j[3(F_i\tilde{H}_j^{(2)} + F_j\tilde{H}_i^{(2)}) - 4\pi(F_i + F_j)]\}^{\frac{1}{2}};
\end{aligned}
$$

$$
\begin{aligned}
(10)\quad &\tilde{m}\{g \in G_3 : gD_j \subseteq D_i \quad \text{or} \quad gD_j \supseteq D_i\} \\
&\geq \frac{1}{N_0}[8\pi^2(V_i + V_j) + 2\pi(F_i\tilde{H}_j + F_j\tilde{H}_i)] \\
&\quad - \pi^2 R\,[3(F_i\tilde{H}_j^{(2)} + F_j\tilde{H}_i^{(2)}) - 4\pi(F_i + F_j)],
\end{aligned}
$$

where R is the radius of the smallest circumscribed ball of D_i, D_j.

LEMMA 1. *If Σ be a simply connected closed surface in the 3-dimensional Euclidean space $\mathbb{R}^3$ and D the domain Σ bounds, then we have the following inequality*

$$
(11)\quad \int_{\Sigma} H^2\, d\sigma \geq \frac{8}{3\,F\,N_0^2}\left(\frac{4V}{F} + \frac{\tilde{H}}{\pi}\right)^2 + \frac{4\pi}{3}.
$$

PROOF. Let $D_i = D_j = D$. Denote by F, V, H, $\tilde{H}$ and $\tilde{H}^{(2)}$ its surface area, volume, mean curvature of boundary ∂D, total mean curvature of ∂D and total square mean curvature of ∂D, respectively. Then the measure on the left hand side of (9) is zero. That is,

$$
(12)\quad \tilde{m}\{g \in G_3 : gD_j \subseteq D_i \quad \text{or} \quad gD_i \subseteq D_j\} = m\{g \in G_3 : gD \subseteq D\} = 0.
$$

Hence by (9) we have

$$
(13)\quad \tilde{H}^{(2)} = \int_{\partial D} H^2\, d\sigma \geq \frac{8}{3\,F\,N_0^2}\left(\frac{4V}{F} + \frac{\tilde{H}}{\pi}\right)^2 + \frac{4\pi}{3}. \quad \square
$$

LEMMA 2. *Let Σ, be as Lemma 1. Denote by R the radius of the circumscribed ball of Σ. Then the following inequality holds:*

$$
(14)\quad \int_{\Sigma} H^2\, d\sigma \geq \frac{2}{3\,R\,N_0}\left(\frac{4V}{F} + \frac{\tilde{H}}{\pi}\right) + \frac{4\pi}{3}.
$$

PROOF. Let $D_i = D_j = D$. Then the measure on the left hand side of (10) is zero. By (10), we have

$$(15) \qquad \int_{\partial D} H^2 \, d\sigma \geq \frac{2}{3 R N_0} \left(\frac{4V}{F} + \frac{\tilde{H}}{\pi} \right) + \frac{4\pi}{3}.$$

Therefore we have proved Lemma 2. □

§4. The total square mean curvature of convex surfaces.

Now we consider convex bodies. Generically, the intersection curve $\partial D_i \cap g\partial D_j$ is a union of simple closed curves. For every rigid motion $g \in G_3$, let $C_g = \partial D_i \cap g\partial D_j = \bigcup_l^{N_g} C_l$, where N_g is always finite and only depends on g and C_i is a simple closed curve.

LEMMA 3. *Let Σ be a convex closed surface in the 3-dimensional Euclidean space $\mathbb{R}^3$. Denote by δ_m the diameter of Σ. Then we have*

$$(16) \qquad \int_\Sigma H^2 \, d\sigma \geq \frac{4}{3}\pi + \frac{4W}{\pi \delta_m} + \frac{16V}{3\delta_m F}.$$

PROOF. In [6] we have the following kinematic measure inequality

$$(17) \quad \tilde{m} = m\{g \in G_3 : gD_j \subseteq D_i \text{ or } gD_j \supseteq D_i\}$$
$$\geq 8\pi^2(V_i + V_j) + 6\pi(F_i W_j + F_j W_i)$$
$$- \frac{\pi^2 \delta_m}{2} \left[3(\tilde{H}_i^{(2)} F_j + \tilde{H}_j^{(2)} F_i) - 4\pi(F_i + F_j) \right],$$

where W_k ($k = i, j$) are *quermassintegrales* of convex bodies D_k.

By letting $D_i = D_j = D$, we have $\tilde{m}\{g \in G_3 : gD \subset D\} = 0$. This leads to

$$(18) \qquad \int_{\partial D} H^2 \, d\sigma \geq \frac{4}{3}\pi + \frac{4W}{\pi \delta_m} + \frac{16V}{3\delta_m F}. \qquad \square$$

For convex body D, we always have $\chi(D \cap gD) \leq N_0 = 1$, for all $g \in G_3$. Hence the following consequences come from *Lemma 1* and *Lemma 2*.

COROLLARY 1. *Let Σ be a convex closed surface in the 3-dimensional Euclidean space $\mathbb{R}^3$. Then we have inequality*

$$(19) \qquad \int_\Sigma H^2 \, d\sigma \geq \frac{8}{3F} \left(\frac{4V}{F} + \frac{3W}{\pi} \right)^2 + \frac{4\pi}{3}.$$

COROLLARY 2. *Let Σ be as Corollary 1. Denote by R the radius of the circumscribed ball of Σ. Then we have*

$$(20) \qquad \int_\Sigma H^2 \, d\sigma \geq \frac{2}{3\pi F R}(4\pi V + 3FW) + \frac{4\pi}{3}.$$

We also have the following

LEMMA 4. *Let Σ be as Corollary 1, then*

$$(21) \qquad \int_\Sigma H^2 \, d\sigma \geq \frac{9W^2}{F}.$$

PROOF. A direct application of Hölder's inequality gives

$$(22) \qquad \int_\Sigma H^2 \, d\sigma \geq \frac{\{\int_\Sigma H \, d\sigma\}^2}{\int_\Sigma d\sigma} = \frac{9W^2}{F} \geq 4\pi.$$

The last inequality is one of Minkowski's inequalities [1]. □

LEMMA 5. *Let Σ be as Corollary 1. Then we have*

$$(23) \qquad \int_\Sigma H^2 \, d\sigma \geq \frac{3\pi^2}{F^3}(4\pi V - WF)^2 + 4\pi.$$

PROOF. In [5] Zhang gave the following kinematic measure inequality

$$(24) \quad \tilde{m} = m\{g \in G_3 : gD_j \subseteq D_i \quad \text{or} \quad gD_j \supseteq D_i\}$$
$$\geq 8\pi^2(V_i + V_j) - 2\pi(F_i W_j + F_j W_i)$$
$$- \frac{2}{3}\left\{2F_i F_j[3(\tilde{H}_i^{(2)} F_j + \tilde{H}_j^{(2)} F_i) - 4\pi(F_i + F_j) - 36W_i W_j]\right\}^{1/2}.$$

Similarly, letting $D_i = D_j = D$, we have $\tilde{m}\{g \in G_3 : gD \subset D\} = 0$. This lead to

$$(25) \qquad \int_{\partial D} H^2 \, d\sigma \geq \frac{3\pi^2}{F^3}(4\pi V - WF)^2 + \frac{6W^2}{F} + \frac{4}{3}\pi$$
$$\geq \frac{3\pi^2}{F^3}(4\pi V - WF)^2 + 4\pi.$$

The last inequality comes from the Minkowski's inequality $9W^2 \geq 4\pi F$. □

§5. Proofs of main results and remarks.

Now we are ready to prove our theorems.

Theorem 1 comes immediately from Corollary 1 and the Minkowski's inequality $9W^2 \geq 4\pi F$.

Theorem 2 comes from the Minkowski's inequality $9W^2 \geq 4\pi F$ and Corollary 2.

Theorem 3 is obtained by the Minkowski's inequality and Lemma 5.

Inequality (22) also gives Theorem 4.

Remark 1. The classical topological proofs for inequality (*) just give the estimate $\mathrm{WDef}(\Sigma, H) \geq 0$. Right now, we are not aware of any other geometric lower bound estimate for the Willmore deficit of convex surfaces. Our inequalities can, at least, for some convex surfaces, give some estimates for the Willmore deficits. For immersed surfaces there is the result of Peter Li and S. T. Yau (see [24]) that if a immersed surface Σ has a double point then $\mathrm{WDef}(\Sigma, H) \geq 4\pi$ and if Σ has a triple point then $\mathrm{WDef}(\Sigma, H) \geq 8\pi$. They also give lower bounds for surfaces of higher topologically type in terms of the conformal area of surface involved. However in the case of convex surfaces these their results all reduce to the well known results $\mathrm{WDef}(\Sigma, H) \geq 0$.

An example: For the ellipsoid Σ_{ellip} of revolution with semiaxis $a, a, \lambda a$, we have, for $0 < \lambda < 1$ [23],

$$(26) \qquad F = 2\pi a^2 \left[1 + \frac{\lambda^2}{\sqrt{1-\lambda^2}} \ln\left(1 + \frac{\sqrt{1-\lambda^2}}{\lambda}\right) \right],$$

$$V = \frac{4}{3}\pi \lambda a^3, \quad W = 2\pi a \left(\lambda + \frac{\arccos \lambda}{\sqrt{1-\lambda^2}} \right),$$

and for $1 < \lambda < \infty$,

$$(27) \qquad F = 2\pi a^2 \left(1 + \frac{\lambda^2 \arccos(1/\lambda)}{\sqrt{\lambda^2-1}} \right), \quad V = \frac{4}{3}\pi \lambda a^3,$$

$$W = 2\pi a \left[\lambda + \frac{1}{\sqrt{\lambda^2-1}} \ln(\lambda + \sqrt{\lambda^2-1}) \right].$$

Theorem 3 gives

$$\text{(28)} \quad \text{WDef}(\Sigma_{\text{ellip}}, H) \geq \frac{2\pi^3}{3\left[1 + \frac{\lambda^2}{\sqrt{1-\lambda^2}} \ln\left(1 + \frac{\sqrt{1-\lambda^2}}{\lambda}\right)\right]^3}$$

$$\times \left\{4\lambda - 3\left(\lambda + \frac{\arccos \lambda}{\sqrt{1-\lambda^2}}\right)\left[1 + \frac{\lambda^2}{\sqrt{1-\lambda^2}} \ln\left(1 + \frac{\sqrt{1-\lambda^2}}{\lambda}\right)\right]\right\}^2,$$

$$\text{for } 0 < \lambda < 1;$$

$$\text{(29)} \quad \text{WDef}(\Sigma_{\text{ellip}}, H) \geq \frac{2\pi^3}{3\left(1 + \frac{\lambda^2 \arccos(1/\lambda)}{\sqrt{\lambda^2-1}}\right)^3}$$

$$\times \left\{4\lambda - 3\left(1 + \frac{\lambda^2 \arccos(1/\lambda)}{\sqrt{\lambda^2-1}}\right)\left[\lambda + \frac{1}{\sqrt{\lambda^2-1}} \ln(\lambda + \sqrt{\lambda^2-1})\right]\right\}^2,$$

$$\text{for } 1 < \lambda < \infty.$$

By Theorem 4, we have

$$\text{(30)} \quad \text{WDef}(\Sigma_{\text{ellip}}, H) \geq$$

$$\frac{9\pi(\lambda\sqrt{1-\lambda^2} + \arccos \lambda)^2}{2\left[1 - \lambda^2 + \lambda^2\sqrt{1-\lambda^2} \ln\left(1 + \frac{\sqrt{1-\lambda^2}}{\lambda}\right)\right]} - 4\pi, \quad \text{for } 0 < \lambda < 1;$$

$$\text{(31)} \quad \text{WDef}(\Sigma_{\text{ellip}}, H) \geq$$

$$\frac{18\pi(\lambda\sqrt{\lambda^2-1} + \ln(\lambda + \sqrt{\lambda^2-1})^2}{\lambda^2 - 1 + \lambda^2\sqrt{\lambda^2-1} \arccos(1/\lambda)} - 4\pi, \quad \text{for } 1 < \lambda < \infty.$$

One would see that (3), (4), (5) and (6) can give some concrete geometric estimations for the Willmore deficit for any C^2-smooth convex surface.

Remark 2. By inspection, the right hand sides of (22), (23), (24) and (25) are well-defined for non-smooth convex bodies. But $\int_\Sigma H^2 d\sigma$ is defined only for the C^2-smooth surface Σ. Still, if we can find some substitutes for $\int_\Sigma H^2 d\sigma$, all results here will applicable for any convex body. This is definitely worthy investigating.

6. Acknowledgement. I would like to thank Professor Eric Grinberg for many suggestions and discussions. I very appreciate Professor R. Howard's many helpful comments. I would also like to thank the organizers of the summer conference at Mount Holyoke College for giving me a chance to stay there a very nice week. Finally, the author thanks referee for valuable comments and suggestions.

References

1. L. A. Santaló, *Integral Geometry and Geometric Probability*, Addison-Wesley, Readings, Math. (1976).
2. S. S. Chern, *On the kinematic formula in the euclidean space of n dimensions*, Amer. J. Math. **74** (1952), 227-236.
3. Delin Ren, *Introduction to Integral Geometry*, Shanghai Press of Sciences and Technology (1987).
4. C-S. Chen, *On the kinematic formula of square of mean curvature*, Indiana Univ. Math. J. **22** (1972-73), 1163-1169.
5. Gaoyong Zhang, *A sufficient condition for one convex body containing another*, Chin. Ann. of Math. **9B(4)** (1988), 447-451.
6. Jiazu Zhou, *Analogues of Hadwiger's theorem–sufficient conditions for one convex body to fit another in $\mathbb{R}^3$ (1991)*, submitted.
7. Jiazu Zhou, *The sufficient condition for a convex body to fit another in $\mathbb{R}^4$*, to appear in Proc. Amer. Math. Soc.
8. Jiazu Zhou, *The analogues of Hadwiger's theorem in space $\mathbb{R}^n$, the sufficient condition for a convex domain to enclose another*, submitted.
9. P. R. Goodey, *Connectivity and free rolling convex bodies*, Mathematika **29** (1982), 249-259.
10. R. Howard, *The kinematic formula in riemannian geometry*, to appear as a Memoir of AMS.
11. Michael Spivak, *A Comprehensive Introduction to Differential Geometry (II)*, Publish or Perish, Inc. (1979).
12. Jiazu Zhou, *When can one domain enclose another in space $\mathbb{R}^3$*, to appear in J. Australian Math. Soc.
13. Jiazu Zhou, *Kinematic formulas for mean curvature powers of hypersurfaces and Hadwiger's theorem in $\mathbb{R}^{2n}$*, to appear in Trans. Amer. Math. Soc.
14. H. Hadwiger, *Genenseitige Bedeckbarkeit zweier Eibereiche und Isoperimetrie*, Viertejsch. Naturforsch. Gesellsch. Zürich **86** (1941), 152-156.
15. H. Hadwiger, *Überdeckung ebener Bereiche durch Kreise und Quadrate*, Comment. Math. Helv. **13** (1941), 195-200.
16. Yu. D. Burago & V. A. Zalgaller, *Geometric Inequalities*, Springer-Verlag Berlin Heidelberg (1988).
17. Jiazu Zhou, *A kinematic formula and analogues of Hadwiger's theorem in space*, Contemporary Mathematics **140** (1992), 159–167.
18. B-Y Chen, *Geometry of Submanifolds*, Marcel Dekker. Inc., New York (1973).
19. P. Goodey, *Homothetic ellipsoids*, Math. Proc. Camb. Phil. Soc. **93** (1983), 25-34.
20. J. Weiner, *On an inequality of P. Wintgen for integral of the square of the mean curvature*, J. London Math. Soc. **(2) 34** (1986), 148–158.
21. T. J. Willmore, *Mean curvature of immersed surface*, Al. I. Cuza Iasi. Sect. I. a. Math. **14** (1968), 99–103.
22. Eric Grinberg, Delin Ren & Jiazu Zhou, *The isoperimetric inequality and the containment problem in a plane of constant curvature*, submitted.
23. H. Hadwiger, *Altes und Neues Über Konvexe Körper*, Birkhauser, Basel and Stuttgart (1955).
24. Peter Li & S. T. Yau, *A conformal invariant and applications to the Willmore conjecture and the first eigenvalue for compact surfaces*, Invent Math **69** (1982), 269–291.

DEPARTMENT OF MATHEMATICS, TEMPLE UNIVERSITY, PHILADELPHIA, PA 19122

E-mail address: zhou@euclid.math.temple.edu